PRACTICAL PROCEDURES IN

Anesthesia

AND CRITICAL CARE

Peter J F Baskett BA MB BCh BAO FRCA MRCP
Chairman European Resuscitation Council
Consultant Anaesthetist
Frenchay Hospital
Bristol, UK

Alasdair Dow MB ChB MRCP FRCA
Consultant Anaesthetist
Royal Devon and Exeter Hospital
Exeter, UK

Jerry Nolan MB ChB FRCA
Consultant Anaesthetist
Royal United Hospital,
Bath, UK

Kimball Maull MD
Formerly Director Maryland Institute for Emergency Medical Services Systems
(M.I.E.M.S.S.) Shock Trauma Center
Baltimore
Maryland, USA

With selected chapters by:
Tom Kneuth MD and
David Tarver MRCP FRCR

M Mosby

London Baltimore Bogotá Boston Buenos Aires Caracas Carlsbad, CA Chicago Madrid Mexico City Milan Naples, FL New York Philadelphia
St. Louis Sydney Tokyo Toronto Wiesbaden

Project Manager:	Linda Kull
Developmental Editor:	Claire Hooper
Designer/Layout Artist:	Marie McNestry
Cover Design:	Mark Willey
Illustration:	Marion Tasker
Production:	Mike Heath
Index:	Nina Boyd
Publisher:	Geoff Greenwood

Copyright © 1995 Times Mirror International Publishers Limited

Published in 1995 by Mosby, an imprint of Times Mirror International Publishers Limited

Printed in Italy by Imago Publishing Ltd.

ISBN 1-56375-606-4

For full details of all Times Mirror International Publishers Limited titles, please write to Times Mirror International Publishers Limited, Lynton House, 7–12 Tavistock Square, London WC1H 9LB, England.

A CIP catalogue record for this book is available from the British Library.

Library of Congress Cataloging-in-Publication Data applied for

Preface

The continuing involvement of technology in acute medicine has required doctors in a variety of specialities to possess a wide spectrum of practical skills. These specialities include anaesthesia, critical care, emergency medicine, cardiology, nephrology and radiology as well as the surgical disciplines. Such is the expectation of enhanced standards that it is incumbent upon doctors in these areas to have a comprehensive repertoire of invasive techniques with which to manage patients with acute illness or injury.

In a number of instances, some of the procedures have moved from the exclusive domain of the doctor to be included in the role of the experienced nurse in the acute sector and the paramedic or operating department assistant. Many of the techniques will also be used by the general practitioner involved with immediate care and, or course, the physician specialising in military and disaster medicine.

In this book, we have tried to bring together the common practical procedures required in the anaesthetic and operating rooms, the emergency department and critical care and high dependency units. We have drawn upon our collective experience of working in these areas in the United Kingdom, the United States and Canada, and mainland Europe and in military, field and sports medicine.

The procedures covered range from the very simple to the relatively advanced – from the placement of the simple intravenous cannula to floatation of the pulmonary artery catheter – from insertion of the urinary catheter to the technique of haemofiltration – and from the passage of an oropharyngeal airway to retrograde tracheal intubation and surgical cricothyroidotomy.

The description of each procedure follows a similar and simple format – beginning with an introductory overview of the technique, a list of indications and contra-indications, the equipment required, the precise and detailed practical steps involved, the special hazards which may be encountered and how to overcome them, and the salient key points which require highlighting. We have been deliberately concise and didactic in putting forward what we believe is a generally accepted and consensus view of a reasonable approach to each procedure. We have been liberal in the number of illustrations to demonstrate the key features of each technique.

Finally we have set out our views on which procedures we consider reasonable for each of the groups and specialists to be familiar with, so that practical training can be targeted primarily on a need-to-know basis.

We sincerely hope that this will be a useful book for the specialist in training, the medical student, the expert nurse and paramedic, and, dare we say, some senior doctors who wish to refresh or broaden their practical skills.

Peter Baskett
Alasdair Dow
Jerry Nolan
October 1994

Acknowledgements

We would like to thank Kathy Graham for help with the manuscript, Marion Tasker for the illustrations, and Linda Kull for her management of the project.

For Fiona, Annie and Sandra

Contents

Abbreviations

ACD:	Active compression–decompression
ACT:	Activated clotting time
ACV:	Assisted control ventilation
APRV:	Airway pressure release ventilation
ARDS:	Adult (acute) respiratory distress syndrome
ATLS:	Advanced Trauma Life Support
AV:	Atrio-ventricular
CAVH:	Continuous arteriovenous haemofiltration
CAVHD:	Continuous arteriovenous haemodialysis
CMV:	Controlled mechanical ventilation
CPAP:	Continuous positive airway pressure
CPR:	Cardiopulmonary resuscitation
CVP:	Central venous pressure
CVVH:	Continuous venovenous haemofiltration
CVVHD:	Continuous venovenous haemodialysis
CPP:	Cerebral perfusion pressure
CRRT:	Continuous renal replacement therapy
CT:	Computerised tomography (scanning)
DBS:	Double burst stimulation
DC:	Direct current
DPL:	Diagnostic peritoneal lavage
EAR:	Expired air respiration
ECC:	External chest compressions
ECG:	Electrocardiogram
EKG:	Electrocardiogram
FG:	French Gauge
FIO_2:	Fractional inspired oxygen
GCS:	Glasgow coma score
HFPPV:	High frequency positive pressure ventilation
HFJV:	High frequency jet ventilation
HFO:	High frequency oscillation
ICP:	Intracranial pressure
ID:	Internal diameter
IMV:	Intermittent mandatory ventilation
IRV:	Inverse ratio ventilation
IVC:	Intraventricular catheter

LFPPV–$ECCO_2$R:	Low frequency positive pressure ventilation with extracorporeal CO_2 removal
LMA:	Laryngeal mask airway
LVEDV:	Left ventricular end diastolic volume
MD:	Medical doctor
N/G:	Naso-gastric
PASG:	Pneumatic anti-shock garment
PAFC:	Pulmonary Artery Flotation Catheter
RAP:	Right atrial pressure
PA:	Pulmonary artery
PAOP:	Pulmonary artery occlusion pressure
PAP:	Pulmonary artery pressure
PCA:	Patient controlled analgesia
PCEA:	Patient controlled epidural analgesia
PCV:	Pressure controlled ventilation
$PÉCO_2$:	Partial pressure of end-tidal CO_2 sample
PEEP:	Positive end expiratory pressure
PSV:	Pressure support ventilation
PTLA:	Pharyngotracheal lumen airway
PTT:	Partial thromboplastin time
RA:	Right atrium
R-on-T:	Event of an R wave on a T wave on the electrocardiogram
RV:	Right ventricle
RVEF:	Right ventricular ejection fraction
RVEDV:	Right ventricular end diastolic volume
SA:	Sino-atrial
SaO_2:	Oxygen saturation of arterial blood
SIMV:	Synchronised intermittent mandatory ventilation
SpO_2:	Oxygen saturation of arterial blood by pulse oximeter
SVC-CPR:	Simultaneous ventilation and compression cardiopulmonary resuscitation
TOF:	Train of four
US:	Ultrasound scanning
VF:	Ventricular fibrillation
VT:	Ventricular tachycardia

Cardiovascular System

Cannulation of peripheral veins (including blood culture sampling)

Indications

Fluid/blood infusion.
Blood sampling.
Drug administration.
Central venous line needed from a peripheral route.
Peripheral venous feeding.

Contra-indications

Absolute
Local sepsis and injury.
Presence of arteriovenous shunt on chosen limb.

Relative
Inexperience with technique.
Damage to more proximal veins, e.g. long saphenous route, is contra-indicated in patients with pelvic fracture.

Peripheral venous cannulation is one of the most commonly performed procedures in medical practice; it can also be one of the most difficult in the shocked or obese patient. This chapter will offer several hints to allow the reader to be more successful with the 'difficult' patient, and to have a range of options available when the conventional routes fail.

Several sites for peripheral cannulation will be described, and the technique of taking blood cultures will be discussed.

There are no absolute contra-indications to peripheral venous cannulation, although care must be taken in a patient with a bleeding diathesis.

Equipment

☐ Antiseptic solution.
☐ Local anaesthetic (e.g. 1% lignocaine with 1:200,000 adrenaline).
☐ Appropriate sized cannula (12–20G in adults, 18–24G in children).
☐ Tourniquet.
☐ Dressing to secure cannula in place.
☐ Intravenous giving set or 'flush' fluid (e.g. heparinised saline).

Technique

Children and babies (over one year old) may benefit from the use of a topical local anaesthetic cream, such as EMLA Cream (TM Astra Pharmaceuticals). This cream may be of value in adults, where cannulation is going to be difficult. In patients with difficult veins, it is helpful to soak the selected limb in warm water for 5 minutes.

The site of insertion depends on the preference of the operator, and the type of patient: ideally a site at the junction of two veins, which does not cross a joint. A possible list of sites is given for three age groups, although this is by no means comprehensive. There is great variability between patients and the list serves only as a reminder of some of the more useful sites.

Adult
Some suitable sites are shown in Fig. 1.1 and listed below:
- Dorsum of hand.
- Cephalic vein at the wrist.
- Cephalic, basilic or cubital vein at the elbow.
- Long saphenous vein at ankle.   ▶ ▶ ▶

▶ ▶ ▶
- External jugular vein.
- Dorsum of foot.

Child

Some suitable sites are shown in Fig. 1.2 and listed below:
- Dorsum of hand.
- Long saphenous vein at ankle.
- Dorsum of foot.
- Antecubital fossa.
- External jugular vein.

Baby (infant or neonate)
- Dorsum of foot.
- Palmar surface of wrist.
- Scalp vein.
- Dorsum of hand.
- External jugular vein. ▶ ▶ ▶

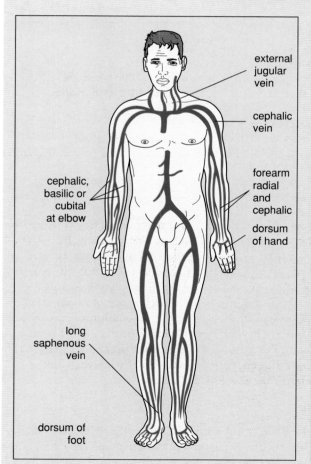

Fig. 1.1 Sites for venous cannulation in the adult

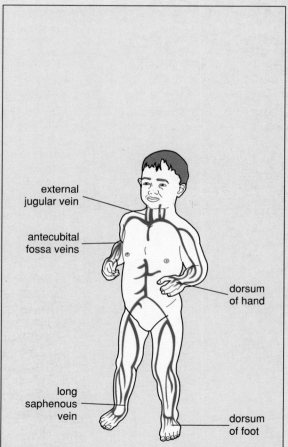

Fig. 1.2 Sites for venous cannulation in a child

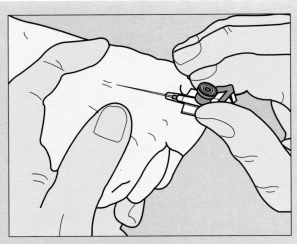

Fig. 1.3 The cannula is held firmly in one hand

▶ ▶ ▶

The vein that has been chosen should be distended by either hanging the limb below the level of the bed, or else applying a tourniquet, or both. The external jugular veins and the scalp veins can be distended by placing the patient head down, and by applying pressure at the root of the neck. Lightly pat the vein, to encourage it to distend.

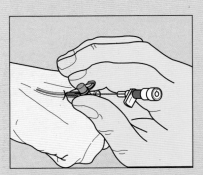

Fig. 1.4 Advance the cannula

1 Clean and drape the area around the chosen vein. The degree of sterility is determined by the urgency of the procedure, and the potential duration of cannula insertion.
2 Infiltrate local anaesthetic into the skin overlying the vein.
3 Grasp the cannula between the thumb and index finger of the dominant hand. Advance the cannula through the skin, applying axial traction distally to stretch the skin with the other hand (Fig. 1.3).
4 When the cannula has penetrated the skin, advance it slowly into the vein. The cannula should be held in a plane parallel to the skin, so as not to 'cut-out' of the vein.
5 As soon as blood fills the hub of the cannula, ensure that the cannula is in the vein, and not just the tip of the needle. Withdraw the needle slightly, and advance the cannula to its hub. This should be done gently, to avoid buckling of the cannula (Fig. 1.4).
6 Withdraw the needle fully, and cap or attach the infusion line onto the exposed end of the cannula (usually a Luer lock connection) (Fig. 1.5). The cannula should be held in place, while an assistant secures it with a sterile dressing.
7 Confirm the cannula is patent, by flushing with infusion fluid. Secure the infusion tubing firmly to the patient.

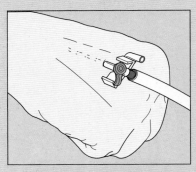

Fig. 1.5 Infusion line connected to cannula

Complications

Failure to cannulate the vessel is the commonest problem, and may be avoided by careful selection of a large vein. Haematoma can occur at the site of insertion, and may be treated by compression dressing. Infection and thrombophlebitis are late complications, and are best managed by removing the cannula.

Key points

- Select the largest straightest vein.
- Apply a tourniquet where possible.
- Do not push the cannula too far into the vein.
- Slight rotation of the cannula and needle may overcome venous valves.
- Grasp the cannula tightly until it is secured in place.
- Flush the cannula with isotonic fluid, before injecting drugs.

TAKING BLOOD CULTURES

This procedure requires venous puncture, using a syringe and needle. The procedure must be done under aseptic conditions, to ensure the validity of the subsequent bacteriology results. There are no contra-indications to blood cultures, although local sepsis demands that an alternative site should be chosen.

Technique

Preparation and equipment are the same as for peripheral venous cannulation. It may be more appropriate to use a needle rather than a cannula, but if the patient has few venepuncture sites, the two procedures can be combined; in this case, the blood must always be drawn off before the cannula is connected up to a giving set.

1 Select an appropriate vein, as discussed above.
2 Put on sterile gloves and gown, and clean and prepare the area, around the vein.
3 Place a sterile towel over the area of the vein. Ask an assistant to apply a tourniquet proximal to the vein, if appropriate.
4 Collect 10–20ml of venous blood in a sterile syringe, and put a sterile dressing over the puncture site. Ask the assistant to release the tourniquet.
5 Open the flip-off tops of the blood culture bottles, and wipe the injection port using a swab soaked with antiseptic cleaning fluid.
6 Put a fresh sterile needle (20G or 18G) onto the blood syringe, and inject 5–10ml of blood into the first bottle. Repeat the procedure for the second bottle. Do not use too large a needle, because air may be introduced into the anaerobic sample bottle.
7 Label the bottles with the appropriate patient details, and then ensure that the bottles are immediately put into an incubator at the correct temperature.

Key points

- Do not use cannulae that are already *in situ*.
- Full asepsis is essential for useful results.
- A second sample requires a second venepuncture site.
- The antecubital fossa is the most practical site.
- Always clean the injection port of the sample bottles.

Central vein cannulation

Central vein cannulation is indicated if peripheral vein cannulation has failed, or if access to the central veins or the right side of the heart is necessary. There are no absolute contra-indications to central vein cannulation, as the condition of the patient may dictate the need; e.g. hypovolaemic shock requiring transfusion, or complete heart block requiring pacing. However, inexperience with a particular technique may favour another route, as will local sepsis or anatomical deformity.

The section will describe several different approaches to the central veins: the preparation and equipment are generally the same for each approach, and will not be repeated for each subsection. Hazards and complications particular to each route will be listed under that approach.

Indications

Fluid infusion.
Infusion of drugs especially vasoactive drugs.
Placement of pulmonary artery flotation catheter (PAFC).
Insertion of pacing wire.
Aspiration of blood/air from heart.
Failure to gain peripheral access.

Contra-indications

Local sepsis or injury.
Severe coagulation disorders.
Unwilling patient.
Inexperience with technique.

Equipment

☐ Patient on tilting bed.
☐ Sterile pack and antiseptic solution.
☐ Local anaesthetic (e.g. 5ml 1% lignocaine with 1:200,000 adrenaline).
☐ Appropriate catheter, with either needle through cannula or Seldinger type kit: size as appropriate for age and purpose. Decide between single, double and triple lumen kits.
☐ Long central venous line for basilic or femoral routes, e.g. Drum cartridge catheter.
☐ Pressure transducer/fluid infusion system with monitor and Luer lock connection.
☐ Heparinised saline for catheter irrigation.
☐ Suture material (e.g. non-absorbable 3/0 suture on straight needle).
☐ Sterile adhesive dressing.
☐ Facilities for post-insertion radiograph.

SUBCLAVIAN VEIN CANNULATION

Sedation or general anaesthesia may be required for those patients who will find the procedure distressing: the young, and the confused or agitated. A qualified assistant should be present to provide any sedation, and also to monitor the ECG during wire insertion.

The patient should be supine with a head down tilt to distend the central veins, and to prevent air embolism. The head should be turned away from the side that is to be cannulated, to allow identification of the landmarks (Fig. 1.6).

Remove any pillows from beneath the patients head, and ask the assistant to draw the right arm down to pull the shoulder out of the way: this last point is very important in the obese patient, as the shoulder may otherwise force the operator into an excessively posterior direction with the needle, thus risking puncture of the pleura.

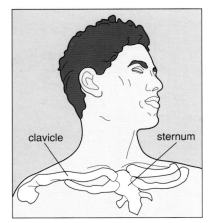

Fig. 1.6 Position for subclavian vein cannulation

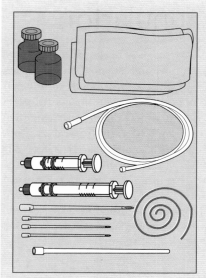

Fig. 1.7 Equipment for subclavian vein cannulation

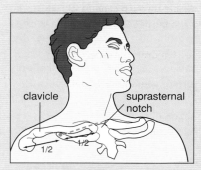

clavicle   suprasternal notch

1/2   1/2

Fig. 1.8 Direction of entry for subclavian vein cannulation

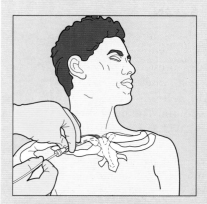

Fig. 1.10 The catheter should not be inserted until the wire has appeared through the hub of the central vein catheter

Technique

This description refers to cannulation of the right subclavian vein.

1 Sterilise and drape the area over the midpoint of the clavicle.
2 Open the appropriate central line kit onto a sterile surface, and check the contents (Fig. 1.7).
3 Infiltrate 5–10ml of local anaesthetic into the skin and subcutaneous tissue overlying the midpoint of the clavicle.
4 Draw an imaginary line joining the midpoint of the clavicle to the suprasternal notch, to represent the direction of insertion (Fig. 1.8).
5 Check that the guide wire will pass down the needle lumen, and that the catheter and dilator will pass over the guide wire. Attach a 5ml syringe to the needle, and advance it into the skin inferior to the midpoint of the clavicle (Fig. 1.9).
6 After the needle has penetrated the skin, aspirate continuously to identify venous puncture. Advance the needle in the horizontal plane just beneath the clavicle, aiming for the suprasternal notch.
7 Aspiration of venous blood confirms entry into the subclavian vein; arterial blood will usually pulse out of the needle. If there is still doubt, compare the blood in colour to a peripheral venous sample.
8 Insert the wire through the needle, and at the same time ask the assistant to watch the ECG for arrhythmias. Withdraw the needle, and make a small incision in the skin, at the point that the wire enters it. Take care not to cut the wire.
9 Pass the dilator over the wire, and insert it up to the hub. This may require some force, although care must be taken not to buckle the dilator or the wire: a rotating movement may be helpful. Remove the dilator, and then insert the catheter over the wire, until the wire extends from the end of the catheter (Fig. 1.10).
10 Remove the wire, and attach Luer lock caps on to the end(s) of the lumen(s) of the catheter. In the average adult, the catheter should be inserted to the 15cm mark.
11 Check that venous blood can be easily aspirated from the central line catheter, and then flush each lumen with heparinised saline.
12 Suture the catheter in place using a non-absorbable suture, and then apply a dry sterile dressing to secure the catheter to the skin.
13 Arrange a chest radiograph, as soon as possible. Ensure that the catheter is about 2cm above the carina, to confirm vena caval position. Check that there is no pneumothorax.

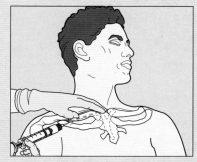

Fig. 1.9 The needle and syringe are advanced beneath the clavicle into the subclavian vein

Hazards

- Beware possible cervical spine fracture in head and neck movement.
- Posterior direction of the needle risks pneumothorax.
- Arrhythmias are rare if wire insertion is slow, and <20cm.
- Arrhythmias are common if wire insertion is rapid, and >20cm.
- Air embolism can occur if the cannula end is left open.

Complications

There are several local complications such as accidental arterial puncture, thoracic duct puncture, and damage to nerve plexuses. These are fortunately rare. The most important complication of this approach to a central vein is a pneumothorax. The chances of this may be reduced by strict attention to the anatomical approach, noting the close supero-posterior relationship of the pleura to the clavicle. The risk of a pneumothorax is 2–5% and so it is important that this route should not be used bilaterally, until a chest radiograph has excluded a pneumothorax on the side that has been first attempted.

Key points

- Head down tilt is essential, especially in the shocked patient.
- If cannulation is unsuccessful, recheck position of entry site.

INTERNAL JUGULAR VEIN CANNULATION

In comparison with the subclavian route, cannulation of the internal jugular vein carries a smaller risk of pneumothorax. Therefore, it is preferred in patients who are obese, or who are scheduled to undergo prolonged surgery. It is also most convenient for the anaesthetist, who is at the head of the table.

The patient positioning is the same as for subclavian cannulation, except that the head should only be turned slightly away from the chosen side.

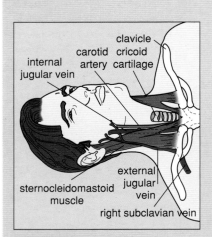

Fig. 1.11 The anatomy of the internal jugular vein

Technique

The technique is described for the right side.

1. Clean and drape the right side of the neck, from mastoid process to sternal notch.
2. In the head down position, the vein may be distended, and can sometimes be seen or balloted; it lies just lateral to the right carotid artery, and is a medial relation of the sternocleidomastoid in this 'high' approach to the internal jugular vein (Fig. 1.11).
3. Identify the midpoint of a imaginary line from the mastoid process to the sternal notch, and then palpate the carotid artery with the fingers of the left hand.
4. Attach a 5ml syringe to the needle, and insert the needle at this point: take care not to enter the external jugular vein, which often crosses the sternocleidomastoid at this point.
5. Aspirating the plunger of the syringe, direct the needle towards the ipsilateral nipple: the vein is not a deep structure, and so the needle should be directed horizontally, and not posteriorly (Fig. 1.12).
6. When venous blood enters the syringe, remove the syringe, and then proceed with the Seldinger technique as described above. ► ► ►

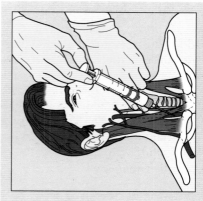

▶ ▶ ▶

7 If the vein is not entered, redirect the needle slightly more medially, taking care to keep lateral to the carotid at all times; it may be helpful to palpate the carotid with the left hand. If this is still unsuccessful, remove the needle, and reassess the landmarks.

Fig. 1.12 Advance the needle into the internal jugular vein

Hazards

- Take care in patients with potential cervical spine injury.
- Too much medial direction risks carotid puncture.
- Too much posterior direction risks vertebral artery puncture.
- In patients with elevated right heart pressures, it may be necessary to attach the cannula to a transducer to distinguish arterial from venous puncture.

Complications

Carotid puncture is the commonest problem, followed by damage to the vagus nerve and its branches in the neck. Rarely, the trachea, vertebral artery or oesophagus may be punctured, particularly if the landmarks are indistinct.

Key points

- The vein can often be seen and palpated in patients who are normo- or hypervolaemic.

EXTERNAL JUGULAR VEIN CANNULATION

The external jugular vein is a useful route for central vein cannulation in the obese, and in children. Its anatomy is relatively constant, and it can be easily distended by digital pressure at the root of the neck. There is little risk of carotid puncture, although haematoma can occur if the vein is transfixed. The main disadvantage of this route is that a valve at the junction of the external jugular and subclavian vein often prevents passage of the catheter into the right side of the heart. The vein also tends to collapse easily, which makes it hard to advance the catheter.

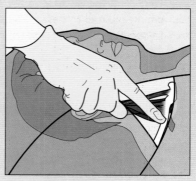

Technique

The procedure is described for the right external jugular vein.

1 Position the patient as for internal jugular vein cannulation; ask an assistant to put gentle pressure at the root of the neck, to distend the vein (Fig. 1.13).
2 Identify the vein, which crosses the sternocleidomastoid at its midpoint.

▶ ▶ ▶

Fig. 1.13 The external jugular vein may be distended by straining or pressure at the root of the neck

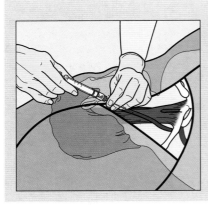

▶ ▶ ▶

3 Prepare the area over the right side of the neck ,as for cannulation of the internal jugular vein. Infiltrate local anaesthetic around the midpoint of the sternocleidomastoid.

4 Attach a 5ml syringe to the needle, and insert the needle, with aspiration on the plunger, in the direction of the vein (Fig. 1.14).

5 As soon as blood enters the syringe, do not advance the needle any further.

6 Remove the syringe, and proceed as for the Seldinger technique for subclavian vein cannulation.

Fig. 1.14 Aspiration of venous blood confirms entry into the external jugular vein

Complications

Local haematoma and bleeding are the commonest problems. It may be difficult to advance the wire or catheter into the vein, but this can often be overcome by gently rotating the wire/catheter as it is advanced. If a valve prevents advance, try flushing a small amount of saline into the catheter, to distend the vein.

Key points

- Select the right side first, as it is usually the more successful route.
- If the vein is not distended, it may be difficult to puncture it correctly: try distending it with pressure at the root of the neck.
- Do not advance the exploring needle too far, as the vein may be damaged.

BASILIC VEIN CANNULATION

The basilic vein is useful in non-obese adults, but may be difficult in the obese and in paediatric patients. This approach suffers from the same disadvantage of all peripheral approaches to the central venous system, in that the catheter may not always reach an intrathoracic central vein; thus it is not always reliable for central venous pressure monitoring.

Technique

1 Select an appropriate long line: either a 50cm central venous line, or else a Drum cartridge catheter (catheter through cannula).

2 Select the non-dominant arm, and apply a tourniquet at mid-humeral level. Position the arm in 30 degrees abduction, and full external rotation.

3 Identify the basilic vein in the antecubital fossa, and prepare the area with antiseptic solution (Fig. 1.15). ▶ ▶ ▶

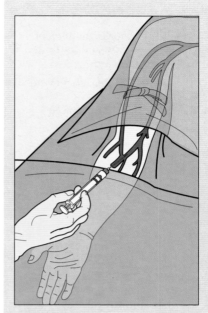

Fig. 1.15 The basilic vein crosses the antecubital fossa

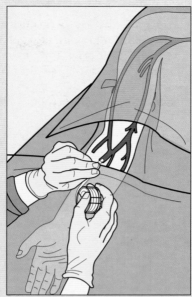

Fig. 1.16 Advance the drum catheter up the cannula, which should be held firmly in the basilic vein

▶ ▶ ▶

4 Seldinger technique: attach a 5ml syringe to the needle, and cannulate the vein with the needle. Grasp the Seldinger wire in the left hand, and then remove the syringe from the needle. Insert the Seldinger wire, and then proceed as for subclavian cannulation above.

5 Drum cartridge catheter technique: cannulate the vein with the introducer cannula, remove the needle and then insert the Drum cartridge catheter into the introducer cannula. Advance the catheter up to about 40cm (Fig. 1.16).

6 Withdraw the introducer cannula out of the vein, leaving the Drum cartridge catheter *in situ*. Lock the hub of the cannula to the proximal end of the Drum catheter.

7 Remove the stiffening wire from the inside of the Drum cartridge catheter.

8 Connect a fluid infusion line to the Luer lock end of the catheter, and check that venous blood drains back into the line when placed below the level of the thorax.

9 Clean and dry the puncture site, and then apply a sterile dressing. Perform a chest radiograph to confirm the catheter site.

Complications

The two most common problems are: a) failure to cannulate the vein, due to a valve or thrombosis; there is little choice, but to try a different site, and b) failure to negotiate the catheter through the axilla. Brachial arterial puncture may occur, if the artery is superficial to the biceps tendon, or if the puncture is too deep. The median nerve may be injured as it crosses the antecubital fossa, and so it is important to identify the vein before puncture, and to keep the needle horizontal to the plane of the arm.

Key points

- Choose the (medial) basilic vein, rather than the (lateral) cephalic vein; the latter often has a valve that prevents cannulation, and turns sharply as it passes through the clavipectoral fascia.
- If the catheter will not advance to 40cm then abduct the arm, and try to advance it again; if this fails, gently flush saline into the cannula, as it advances.
- Perform a chest radiograph.

FEMORAL VEIN CANNULATION

The femoral vein is not a first line approach to the central venous system, but is useful in certain situations. It is appropriate for patients with suspected upper body injuries, where upper limb infusion is contra-indicated. It can also be used where there is local injury or sepsis to the neck and clavicle.

The patient should be supine, and the groin should be shaved.

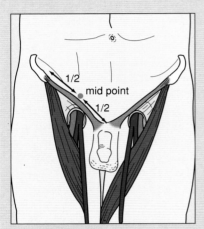

Fig. 1.17 The femoral vein lies medial to the pulse of the femoral artery

Technique

The technique is described for the right side.

1 Clean and drape the area at the midpoint of the inguinal region.
2 Palpate the femoral artery with the fingers of the right hand: the femoral vein lies directly medial to the artery. When the artery has been located, change hands, and keep a finger of the left hand on the femoral arterial pulse for reference (Fig. 1.17).
3 Insert the needle with a 5ml syringe attached medial to the femoral artery, directing it towards the umbilicus.
4 The needle should be kept horizontal, with only a slight posterior direction; aspirate the syringe at all times (Fig. 1.18).
5 When venous blood enters the syringe, remove the syringe, and occlude the needle end with a finger. Advance the catheter over the needle (Drum Cartridge Catheter technique) or introduce a Seldinger wire through the needle (Seldinger technique).
6 Proceed as for basilic vein cannulation (Drum cartridge technique) or for subclavian cannulation (Seldinger technique).

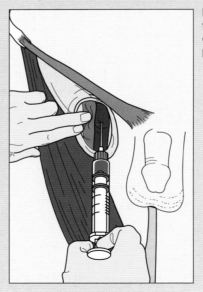

Fig. 1.18 The needle is advanced into the femoral vein: the fingers of the opposite hand remain on the femoral pulse

Complications

Haematoma and infection are the commonest local complications, and may be avoided by close attention to detail. Accidental arterial puncture can be reduced by keeping a finger on the femoral pulse at all times. The femoral nerve is a lateral relation of the femoral artery, and may be damaged by inaccurate lateral direction of the needle.

Key points

- Always keep a finger on the femoral pulse.
- Always puncture the skin medial to the femoral pulse.
- Direct the needle more laterally with each attempt.
- Keep the wire/catheter close to hand on the sterile tray.

Tunnelled central venous feeding lines

Feeding lines are used for patients requiring parenteral nutrition. The indications for parenteral feeding are listed below. The site of the feeding line is not critical, but it is essential that the site can be easily observed and dressed. These lines should be used for feeding only, and are not for drugs or other fluids.

The most common route used, the subclavian, will be described, although it is possible to use any of the other routes listed in the section under central venous cannulation.

Indications

Protein and/or calorie malnutrition due to:
- Hypermetabolic state.
- Failure or contra-indication to enteral feeding, such as: short gut syndrome, paralytic ileus, intestinal sepsis or haemorrhage.
- Prolonged unconsciousness or immobility.
- Bulbar or pseudo-bulbar palsy.

Contra-indications

Absolute
Enteral feeding possible.
Local sepsis or injury.
Inexperience with technique.
Absence of aseptic facilities.

Relative
Coagulation defects.
Need for short term (<48 hours) feeding only.

Equipment

See Fig. 1.19.
- ☐ Patient on tilting bed.
- ☐ Local anaesthetic: 1% lignocaine with 1:200,000 adrenaline.
- ☐ Full aseptic preparation kit with antiseptic solution.
- ☐ Appropriate intravenous line with hub for connection to feeding bag.
- ☐ Scalpel and metal dilator.
- ☐ Suture material.
- ☐ Sterile adhesive dressing.

Technique

The line should be inserted under full aseptic conditions, ideally in an operating theatre with a circulating air-exchange system. The line chosen should have an appropriate hub for connection to a feeding bag. In some patients it may be necessary to administer general anaesthesia for the procedure, as the insertion can be lengthy and uncomfortable.

The patient should be positioned head down, with the head turned away from the side of insertion. The arm on the chosen side should be allowed to relax, and it may be necessary to ask an assistant to pull the arm down to depress the shoulder.

1 Full aseptic precautions should be observed: therefore scrub up, and put on sterile gloves and gown.
2 Clean and drape the area around the shoulder and clavicle with sterile towels.
3 Open the chosen feeding line, and check that the hub has a suitable connection (usually Luer lock).
4 Identify the midpoint of the clavicle on the chosen side. Infiltrate 20ml of local anaesthetic along a line about 6cm caudad along the chest wall.
5 Attach a 10ml syringe to the locating needle, and advance the needle through the skin below the midpoint of the clavicle. ► ► ►

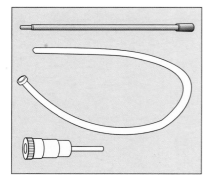

Fig. 1.19 Central venous feeding cannula

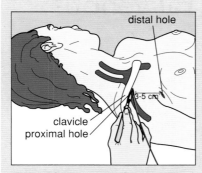

Fig. 1.20 An incision is made around the wire

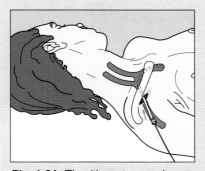

Fig. 1.21 The dilator is passed over the wire

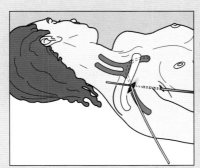

Fig. 1.22 The metal dilator is pushed through the skin to emerge beside the line insertion point

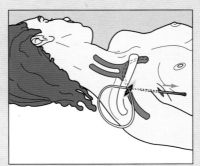

Fig. 1.23 The metal dilator is retracted with the feeding line attached to the distal end

▶ ▶ ▶

6 Direct the needle parallel to the surface of the skin, towards the suprasternal notch, and aspirate gently.

7 When the venous blood enters the syringe, remove it from the needle, and advance the wire through the hub of the needle. Remove the needle, and make a small incision around the wire, to allow the dilator to enter (Fig. 1.20).

8 Pass the dilator over the wire (Fig. 1.21), remove it, and then pass the introducer cannula over the wire. Remove the wire, and occlude the end of the introducer cannula. Push the feeding line through the introducer cannula, until about 12–14cm of line remains outside. Remove the introducer cannula.

9 Make an incision in the skin about 4–6cm below the needle insertion, and push the blunt tapered end of the metal dilator up from here, until it emerges beside the feeding line (Fig. 1.22).

10 Attach the open end of the feeding line to the end of the metal dilator, and then gently pull the metal dilator out of the second incision site (Fig. 1.23).

11 Remove the metal dilator, and attach the hub of the connector to the feeding line. Check that the line is not kinked at the first puncture site, and that the feeding line is not pulled too tight.

12 After aspiration to confirm venous blood, attach a cap to the proximal end of the feeding line connector, and flush the line with heparinised saline.

13 Suture the line in place, and also carefully suture the first incision, to close the insertion site. Take care not to catch the feeding cannula in the stitch.

14 Apply a sterile dressing, and perform a chest radiograph to confirm correct line placement.

Complications

All the complications of central vein cannulation via the subclavian route apply to this technique: pneumothorax, puncture of the subclavian artery, damage to the thoracic duct, and haematoma formation. Aspiration of air is possible if the open end of the feeding line is elevated above the thorax, and it is therefore crucial that the end is occluded or connected at all times. Subsequent use of the line may

Hazards

- The hub mechanism of the feeding line must be tightly secured to prevent air embolism.
- Do not put the feeding line under tension following complete insertion.
- Check that the feeding line is not kinked before closing the insertion site.
- Do not allow the line to be used for anything other than feeding.

be followed by sepsis, either local or systemic, and air or clot may be accidentally injected via the line during long term use.

Key points

- Check the line to make sure that it fits onto the hub of the feeding set, usually by a Luer lock connection.
- Make sure that you understand how to assemble the feeding line before you insert the subclavian cannula.
- The metal dilator must make a clear and patent passage between the two incision sites in the subcutaneous tissues.

Cut-down venous cannulation

Cut-down on to a peripheral vein is required when more conventional approaches to cannulation have failed. There are many reasons for failed percutaneous cannulation; the most common are venous constriction due to severe hypovolaemic shock and cold, or obesity.

Indications

Intravenous fluid and/or drug administration with failed percutaneous peripheral/central cannulation.

Contra-indications

Absolute

Local sepsis or injury.
Lack of aseptic facilities.
Suspected injury to the pelvic veins or inferior vena cava (in this situation use upper body veins, e.g. cephalic or basilic).

Relative

Known bleeding diathesis.

Equipment

See Fig. 1.24.
- ☐ Tilting bed.
- ☐ Antiseptic solution.
- ☐ Local anaesthetic; 1% lignocaine with 1:200,000 adrenaline.
- ☐ Cut-down set.
- ☐ Scalpel with no. 10 blade.
- ☐ Small haemostatic forceps.
- ☐ Suitable size cannula (e.g. 10–14G).
- ☐ Intravenous giving set and fluids.
- ☐ Ties 3/0.
- ☐ Non-absorbable 4/0 sutures on cutting needle.
- ☐ Sterile adhesive dressings.

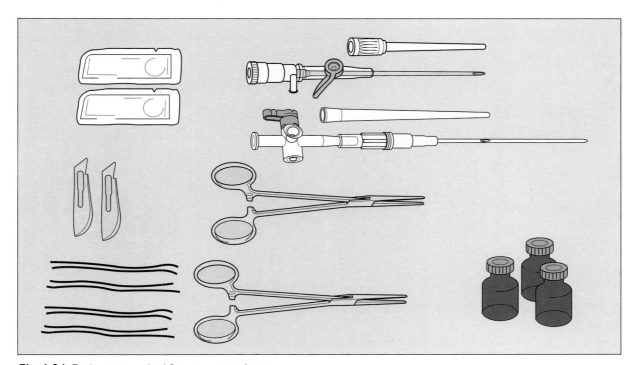

Fig. 1.24 Equipment required for venous cut-down

Technique

The patient should be supine, on a tipping trolley or bed. The long saphenous vein at the ankle is the commonest site, although the same vein can be cannulated at the groin. If the saphenous vein is palpable or visible at the ankle (Fig. 1.25) and will admit a cannula of suitable diameter, then choose this route; otherwise, choose the groin. In severely hypovolaemic patients, more than one route may be attempted simultaneously. In extreme circumstances, where the patient is unconscious, local anaesthesia is not required. However, it is usual to explain the procedure to the patient and to infiltrate with local anaesthetic.

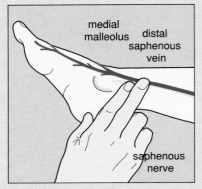

Fig. 1.25 The site of the saphenous vein

1 Put on sterile gloves.
2 Clean and drape the area with antiseptic cleaning fluid.
3 Infiltrate local anaesthetic into the skin and subcutaneous tissues.
4 Ankle: make a 2.5cm transverse incision over the vein, as it runs anterior to the medial malleolus (Fig. 1.26a). Groin: palpate the femoral artery in the skin crease, and then drop down 3cm. Make a shallow 4cm transverse incision at this point (Fig. 1.26b).
5 Expose and isolate the vein using blunt dissection with the points of the haemostatic forceps. Make sure that you are below the sapheno-femoral junction in the groin. Dissect out the vein for a length of 2cm and then tie a ligature round the distal end, leaving long cut ends for traction (Fig. 1.27).
6 Put a second ligature loosely around the proximal end of the vein, and put gentle traction on this.
7 Make a small transverse venotomy and gently dilate the venotomy with the tip of a closed haemostatic forceps. Insert the largest cannula possible into the vein. Venous blood will flow back if the traction on the proximal end is released slightly (Fig. 1.28).
8 Tie the proximal ligature tightly around the vein, to secure the cannula.
9 Close the wound with interrupted sutures, and apply a sterile dressing.

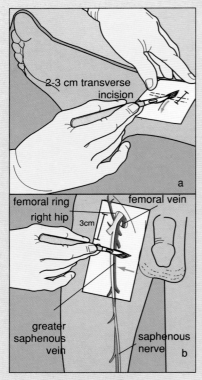

Fig. 1.26 Sites of incision for the saphenous vein at the ankle and the groin

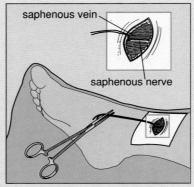

Fig. 1.27 A ligature is tied around the distal part of the vein

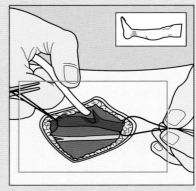

Fig. 1.28 The cannula is inserted into the vein

Complications

Local haemorrhage and sepsis are the most frequent complications. Less often, the cannula may dislodge, and may be followed by haemorrhage into the wound; this can be prevented by ensuring that an adequate (3–4cm) length of cannula is inserted in the vein, before tying the proximal ligature.

Ensure that the structure that is cannulated is indeed a vein: this can be checked by tightening and releasing the proximal tie, and observing the flow of venous blood. It is important that if the groin approach is used, the incision is not made close to the inguinal skin fold for the femoral vein may be mistaken for the saphenous vein. The femoral vein must never be tied off for cannulation.

Hazards

- Attempted cannulation of a non-venous structure, e.g. nerve or artery.
- Mistaken ligation of the femoral vein.

Key points

- Gentle blunt dissection is safer than an initial deep incision.
- The distal ligature should be firmly tied, to prevent bleeding.
- The proximal ligature must be tested before the venotomy is performed.
- In severe hypovolaemia, insert the cut end of the intravenous giving set tubing itself into the vein, to ensure the highest possible flow rates.

Intraosseous cannulation and infusion

Indications

Failure to cannulate vein for:
- Emergency drugs and fluids in cardiac arrest, hypovolaemic shock, major burns and status epilepticus.
- Obtaining blood sample for grouping and cross-matching.

Contra-indications

Infection at intended insertion site.
Ipsilateral fractured extremity.
Osteogenesis imperfecta.
Osteopetrosis.

Rapid intravascular access is required for the appropriate management of the majority of medical emergencies. Occasionally, particularly in young children and hypovolaemic patients, intravenous cannulation can be extremely difficult. In these circumstances, intraosseous infusion represents an excellent alternative method of administering drugs until it can be replaced by a cannula placed intravenously.

Substances injected into the bone marrow are absorbed almost immediately into the systemic venous system, via medullary venous channels and nutrient and emissary veins. Any drug that can be infused intravenously can be infused through an intraosseous needle. The intraosseous route is usually associated with paediatric resuscitation where, in addition to drug administration, typical flow rates of 10ml/min contribute towards effective restoration of intravascular volume. Drugs can effectively be given to adults through an intramedullary needle but, with the exception of hypertonic saline, the volume of fluid given via this route is unlikely to be effective for volume resuscitation.

Equipment

☐ Antiseptic solution.
☐ 1% lignocaine.
☐ Intraosseous infusion needle, e.g. Sur-Fast® (Fig. 1.29) or bone marrow aspiration needle, e.g. Osenthal or Osgood.
☐ 5ml syringe.
☐ Bag of crystalloid and standard intravenous infusion set.

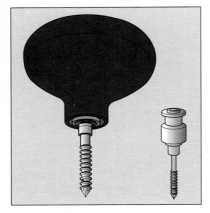

Fig. 1 29 Sur-Fast® intraosseous infusion needle (with detachable handle)

Technique

This procedure is only performed in emergencies and should be completed simply and rapidly. The unconscious patient will not require local anaesthetic. In infants, and children under six years, the best insertion sites are the proximal tibia or distal femur. In adults, the best site is in the distal tibia. Place the patient supine, place a sandbag behind the knee for support, and restrain the leg.

1 Clean the insertion site with antiseptic solution.
2 If the patient is conscious, infiltrate the skin and periosteum with lignocaine.
3 If using a needle with a screw thread (e.g. Sur-Fast®), make a small incision in the skin with the scalpel supplied.
4 If using the proximal tibial site, palpate the tibial tuberosity with your index finger and grasp the medial aspect of the tibia with your thumb.

► ► ►

The optimal insertion site is halfway between these points and 1–2cm distally (Fig. 1.30). Direct the needle slightly distally (about 15° from the perpendicular) to avoid the growth plate (Fig. 1.31). In children under one year, insert the needle just distal to the line of the tibial tuberosity; the bone is very narrow distal to this, increasing the possibility of fracture.

5 If using the distal tibial site, insert the intraosseous needle 2cm proximal to the tip of the medial malleolus, in a slightly cephalad direction (Fig. 1.32).

6 Using moderate pressure, insert the intraosseous needle into the bone using a to-and-fro twisting motion. In the case of a needle with a screw thread, once the cutting tip is 2–3mm into the bone, continue to advance with a screwing motion.

7 Stop advancing the needle when there is a slight decrease in resistance.

8 Aspirate blood or bone marrow to confirm placement, and flush with crystalloid. The needle should stay upright without support.

9 Connect intravenous giving set to the needle. Higher flow rates can be obtained by pressurising the fluid up to 300mmHg.

10 Apply a simple sterile dressing.

11 Discontinue the intraosseous infusion as soon as reliable venous access has been established.

12 When stable, obtain a radiograph of the insertion site in children to exclude fracture.

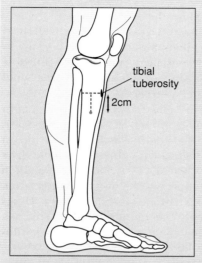

Fig. 1.30 Insertion site in proximal tibia

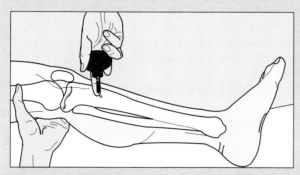

Fig. 1.31 Insertion of intraosseous needle in proximal tibia

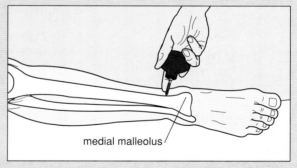

Fig. 1.32 Insertion of intraosseous needle in distal tibia

Complications

The most common complication is misplacement of the needle, resulting in incomplete penetration of the anterior cortex or over penetration with the needle passing through the posterior cortex. The relatively common problem of subcutaneous and subperiosteal extravasation is significantly reduced with the use of a Sur-Fast® needle. Tibial fractures have been reported in an infant, probably as a result of inserting a relatively large intraosseous needle too distally. Localised cellulitis occurs in 0.7%, and the more serious problem of osteomyelitis has been reported in 0.6%. Long-term effects on the growth plate have not been identified.

Hazards

• In the infant, insertion too distally in the tibia may fracture the bone.

Temperature controlled rapid fluid infusion

Indications

Following major haemorrhage:
- Trauma.
- Obstetric complications.
- Gastrointestinal bleeds.

Where major haemorrhage is expected:
- Major vascular surgery.
- Liver transplantation.

Contra-indications

None.

Factors that determine the maximum possible flow during intravenous infusion include: the cannulation site, the cannula, the type of administration set, the infusion pressure, and the temperature of the fluid. Rapid infusion techniques incorporate short, large-bore cannulae placed in large veins in combination with wide-bore infusion sets. Flow rates can be increased by pressurising the system with automatic pressure infusors enclosed in rigid boxes.

Massive transfusion of cold fluids, especially blood, may cause hypothermia and its accompanying adverse physiological effects. A very efficient fluid warmer, the Level 1 (Fig. 1.33), helps to overcome these problems. Water heated to 40°C at the base of the warmer is circulated through a closed-flow, aluminium counter-current heat exchanger which forms an integral part of disposable giving sets. It is able to warm cold (10°C) packed red cells to temperatures >35°C at flows of 500ml/min. The most efficient warming and infusion device currently available is the Rapid Infusion System. It comprises a roller pump mechanism and heat exchanger and can deliver blood products at precise rates and under normothermic conditions at up to 1500ml/min.

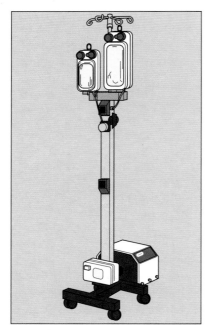

Fig. 1.33 The Level 1 fluid warmer

Equipment

- ☐ Sterile pack and antiseptic solution.
- ☐ 1% lignocaine.
- ☐ Syringes, 5ml and 10ml.
- ☐ Large-bore cannula e.g. pulmonary artery catheter introducer set.
- ☐ Scalpel blade.
- ☐ Suture, e.g. 2/0 silk on a straight needle.
- ☐ Sterile adhesive dressing, e.g. Op-Site.
- ☐ Level 1 fluid warmer.
- ☐ Disposable giving set for Level 1 warmer.
- ☐ Litre bag of Hartmann's solution x2.

Technique

For the purposes of rapid fluid infusion, the best sites for placing a pulmonary artery catheter introducer are the subclavian, internal jugular or femoral veins. The femoral route will be described as this is a particularly good choice in the hypovolaemic patient.

Position the patient supine and, assuming that the right femoral vein is to be used, place the right leg in external rotation and 30° abduction.

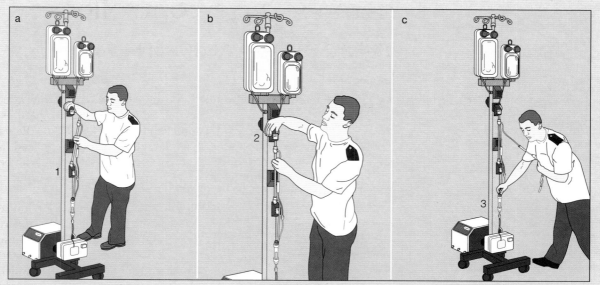

Fig. 1.34 Attaching the disposable to the Level 1 fluid warmer

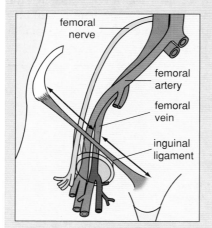

Fig. 1.35 Anatomy of the femoral vein

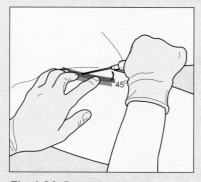

Fig. 1.36 Femoral venepuncture

► ► ►

1 Open the pack containing the Level 1 disposable giving set (e.g. D-100) and attach it to the infusion stand holding the warmer. First, plug in the lower end of the heat exchanger, then secure the top end before finally mounting the air eliminator (Fig. 1.34).

2 Prime the giving set with Hartmann's and switch on the warmer.

3 If the cannulation is being performed electively, shave the hair around the area.

4 Clean the insertion site thoroughly with antiseptic solution and drape the area.

5 Palpate the femoral arterial pulse at the midpoint of a line drawn between the anterior superior iliac spine and the symphysis pubis. The femoral vein lies in the femoral sheath, medial to the femoral artery just below the inguinal ligament (Fig. 1.35). Infiltrate 5ml of local anaesthetic at the insertion site 3cm below the inguinal ligament and 1cm medial to the maximal femoral pulsation .

6 Attach a 5ml syringe to the thin-wall needle supplied in the introducer kit; the guidewire will be passed through this. Puncture the skin and advance the needle at 45° and cephalad, while gently aspirating on the syringe (Fig. 1.18, 1.36).

7 On puncturing the femoral vein, continue placement of the introducer as described under 'Pulmonary artery catheterisation', p. 26.

8 Connect the infusion set directly to the introducer sheath. Do not use the side port and valve included in the introducer set, as it significantly reduces the maximum rate of infusion (Fig. 1.37).

9 Increase the rate of infusion by placing the fluid bags in the automatic pressure infusor boxes at the top of the Level 1 infusion stand and pressurise up to 300mmHg.

10 If using packed red blood cells, increase the rate of infusion by first haemodiluting with crystalloid, hence reducing the viscosity.

Complications

Accidental puncture of the femoral artery is the commonest complication associated with attempted cannulation of the femoral vein. This is not normally a major problem as direct pressure can easily be applied at this site.

If there is leakage at the cannulation site, it is possible for large volumes of fluid or blood to be infused under pressure into the perivascular tissues. Ideally the infusion site should be kept in view.

Key Points

- The rate of infusion can be maximised by using large-bore short cannulae in combination with large-bore giving sets (internal diameter of 4.8mm or more) to infuse fluids under pressure warmed to near normal body temperature.

Hazards

- If arterial puncture (femoral, subclavian, or carotid) goes unrecognised, it is possible for a large-bore cannula to be placed in the artery with risk of significant vascular damage.

Pulmonary artery catheterisation

Pulmonary artery floatation catheters (PAFC) are available with varying degrees of complexity and versatility. The most basic catheter allows measurement of right atrial pressure (RAP), pulmonary artery pressure (PAP), and pulmonary artery occlusion pressure (PAOP). The more sophisticated, thermistor equipped PAFC permits determination of cardiac output by thermodilution and, with measurements of arterial and mixed venous oxygen content, calculation of oxygen supply and demand. Other catheters are equipped with fibre-optics enabling continuous estimation of mixed venous oxygen saturation (SvO_2), while others have electrodes on the catheter surface or lumina for passing electrodes to diagnose dysrhythmias or for cardiac pacing. The right ventricular ejection fraction (RVEF) catheter, equipped with a fast response thermistor, is able to measure RVEF and right ventricular end diastolic volume (RVEDV).

The PAFC provides considerable physiological information to help with the management of critically-ill patients but whether this actually contributes to improving patient outcome is controversial. The assumption that PAOP is a reliable indicator of left ventricular end diastolic volume (LVEDV) is not always correct. Furthermore, the PAFC is associated with significant morbidity and occasionally mortality. Thus, the precise indications for inserting a PAFC vary greatly from one physician to another, and between centres and countries. Having decided to subject a patient to the risk of PAFC insertion, the derived data should be obtained frequently and acted upon promptly and appropriately.

Indications

The European Intensive Care Society have published guidelines on the indications for a PAFC:
- Myocardial infarction complicated by shock.
- Severe acute left ventricular failure.
- Predominant right ventricular failure.
- Unexplained sinus tachycardia.
- To confirm pulmonary oedema is truly due to cardiac disease.
- Pulmonary oedema which fails to respond to initial therapy.
- Heart failure associated with oliguric renal failure.
- Pulmonary embolism associated with shock.
- Anticipated complicated cardiac surgery.
- Acute respiratory failure associated with left heart failure.
- Therapeutic PEEP manoeuvres which can influence cardiac output.
- Sepsis and/or multiple organ dysfunction with capillary permeability.
- Unstable patients during renal replacement therapy.
- ARDS when respiratory function is deteriorating.
- Patients with impaired left ventricular function who fail to wean from mechanical ventilation.
- Major trauma and severe sepsis to ensure a hyperdynamic state.

In addition the following indications may apply:

- Perioperative monitoring of high-risk surgical patients.
- Severe pre-eclampsia and heart disease in pregnancy.
- Severe systemic disease, e.g. pancreatitis.

Contra-indications

If the information to be derived is considered essential, there are no absolute contra-indications.

Relative

Untreated severe coagulopathy or thrombocytopenia

(if necessary, proceed via ante-cubital, external jugular, or internal jugular venous routes).
Endocardial pacemaker or defibrillator *in situ*.
Prosthetic tricuspid or pulmonary valve.
Pulmonary valvular disease.
Severe mitral regurgitation (makes PAOP difficult to interpret).
Primary pulmonary hypertension (increased risk of pulmonary artery rupture).
Cardiac septal defects.
Left bundle-branch block.

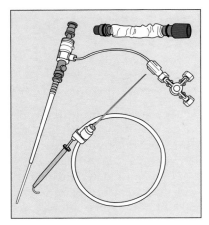

Fig. 1.37 Pulmonary artery catheter introducer kit

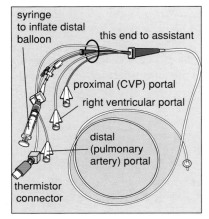

Fig. 1.38 Pulmonary artery catheter

Equipment

- ☐ Sterile pack and antiseptic solution.
- ☐ 1% lignocaine.
- ☐ Syringes, 5ml and 10ml.
- ☐ 25 gauge needle for local anaesthetic.
- ☐ One or two pressure transducers and appropriate monitor.
- ☐ 500ml bag normal saline with 500 units heparin and pressure infusor.
- ☐ PAFC introducer set (Fig. 1.37)
  thin-wall needle
  introducer sheath
  haemostatic valve and sidearm
  J guide wire
  dilator and external catheter sheath.
- ☐ Scalpel blade.
- ☐ Suture, e.g. silk on a straight needle.
- ☐ Sterile adhesive dressing.
- ☐ 1 litre bag of crystalloid and primed drip set .
- ☐ PAFC (Fig. 1.38).
- ☐ Cardiac output computer.
- ☐ Injectate giving set, ice container, ice and in-line temperature probe .
- ☐ Facilities for post-insertion radiograph.

Technique

All the sites for CVP line insertion can be used for the placement of a PAFC (internal and external jugular, subclavian, femoral and basilic veins), but the right internal jugular vein or left subclavian allow best use of the natural curve of the PAFC. Position the patient as previously described for central line insertion (p. 6). Do not use excessive head down tilt in patients with cardiac failure. In the presence of a coagulopathy, the basilic route is safest.

Make sure a defibrillator and resuscitation drugs are immediately available.

Flush the pressure transducer and manometer lines with heparinised saline. Zero and calibrate the transducer. In most cases RA pressures are measured only intermittently thus, using a 3-way tap, one transducer can be used for both PA and RA lumina.

Put on sterile gloves and gown.

Insertion of the PAFC introducer
PAFC insertion into the right internal jugular vein:
1 Open the sterile pack. Clean and drape the skin as described in 'Central vein cannulation' p. 6. Make sure the patient is well covered with drapes; it is easy to desterilise the long PAFC.
2 Open the introducer kit and prepare guidewire by withdrawing the J end into its sheath. ► ► ►

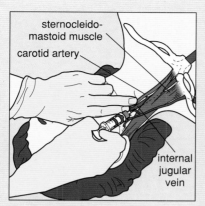

Fig. 1.39 Approach to right internal jugular vein

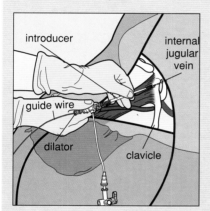

Fig. 1.40 Insertion of pulmonary artery introducer

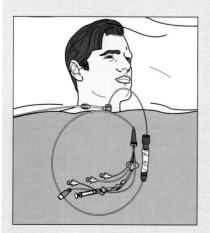

Fig. 1.41 Pulmonary artery catheter ready for insertion

▶ ▶ ▶

3 Screw the sidearm and valve onto the introducer sheath and mount them both on the dilator (Fig. 1.37).

4 Infiltrate the insertion site with 1% lignocaine. For an approach medial to the sternocleidomastoid, this site is level with the cricoid cartilage and just lateral to the pulsation of the carotid artery.

5 Mount the thin-wall needle on a 5ml syringe, puncture the skin, and advance while gently aspirating, aiming at the ipsilateral nipple (Fig. 1.39).

6 On aspirating venous blood freely, steady the needle, disconnect the syringe and insert the J guide wire up to 20cm before carefully removing the thin-wall needle.

7 Using the scalpel blade, enlarge the skin entry site to accommodate the PAFC introducer.

8 Slide the introducer/dilator over the wire and, with a twisting motion, advancing all three parts together with both hands, one proximal and one distal (Fig. 1.40).

9 Remove the vein dilator and wire, aspirate blood from the sidearm and flush with heparinised saline. Secure the introducer with a suture.

Insertion of the PAFC

10 Remove the PAFC from its pack and pass it through the external catheter sheath. Some PAFCs are packaged with this protective sheath already mounted.

11 Inflate the PAFC balloon (1.5ml) and check that it inflates evenly and that it deflates passively. Active deflation, at any time, can invaginate a small part of the balloon into the lumen of the catheter which may cause rupture of the balloon.

12 Attach a 3-way tap to the proximal port; attach the pressure transducer to the distal port, flush both ports with heparinised saline, and check that the transducer is level with the patient's left atrium. Shake the distal end of the PAFC and confirm correct assembly by the appearance of spiky waveforms on the monitor.

13 Lay out the catheter on top of the drapes on the patient's chest, so that the natural curve of the catheter will result in the tip being advanced in an anticlockwise direction through the right heart into the right pulmonary artery (Fig. 1.41).

14 Pass the PAFC through the introducer up to the 20cm mark; a central venous pressure waveform should be displayed on the monitor. Inflate the balloon with the volume of air recommended for the particular catheter (typically, 1.0–1.5ml), and close the gate valve to maintain inflation.

15 With continuous monitoring of the distal waveform (Fig. 1.42) and ECG, advance the catheter through the right atrium (typical distance from right internal jugular 20–30cm) and right ventricle (30–40cm) into the pulmonary artery (40–50cm). Typical distances to the RV from other access sites are: 45cm from the left internal jugular or left subclavian veins, 50cm from the femoral veins, 60cm from the right basilic vein, and 70cm from the left basilic vein. ▶ ▶ ▶

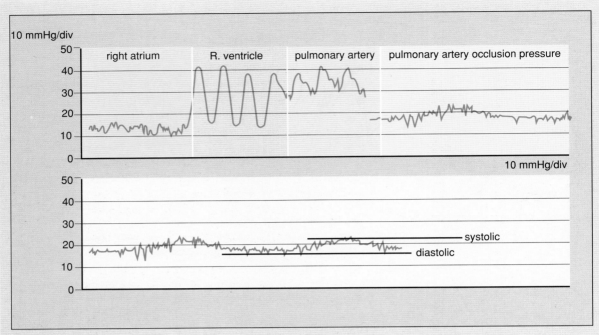

Fig. 1.42 Pressure waveforms during insertion of pulmonary artery catheter

▶ ▶ ▶

16 If the PA is not entered within 15cm of the first entering the RV, the catheter is probably coiling and should be withdrawn back to the RA. *Always deflate the balloon before withdrawing the catheter,* and reinflate before re-advancing. If ventricular ectopics occur (usually while the tip is in the RV), withdraw the catheter from the right heart and try again. Give lignocaine 50mg if ventricular ectopics persist.

17 If the catheter will not pass into the PA, place the patient in the right lateral position and try again. Once in the PA, slowly advance the catheter until a pulmonary artery occlusion pressure (PAOP) waveform (Fig. 1.42) is obtained (usually at 45–55cm). Record the PAOP at the end of the expiratory phase of respiration (the diastolic value when the monitor is set on systolic/diastolic mode).

18 Deflate the balloon passively and observe immediate return of the PAP waveform. Slowly reinflate the balloon; it should require 0.8–1.2ml to obtain a PAOP waveform; if it requires less than 0.7ml, deflate the balloon, withdraw the catheter 1cm and recheck. The PAOP should be less than the mean PAP. A PA blood gas taken when wedged should have a higher PaO_2 than that taken with the balloon deflated.

19 Record the depth of insertion of the catheter, extend the external catheter sheath and secure it to the introducer.

20 Obtain a chest radiograph to confirm correct positioning and to exclude a pneumothorax. ▶ ▶ ▶

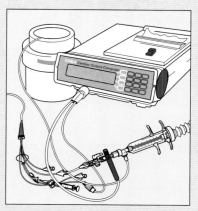

Fig. 1.43 Set up for estimation of cardiac output by thermodilution

▶ ▶ ▶

Determination of cardiac output by thermodilution

21 Attach the thermistor wire from the PAFC to the appropriate lead from the cardiac output computer.

22 Run through an i.v. giving set and coil with normal saline (the injectate solution) and connect it to the 3-way tap on the proximal port of the PAFC. Place the coil in an insulated container full of ice. Attach a 10ml syringe to the remaining port of the 3-way tap. When filling the injectate syringe, the saline will be cooled as it passes through the coil. Position the temperature probe to measure the temperature of the iced injectate; it is best placed in-line at the proximal injection port and a specific adapter is available for this purpose. (Fig. 1.43).

23 Aspirate 10ml of injectate solution into the syringe, press the start button on the computer, and immediately, smoothly inject the syringe contents into the patient. Inject the 10ml in less than four seconds. The computer will display the calculated cardiac output.

24 Repeat the measurement three times, injecting the saline at the same phase in the respiratory cycle, and record the cardiac output as the average of these three.

25 Many clinicians claim that the use of injectate at room temperature provides an accurate estimation of cardiac output, except where the cardiac output is very high (>10litres/min). However, ice cold injectate is the gold standard and should be used whenever the appropriate equipment is available.

Complications

The complications associated with insertion of the introducer are those listed for internal jugular cannulation in 'Central vein cannulation' p. 6. There are, in addition, a number of complications associated with the PAFC itself. In over 70% of cases dysrhythmias (atrial and ventricular ectopics, atrial fibrillation, ventricular tachycardia and occasionally ventricular fibrillation) occur during catheter insertion. Patients with coronary artery disease will be at risk of stress-induced myocardial ischaemia. The risk of coils, kinks, and knots that may occur during placement of the PAFC may be reduced by not inserting excessive lengths of catheter. Pulmonary artery rupture occurs in up to 0.2% of insertions and may be caused by over-inflating the balloon or inflating the balloon when the catheter is already in a wedged position. Direct catheter trauma can also result in valvular incompetence and cardiac perforation. PAFCs commonly cause pulmonary emboli. Pulmonary infarction can result from emboli or from direct occlusion of flow by the catheter. Catheter sepsis, which may result in endocarditis, is a significant concern and for this reason the PAFC should not be left *in situ* for more than three days.

Hazards

- Life-threatening dysrhythmias may occur during PAFC insertion. Have lignocaine and a defibrillator available beforehand.
- Withdrawing the catheter with the balloon inflated may rupture cardiac valves.
- Pulmonary artery rupture may result from over or prolonged inflation of the balloon.
- Whenever a PAFC is *in situ*, monitor the PA trace continuously in order to detect spontaneous wedging.

Key point

- Use the natural curve of the catheter to direct it into the pulmonary artery. Remember the typical distances from the insertion point to the RV and PA and do not insert excessive lengths of catheter.

Arterial cannulation

Peripheral arterial cannulation is one of the most common procedures performed in the critical care unit and is frequently performed in the operating room. The artery selected for cannulation should be large enough to measure pressure accurately without occlusion of the vessel or there should be good collateral circulation. Ideally, the site should be readily accessible for nursing care and should not be in an area prone to contamination. The most commonly used site is the radial artery at the wrist but there are a number of other suitable arteries: the ulnar, dorsalis pedis, and posterior tibial arteries are, like the radial artery, relatively small distal vessels, but each has a collateral vessel. The brachial, femoral, and axillary arteries do not have collaterals but are much larger and less likely to thrombose.

Indications

Continuous monitoring of arterial blood pressure

Where haemodynamic instability is anticipated:
- Major surgical procedures, e.g. cardiac, vascular.
- Large fluid shifts, e.g. major trauma.
- Medical problems, e.g. valvular heart disease.
- Drug therapy, e.g. inotropes, sodium nitroprusside.

For neurosurgical procedures.

Where non-invasive blood pressure monitoring is difficult, e.g. burns, obesity.

Sampling

Blood gases.

Repeated blood sampling (to prevent the need for multiple punctures).

Contra-indications

Local infection.

Coagulopathy is a relative contra-indication.

Equipment

- ☐ 500ml fluid bag or cushion (to support the wrist during radial artery cannulation).
- ☐ Antiseptic solution.
- ☐ 2ml syringe of 1% lignocaine with 25G needle.
- ☐ 5ml syringe.
- ☐ 18G needle.
- ☐ Arterial cannula 20G or appropriate Seldinger cannula with guidewire and thin-wall needle.
- ☐ Adhesive tape.
- ☐ Transducer and pressurised flushing device, run through with heparinised saline, and connected to direct pressure monitor. Place a 3-way tap near the distal end of the transducer tubing.

Technique

Cannulation of the radial artery is described in detail, followed by a summary of the approaches to other commonly used sites.

A modified Allen's test may be performed to assess the adequacy of collateral blood flow to the hand before cannulating the radial artery: the radial and ulnar arteries are compressed; the patient clenches his fist until it blanches and then relaxes his hand; pressure on the ulnar artery is released; if collateral flow is adequate, the skin immediately becomes hyperaemic. Whether this test accurately predicts the risk of ischaemic damage after cannulation is controversial. If there is any doubt about the perfusion of the hand after radial cannulation, remove the cannula immediately.

The patient is usually supine for this procedure. Place the patient's arm on an arm-board and hyperextend the wrist over a 500ml bag of fluid (Fig. 1.44). Loosely tape the patient's hand to the arm-board.

 ► ► ►

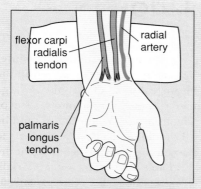

Fig. 1.44 Position of the wrist for radial artery cannulation

flexor carpi radialis tendon

radial artery

palmaris longus tendon

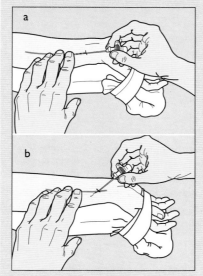

Figs. 1.45 Palpation and cannulation of the radial artery: **(a)** direct; **(b)** transvascular

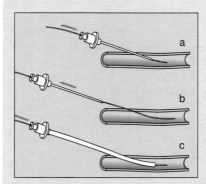

Figs. 1.46 Insertion of arterial cannula using the Seldinger technique

▶ ▶ ▶

Although a Seldinger technique can be used, an ordinary cannula is usually quicker and easier.

1 Put on sterile gloves and clean the overlying skin with antiseptic solution.
2 Palpate the artery proximal to the proximal wrist crease, lateral to the tendon of flexor carpi radialis.
3 Infiltrate local anaesthetic at the site of the intended puncture. This can be omitted in the unconscious patient.

Insertion of catheter-over-needle cannula
4 Make a small hole in the skin with the 18G needle; this prevents a skin plug occluding the arterial needle/catheter.
5 While palpating the artery with the left hand, advance the needle and cannula with the right hand, through the skin at 30° to the horizontal along the line of the artery (Fig. 1.45a). Do not use a ported cannula; this increases the risk of inadvertent intra-arterial injection of irritant drugs.
6 When blood flashes back into the hub of the needle, reduce the angle of entry, advance the needle and cannula a further millimetre, then slide the cannula off the needle into the artery.
7 Alternatively, advance the needle and catheter through the back wall of the artery (Fig. 1.45b), withdraw the needle partially, then slowly withdraw the cannula until blood pours freely from it. Advance the cannula up the artery and remove the needle.

Insertion of arterial cannula with the Seldinger technique
4 Mount the needle on a 5ml syringe. While palpating the artery with the left hand, advance the needle through the skin at 30° along the line of the artery.
5 When blood flashes back into the hub of the needle, detach the syringe and pass the guide wire through the needle and a few centimetres up the artery (Fig. 1.46a).
6 Remove the needle, taking care not to displace the wire (Fig. 1.46b).
7 Thread the arterial cannula over the wire and into the artery. Finally, withdraw the wire (Fig. 1.46c).
8 Compress the artery proximal to the cannula to reduce blood loss or, alternatively, if the cannula has a flow switch, turn it off. Connect the cannula to the transducer tubing and, having first excluded any air bubbles, flush with heparinised saline.
9 Carefully secure the cannula with adhesive tape. Considerable blood loss can occur if an arterial cannula is accidentally dislodged. Mark the transducer tubing as an arterial line (Fig. 1.47). ▶ ▶ ▶

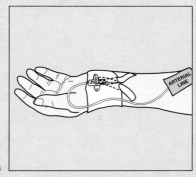

Fig. 1.47 Secure and label arterial line

▶ ▶ ▶

10 Zero the transducer system by opening the 3-way tap to atmosphere and pushing the zero button on the pressure monitor. Return the 3-way tap to the patient position and check for an arterial waveform on the monitor.

11 If there is no waveform, check the cannula, tubing and transducer in turn.

ALTERNATIVES TO RADIAL ARTERY CANNULATION

- The *ulnar artery* can be cannulated using the position and technique described above. If multiple attempts at cannulation of the radial artery have been unsuccessful, do not attempt to cannulate the ipsilateral ulnar artery.
- The *brachial artery* may be cannulated just proximal to the skin crease of the antecubital fossa, medial to the biceps tendon and lateral to pronator teres. Stabilise the elbow in extension and use an 18G cannula (Fig. 1.48).
- Although a difficult site for nursing care, the *axillary artery* has the advantage of extensive collateral flow, making ischaemic complications rare. Position the patient's arm in abduction and external rotation and shave the site. Palpate and cannulate the artery as high as possible in the axilla (Fig. 1.49). Use the catheter-over-needle or Seldinger technique, and an 18G cannula.
- If perfusion to the foot is satisfactory, the *dorsalis pedis artery* or *posterior tibial artery* may be cannulated safely with a 20G catheter (Fig. 1.50).
- The femoral artery may be cannulated 1–2cm distal to the inguinal ligament at the midpoint of a line drawn between the superior iliac spine and the symphysis pubis (Fig. 1.51). Insert an 18G central venous

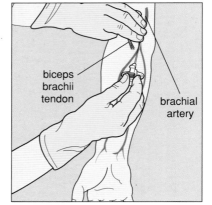

Fig. 1.48 Cannulation of the brachial artery

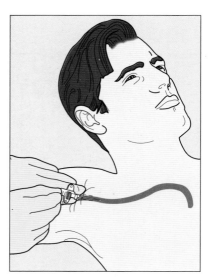

Fig. 1.49 Cannulation of the axillary artery

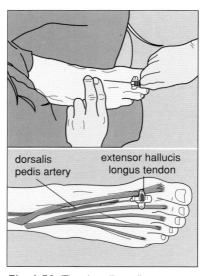

Fig. 1.50 The dorsalis pedis artery

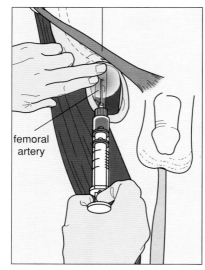

Fig. 1.51 Cannulation of the femoral artery

cannula into the artery using the Seldinger technique. A standard 20G arterial cannula is too short for reliable femoral access.

Complications

The most significant complications are ischaemia and infection but overall, the incidence of serious complications is low. Thrombosis is more likely to occur when the cannula is large relative to the artery, particularly if it is left in place for longer than 72 hours. In some series, 50% of radial artery cannulations have resulted in thrombosis but few of these cause ischaemia. When using the Seldinger technique it is possible to cause a small dissection and arterial occlusion by passing the guidewire between the intima and media. Thrombi at the catheter tip can embolise periph-erally. Flushing the arterial catheter can cause retrograde clot or air emboli. Disconnection can cause extensive haemorrhage, and bleeding around the catheter site can cause haematomas, particularly in patients with a coagulopathy. Infection is extremely rare in patients who have arterial catheters solely for intra-operative monitoring, but it is a significant risk in the critical care unit, particularly after about 4 days. An arterial catheter should be removed immediately there is any local inflammation. Aneurysm and pseudoaneurysm formation are rare, late complications.

Key points

- For most adults, the radial artery is the preferred location for an indwelling cannula. In patients with marked peripheral vaso-constriction, the femoral artery is a good alternative.

Hazards

- Do not use cannulae with injection ports for arterial cannulation.
- Clearly label all arterial lines.
- Remove any arterial cannula that is thought to be compromising distal circulation.

Pericardiocentesis

There are many causes for an acute or chronic collection of fluid in the pericardial space. The removal of this fluid, by the technique of pericardiocentesis, may be for diagnostic or therapeutic reasons and can be performed percutaneously or by open surgery. Cardiac tamponade occurs when the pressure of fluid accumulating in the pericardium impairs ventricular filling (particularly the right ventricle), and results in a critical drop in cardiac output. When the fluid accumulates rapidly, usually blood following penetrating or blunt injury, a small volume can result in tamponade. This is a medical emergency and the immediate removal of even small amounts of blood (20ml) from the pericardium may benefit the critically ill patient. Accumulation over a long period allows the pericardium to distend and accommodate a much larger volume before impairing ventricular filling.

An inconsistent variety of clinical signs are associated with cardiac tamponade. The classic Beck's triad comprises distended neck veins, hypotension, and muffled heart sounds. Pulsus paradoxus, a decrease in systolic pressure during inspiration in excess of 10mmHg, is often, but not always present. Kussmaul's sign, a rise in jugular venous pressure with inspiration when breathing spontaneously, is more typical of constrictive pericarditis rather than acute tamponade. In the case of chronic pericardial effusions, with or without tamponade, the diagnosis can be confirmed by echocardiography.

Percutaneous needle pericardiocentesis is associated with significant morbidity and a number of specialists prefer to use an open technique. This chapter is concerned with the former only.

Equipment

- ☐ Defibrillator.
- ☐ Antiseptic solution.
- ☐ 5ml 1% lignocaine.
- ☐ 5ml syringe and 23G needle.
- ☐ 10ml syringe.
- ☐ 30ml syringe.
- ☐ Thin-wall 9–15cm needle, appropriate guidewire and introducer, and 8–9FG catheter with side-holes (or pig-tailed catheter for chronic drainage) or 16G 9–15cm over-the-needle catheter and 3-way tap or long spinal needle.
- ☐ ECG electrodes, leads and monitor.
- ☐ Double crocodile clips.

Technique

The pericardium is attached anteriorly to the manubrium and inferiorly to the diaphragm. When the patient is supine, pericardial fluid usually accumulates anterior to the right ventricle. Of the three main approaches for aspiration: anterior, apical, and subxiphoid, the latter is the most popular and will be described here. If pericardiocentesis is being performed to drain a suspected acute tamponade in a patient who is *in extremis*, do not waste time trying to find ideal equipment or an ideal location. However, in the case of chronic effusions, the procedure should be performed under sterile conditions and with full resuscitative facilities available.

There are a few needles and kits designed specifically for pericardiocentesis. Often, these include a 9–15cm thin-wall, short-bevel needle, guidewire and large-bore catheter with side holes. An ECG lead can be connected to the metal needle and provides early warning of contact with the myocardium (see below). However, electrical contact between an ECG lead and a standard catheter-over-needle assembly is not possible. Some clinicians use long spinal needles for pericardiocentesis. Direct ECG monitoring is possible via a spinal needle but the internal diameter is relatively small making drainage slow.

The patient should have an intravenous cannula in situ and should be placed in a semi-sitting position at about 20°. A defibrillator should be available.

1 Attach the ECG leads to the patient. If using a thin-wall or spinal needle, attach the V lead to one end of the double crocodile clip.
2 Clean and drape the subxiphoid area, and infiltrate the entry site (2cm below the xiphoid and 2cm left of the midline) with lignocaine (Fig. 1.52).
3 Attach the 30ml syringe to the pericardiocentesis needle. Attach the crocodile clip from the V lead of the ECG to a proximal part of the pericardiocentesis needle. Set the ECG to record from the V lead. If using a catheter-over-needle assembly, continue to monitor the ECG through the standard lead positions. ► ► ►

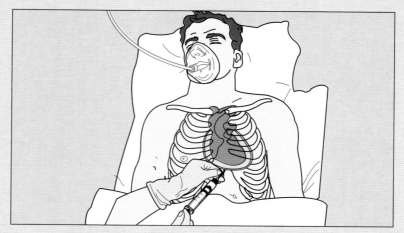

Fig. 1.52 Subxiphoid entry site for pericardiocentesis

▶ ▶ ▶

4 While gently aspirating on the syringe, advance the needle from the point of entry, at angle of 45° to the skin and aiming at the left shoulder (Fig. 1.53).

5 Watch the ECG monitor which shows a standard V lead trace. If the ventricle is touched, an injury pattern of S–T elevation and ectopic beats will be seen (Fig. 1.54). If the atria are touched, the amplitude of the P wave will change. If either of these appear, withdraw the needle slightly.

6 Successful aspiration of fluid identifies the pericardial space.

7a If being performed for diagnosis solely, or if using a spinal needle, now remove the needle.

7b If using a catheter-over-needle, and further drainage is likely to be required urgently (while waiting for definitive surgery), remove the needle leaving the catheter in position and attach a 3-way tap to the catheter.

7c If using a thin-wall needle, detach the syringe and thread a J-tipped guidewire into the pericardium. Remove the needle without displacing the wire. If the catheter kit is supplied with a dilator, use it before threading the catheter over the wire. The ideal catheter is a size 8–9FG with side holes. ▶ ▶ ▶

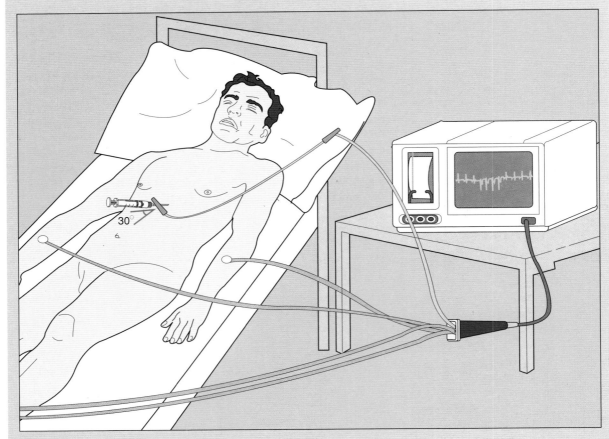

Fig. 1.53 Direction of insertion of pericardiocentesis needle, with ECG monitoring

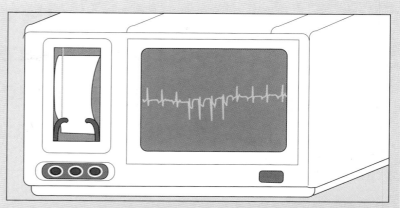

Fig. 1.54 An injury pattern appears on the ECG if the ventricle is touched

▶ ▶ ▶

7d For large, chronic pericardial effusions, where prolonged drainage may be required, use this technique to place a pigtail catheter in the pericardial space. This can be left in place for several days.

8 In the case of acute tamponade following trauma, aspirate as much fluid as possible. Unlike intracardiac blood, fluid from the pericardium usually does not clot. Check for immediate improvement in the patient's clinical condition (e.g. increased blood pressure, better peripheral perfusion). Close the 3-way tap, remove the syringe and secure the catheter with tape. Reaspirate fluid if tamponade recurs before the patient undergoes appropriate surgery.

9 Obtain a chest X-ray to exclude a haemo- or pneumothorax.

Hazards

- Use fully isolated ECG equipment; leaking micro-currents can cause ventricular fibrillation.
- Patients with small pericardial effusions or those who have had previous cardiac surgery are at increased risk for perforation of the right ventricle during pericardiocentesis.
- Thin-wall intravenous-type cannulae have a tendency to break and should be left in the pericardial space for a short time only; for example, to drain an acute tamponade while awaiting thoracotomy.

Complications

The most common complications of pericardiocentesis include: perforation of the right ventricle or atrium, perforation of the left ventricle, laceration of the right coronary artery (particular the marginal branches), pneumothorax, and puncture of the peritoneum with infection and trauma to the abdominal organs. Damage to the thin-walled chambers (right atrium and ventricle) is particularly hazardous, and the associated profuse bleeding may require urgent surgery. Ventricular dysrhythmias occur frequently when the needle touches the myocardium, and pericardial puncture can cause vasovagal reactions with accompanying bradycardia.

External chest compression, active compression/ decompression and the precordial thump

EXTERNAL CHEST COMPRESSION

External chest compressions (ECC) is a proven method of providing some temporary circulation in patients with cardiac arrest and a modest enhancement of perfusion in patients with a profoundly low cardiac output.

The technique can be taught to lay members of the public as well as health-care professionals. The term 'external chest compressions' is to be preferred to the older term 'external cardiac massage' as it describes the procedure more accurately.

ECC consists of rhythmical compressions applied to the lower half of the sternum with the supine patient placed on a flat firm surface. The heart is squeezed between the back of the sternum and the spinal column (Fig. 1.55). ECC must be combined with some form of artificial ventilation to ensure gas exchange as the blood passes through the lungs.

There remains considerable academic debate as to the best application of chest compressions in relation to ventilation. Conventional opinion proposes a relatively physiological sequence of five compressions with a short pause for an interposed ventilation when two rescuers are taking part. For a single rescuer, a sequence of 15 compressions and a pause for 2 ventilations is advocated to minimise the delay imposed by the rescuers change of position.

There is some evidence that cardiac output is enhanced if there is an intermittent increase in intra-thoracic pressure timed to coincide with the compression stroke. This has been termed the 'thoracic pump effect' and has led to experimentation with a technique known as simultaneous ventilation and compression cardiopulmonary resuscitation (SVC–CPR).

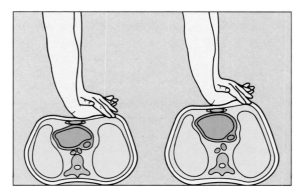

Fig. 1.55
Compression of heart between back of sternum and spinal column

Some support for the thoracic pump effect is given by the fact that rhythmical coughing alone can provide a circulation for a short period during cardiac arrest. Studies of SVC–CPR under controlled conditions have provided some evidence of enhanced circulation when compared with conventional CPR but unfortunately outcome was not as good as conventional CPR in clinical practice. Clearly SVC–CPR can only be applied in intubated patients using a sophisticated system to ensure precisely simultaneous application of ventilation and compression which makes the technique generally impractical in the clinical management of cardiac arrest.

However, interest in the thoracic pump effect has been rekindled by a chance attempt at CPR by a lay bystander, using only a domestic drain plunger applied forcibly and rhythmically to a patient's chest for some 15 minutes prior to conventional CPR, which was rewarded with recovery.

As a consequence of this event, a modified device (the CardioPump, Ambu Int) has been produced commercially which is capable of providing active compression and decompression (ACD) (Fig. 1.56). Early results using the device have been promising and the outcome of further studies are awaited.

External chest compressions (ECC) can be provided manually, with a mechanical piston (chest thumper) or using the CardioPump.

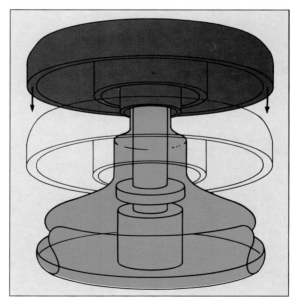

Fig. 1.56 The active compression and decompression CardioPump

---

Indications

Cardiac arrest.
Profoundly low cardiac output.

Contra-indications

Adequate cardiac output.
Resuscitation not appropriate.

Equipment

☐ No equipment is required for conventional manual ECC.
☐ The appropriate device is required for mechanical chest thumping or ACD resuscitation.

Technique

Make sure that there are no hazards to either victim or rescuer. Summon help if you have not already done so.

Manual external chest compressions

1 Place the patient supine on a firm surface.
2 Elevate the legs, if possible, to maximise venous return.
3 Kneel by the side of the patient's chest and locate the site of chest compression which is at the junction of the upper two-thirds and lower one third of the sternum. This approximates with the nipple line and can also be found by placing two fingers on the xiphisternum and aligning the heel of the other hand alongside above them (Fig. 1.57a).
4 Place one hand on top of the other hand in the correct location intertwining the fingers or grasping the wrist of the hand on the sternum (Fig. 1.57b).
5 Ensure that only the heel of the hand is applied to the sternum. Keep the fingers off the rib cage to reduce the risk of fracture (Fig. 1.57c).
6 Keep the elbows locked straight and place the shoulders over the patient's sternum (Fig. 1.57c).
7 Apply rhythmical compressions to the patient's sternum with a force sufficient to depress the sternum 4–5cm. ► ► ►

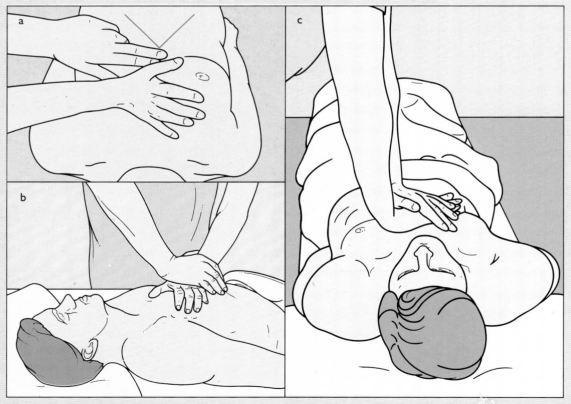

Fig. 1.57 Technique of external chest compressions

▶ ▶ ▶

8 The compression rate should be 80–100/min and compression should occupy 50% of the cycle.

9 Continue compressions until signs of a spontaneous circulation return or until the patient is deemed unrevivable.

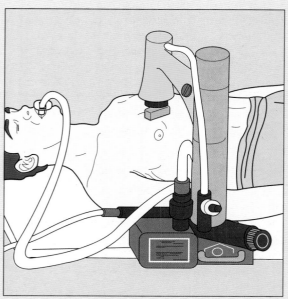

Fig. 1.58 Mechanical chest compressions

Mechanical chest compressions

1 With the patient supine on a firm surface and legs elevated if possible, insert the back plate of the mechanical device beneath the patient's chest so that it is centred on the two thirds/one third junction of the sternum (Fig. 1.58).

2 Fold the hinged anterior plate over the front of the patient's chest, locating the piston precisely in the midline at the approved compression point, and lock it into the back plate.

3 Turn on the compressed gas driving the piston and adjust the stroke to provide 4–5cm sternal depression at a rate of 80–100/min, using 50% of the cycle for the compression phase.

Active compression decompression

1 With the patient supine on a firm surface and legs elevated if possible, apply the suction cap of the ACD device in the midline over the approved compression point.

2 Apply rhythmical compressions by alternately pressing on the device with active decompressions to lift the lower thorax with suction cup applied to the chest. The initial compression should ensure that the suction cup forms an effective vacuum seal with the chest wall (Fig. 1.59a).

3 Compression and decompression force should be monitored by the meter incorporated in the handle of the device (Fig. 1.59b). In adults the compression force should be of the order of 40–50kg (90–110lbs) to produce a sternal depression of 4–5cm and the decompression force should be 10kg (20lbs) (Fig. 1.59c). The rate should be 80–100/min with compression occupying 50% of the cycle.

Children, infants and neonates

In children, infants and neonates, the principle of external chest compressions is precisely the same. However, the rate should be faster: >100/min in children under five years and infants and neonates. The compression force should provide equivalent sternal depression compared with the adult. In infants younger than one year and neonates, external chest compressions should also be applied with spontaneous pulse rates below 60/min respectively. ▶ ▶ ▶

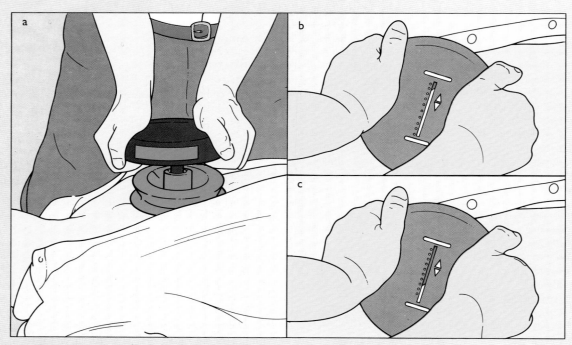

Fig. 1.59 Active compression decompression

▶ ▶ ▶

Children under 10 years (Fig. 1.60a):
- Use the heel of one hand applied in the adult position to apply the compression force.

Neonates and infants (Fig. 1.60b):
- Use two fingers applied to the midsternal point to apply the compression force.

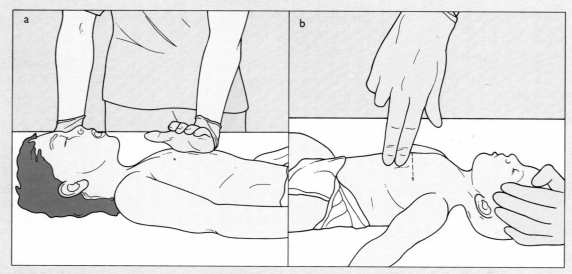

Fig. 1.60 External chest compression in neonates and small children

Complications

- Fractured ribs and/or sternum.
- Laceration to the spleen and/or liver.
- Rupture of a distended stomach.
- Barotrauma to the lungs leading to a pneumothorax or pneumomediastinum.

These traumatic complications occur more frequently with SVC–CPR.

Key points

- To prevent major hypoxic damage to vital organs, ECC must be started as soon as possible after cardiac arrest has been diagnosed and must be accompanied by adequate ventilation, preferably with added oxygen.
- ECC provides, at best, a very modest cardiac output (20–40% of normal values). Interruption of ECC for procedures such as defibrillation, intravenous cannulation and tracheal intubation should be kept to an absolute minimum for it is hard to re-establish a circulation from a zero output state.

THE PRECORDIAL THUMP

The precordial thump is recommended as a preliminary measure prior to ECC in witnessed cardiac arrests believed to be of primary cardiac origin. There have been a number of reports of conversion of ventricular fibrillation and asystole to a rhythm producing a spontaneous cardiac output after the precordial thump. Conversely, it has been unsuccessful in many cases and on occasion ventricular fibrillation has been converted to asystole.

Hazards

- Inappropriate application. Always check the pulse in a major artery prior to applying ECC.
- Profuse haemorrhage may occur from relatively minor trauma if thrombolytic therapy is given before or after ECC.

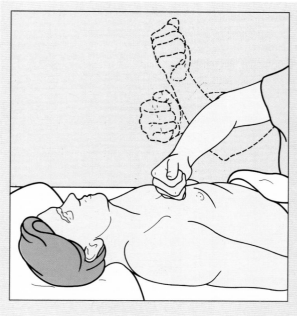

Technique

1 Place the patient supine on a firm surface immediately cardiac arrest is detected.
2 Deliver a blow with the ulnar aspect of the clenched fist to the sternum in the midline at the junction of the upper two thirds and lower one third of the distance between the manubrium and the xiphoid process (Fig. 1.61).
3 If the thump is temporarily effective but cardiac arrest recurs, deliver a series of thumps for up to 30 seconds at a rate of 60–80/min (fist pacing).
4 If the single thump or fist pacing is not effective immediately proceed with ECC and artificial ventilation.

Fig. 1.61 The precordial thump

Internal cardiac massage
(Tom Kneuth MD)

Internal cardiac massage is a component of open chest resuscitation that is used as a last resort in dire situations. Although it appears dramatic and sometimes overly aggressive, in some situations open cardiac massage provides the patient with the best chance of survival. Opening the chest offers the most effective means to control life-threatening haemorrhage from the chest or abdomen, and the quickest opportunity to relieve cardiac tamponade. It allows direct assessment of resuscitative interventions and volume replacement. Direct cardiac compressions produce better arterial flow than indirect, sternal compressions, and internal direct defibrillation may be more effective. The chances of maintaining myocardial and cerebral viability and restoring spontaneous circulation are thereby increased in patients who would otherwise have died using only closed cardiopulmonary resuscitation (CPR). The complications, on the other hand, are relatively minor. Infection occurs rarely and is usually not life-threatening.

Although open chest resuscitation is best performed by a surgeon who is also capable of repairing the injury that caused the arrest, it should be within the capabilities of all physicians practising emergency care. Surgeons should be immediately available, however, because the patient will require transfer to the operating theatre for definitive treatment and closure of the chest wall.

Indications

Penetrating chest injury in patients who are about to arrest or who have arrested.

As an immediately life-saving manoeuvre, open chest resuscitation with internal cardiac massage is indicated for:

- The patient who develops cardiac arrest when the chest is already open, in the operating room.
- Cardiorespiratory arrest or imminent exsanguination arrest due to intrathoracic blood loss from penetrating trauma to the chest.
- Imminent exsanguination arrest from penetrating or blunt trauma to the abdomen, to control bleeding by temporary cross-clamping of the aorta.
- Alleviation of life-threatening pericardial tamponade by rapid pericardiotomy.
- Rapid access to repair life-threatening penetrating cardiac injuries.
- Suspected massive pulmonary embolism, in order to perform direct break-up or removal of the thrombus and as well as prompt initiation of internal cardiac massage.

Contra-indications

Hypotensive patient with inadequate fluid resuscitation.

A patient with obvious mortal head injuries.

Equipment

- ☐ Antiseptic solution.
- ☐ Scalpel with no. 10 blade.
- ☐ Mayo and Metzenbaum scissors.
- ☐ Rib spreaders.
- ☐ Aortic vascular clamp.
- ☐ Defibrillator with internal electrodes.

Technique

Place the patient in a supine position with the left arm abducted (Fig. 1.62). Minimal skin preparation is required. Pour antiseptic solution over both sides of the chest. Don sterile gloves and protective gear (goggles, face mask, gown).

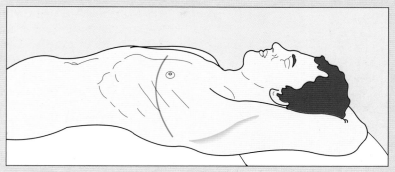

Fig. 1.62 Incision for internal cardiac massage

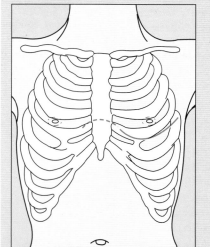

Fig. 1.63 Incision line for extending left thoracotomy to the right hemithorax

1 Ensure that the anaesthetist has obtained a secure airway by endotracheal intubation and apply 100% oxygen by intermittent positive pressure ventilation.
2 Make a left thoracotomy incision over the left fourth or fifth intercostal space (in the male, just below the nipple; in the female, in the infra mammary fold) beginning anteriorly at the midline and ending at the posterior axillary line (Fig. 1.63). Use the body of the rib as a 'cutting board' to avoid inadvertent injury to the lung in a hasty entry.
3 Enter the pleural cavity bluntly with the scalpel handle or large Mayo scissors. Avoid injury to the heart and coronary vessels.
4 Incise the intercostal muscle by sliding partially opened Mayo scissors along the superior border of the lower rib to avoid the neurovascular bundle.
5 Insert the rib spreaders with the handle in the inferior position so that they do not interfere with the possibility of extending the incision across the midline. Pull the intercostal space open as far as needed. Incise the two superior costal cartilages with the scalpel to achieve greater exposure.
6 Retract the lung posteriorly to expose the heart. Retract the lung anteromedially and inferiorly to visualise the major thoracic vessels.
7 Direct attention to the origin of blood loss and place a vascular clamp on any bleeding vessels with an atraumatic vascular clamp.
8 If there is no bleeding into the left chest, cross-clamp the descending aorta using the following technique:
   • Follow the posterior curve of the rib cage to the costovertebral junction and locate the aorta using the forefinger of the non-dominant hand.
   • Bluntly dissect through the parietal pleura to completely surround and isolate the aorta with the thumb and forefinger. ▶ ▶ ▶

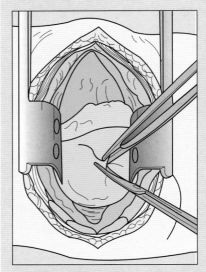

Fig. 1.64 Incision of the pericardium

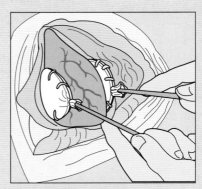

Fig. 1.65 Internal defibrillation

• Using an atraumatic vascular clamp, and fingers as a guide, cross-clamp the aorta. For effective cross-clamping, the entire diameter of the aorta should be within the clamp, but ensure that the tips of the clamp do not injure the oesophagus.

9 If unsure of the bleeding site, insert a chest tube into the right chest. If bleeding is into the right chest, extend the thoracotomy incision across the midline by cutting through the sternum with bone cutters, heavy scissors, or a Gigli saw and make a mirror-image thoracotomy incision on the right. Cross-clamp bleeding vessels in that side of the thorax.

10 Assess pericardial fullness. If tamponade is present, open the pericardium in the coronal plane, parallel to and 1cm above the phrenic nerve (Fig. 1.64).

11 Assess intravascular volume by fullness of the heart.

12 Assess myocardial motion. If fibrillation is present, defibrillate using internal electrodes and 5–20 J of delivered energy (Fig. 1.65). Since low-energy voltage is delivered, it is not necessary to interrupt other surgical procedures during defibrillation.

13 If air bubbles are seen in the coronary arteries, immediately clamp the hilum of the injured lung using a Satinsky clamp and place the patient in a Trendelenburg position.

14 If the heart is beating feebly or is in asystole, give adrenaline, 1mg, by intracardiac injection into the tip of the left ventricle. Avoid laceration of the coronary vessels.

15 If the heart appears to be contracting well but no pulse is appreciable, compression is required to establish flow. Squeeze the heart inside the pericardium at a rate of 60 times per minute. Several techniques are acceptable. Use two hands with the left hand over the right ventricle and the right hand over the left ventricle posteriorly (Fig. 1.66). Alternatively, with the right hand in the oblique sinus posteriorly, compress the heart against the sternum anteriorly (Fig. 1.67). The heart can also be compressed effectively by placing it in the palm of one hand and squeezing with the outstretched fingers and thumb or thenar eminence. Avoid compression with the tips of the fingers, since it is possible to perforate the myocardium. ▶ ▶ ▶

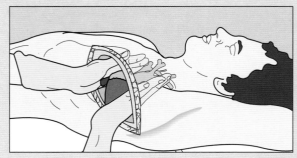

Fig. 1.66 Bimanual internal cardiac massage

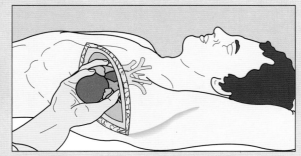

Fig. 1.67 Internal cardiac massage with one hand

16 Discontinue cardiac compressions when a strong, sustained beat returns. Remove cross clamps as soon as more precise haemostasis is obtained.

Complications

- Injury to the lung parenchyma or heart during uncontrolled entry.
- Post-resuscitative bleeding (remember to ligate the transected internal mammary artery).
- Injury to the oesophagus during aortic cross-clamping.
- Injury to the phrenic nerve during pericardiotomy.
- Perforation of the myocardium.
- Infection.

Key points

- Indications for internal cardiac massage need to be identified early in the resuscitation.
- Entry into the chest should be rapid but controlled.
- More success with this procedure will be seen with penetrating trauma patients; blunt trauma patients are almost never revived successfully.

Defibrillation and cardioversion

The use of a direct current (DC) shock for conversion of haemodynamically important cardiac arrhythmias has been practised for many years. The application of an asynchronous DC shock is the treatment of choice for ventricular fibrillation (VF), and pulseless ventricular tachycardia (VT). A synchronous DC shock is a useful technique in the conversion of less serious rhythm disturbances; atrial fibrillation, supraventricular and ventricular tachycardia, and re-entrant tachydysrhythmias being the commonest examples. The device and technology to apply such a shock are similar for both types of defibrillation and cardioversion: they will therefore be considered together.

Cardioversion (which includes defibrillation in the following discussion) is the technique of the application of a DC electrical shock across the heart. This shock has the effect of depolarising all the fibres of the heart simultaneously, after which they remain in an absolute refractory phase for a short time. At this point, the fibres that have the shortest absolute refractory phase will begin the slow phase of spontaneous depolarisation, phase 0. This spontaneous depolarisation distinguishes it from skeletal muscle. Generally the sinoatrial (SA) node has the shortest absolute refractory period and the fastest rate of spontaneous depolarization. After a successful DC shock the SA node will become the pacemaker, and initiates a wave of co-ordinated electrical pattern of depolarisation through the heart.

In VF and pulseless VT (Fig. 1.68), the shock is applied without synchrony, as it is not important when the massive depolarisation occurs. In all other rhythms, application of a shock during the phase of ventricular repolarisation (represented by the T wave on the ECG) may result in ventricular fibrillation. Therefore, in all rhythms except VF and pulseless VT, the shock must be synchronised to the ECG. When the synchronous mode is selected, the defibrillator will read the ECG and

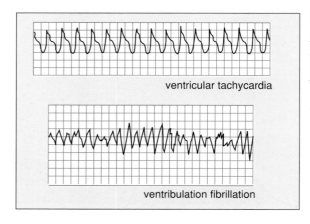

ventricular tachycardia

ventribulation fibrillation

Fig. 1.68 The traces show ventricular tachycardia (VT) and ventricular fibrillation (VF): these are the two rhythms that will require emergency cardioversion

attempt to detect R waves. If the R waves are of insufficient amplitude, they will not be recognised by the defibrillator, and the machine will not deliver a shock. Rarely, the T wave may be the tallest complex on the ECG, especially in hyperkalaemia, and the machine will incorrectly interpret this as an R wave. This can be overcome by switching the electrodes around, and checking that the marked complex is indeed an R wave. (No such recognition is possible in VF and pulseless VT). The synchronous mode is selected, and the shock is delivered as soon as the defibrillator button(s) is pressed.

Four factors must be considered before cardioversion.

Type of shock to be delivered

Synchronous cardioversion requires the use of ECG electrodes; asynchronous defibrillation does not.

Type of defibrillator to be used

Manual defibrillators are used for all synchronous shocks, and may, of course, be used for defibrillation. They require the operator to recognise the rhythm, select the correct energy level, and deliver the shock. Semi-automatic defibrillators incorporate computer technology to interpret the ECG, and inform the operator if defibrillation is required. If this is the case, the operator has to press the defibrillate button, and the machine delivers a shock of the appropriate energy (200J, 200J, 360J etc.). Fully automatic defibrillators are similar to the semi-automatic machines, except that the machine, having warned the operator to stand clear, will deliver the shock automatically. The operator has only to connect up the large sensing electrodes which detect the ECG and conduct the shock.

The manual defibrillator is most useful for fully-trained hospital personnel, but carries the disadvantage that a shock may be incorrectly delivered.

The semi-automatic types do not have this problem, and so are useful for less trained operators, such as ambulance personnel or first aid workers. In many models manual override is possible. A further disadvantage is that fine VF may be of such small amplitude that it is unrecognised as such. Automatic defibrillators are designed for use by untrained personnel such as sports officials and transport workers, and have the same disadvantage as the semi-automatic models with respect to energy size.

Size of shock to be delivered

This is measured in energy delivered by the apparatus (Joules). The shock actually delivered is about 10% less than the stored energy. Defibrillation in an adult requires about 200J delivered, and after two or more attempts, 360J: lower energy levels may not reach the threshold for defibrillation, while higher levels may cause myocardial damage.

Synchronous cardioversion of other rhythms requires energy levels of 25–100J.

Paediatric defibrillation, which is uncommon because VF is rare in children, requires a shock of about 2J/kg.

Internal defibrillation requires an energy of 10% of the above values.

Site of the shock

External cardioversion is usually applied from below the outer half of the right clavicle to apex (see below), although it may be performed from front of sternum to back, especially in small children. It requires paddles (or special adhesive electrodes) of 10cm diameter (4.5cm for infants).

Internal defibrillation requires an open chest, to allow direct application of the paddles to the heart, and so may be useful in operating theatres. Paddle sizes are 6cm for adults, and 2cm for infants for internal defibrillation.

Indications

Asynchronous cardioversion (defibrillation): ventricular fibrillation or pulseless ventricular tachycardia.

Synchronous cardioversion: other tachydysrhythmias, especially those associated with haemodynamic compromise.

Contra-indications

Conscious patient.

Moisture or conducting jelly spread across chest.

Equipment

☐ Defibrillator of appropriate type.
☐ Paddles or adhesive electrodes for shock application.
☐ ECG electrodes (for synchronous cardioversion).

Technique

Defibrillation requires no preparation, since it is the most immediate medical emergency, and delay rapidly reduces the chance of successful conversion. In situations where the ECG analysis is unavailable, or is not functioning correctly, VF should be assumed to be present in cardiac arrest, and the patient should be promptly defibrillated.

1 Lay the patient supine on a flat dry surface. Remove the clothes from the upper half of the body, and ensure that the chest is dry. Remove glyceryl trinitrate patches if present as they may explode.

Manual defibrillators

2 If the patient has an ECG monitor attached, and VF or VT is confirmed, go to step 5. If the patient has no ECG attached, remove the paddles from the defibrillator, and turn on the power. Discontinue chest compressions and ventilation.

3 Apply one paddle with a force equal to 10kg weight, over the apex of the heart and the other under the right clavicle (Fig. 1.69).

4 Confirm VF or VT on the ECG trace. Remove the paddles, and recommence cardiac resuscitation.

5 Apply defibrillator contact pads to the sites above or apply electrode jelly to the paddles.

6 Select the appropriate energy level (p. 278), and press the charge button.

7 Discontinue chest compressions and ventilation. Order everybody to stand clear, and make sure that you are clear of the patient.

8 Press the defibrillate buttons on the paddles.

▶ ▶ ▶

9 Restart ventilation and feel for a pulse immediately. If no pulse is palpable, repeat the sequence from step 6.

10 If defibrillation has been unsuccessful after 3 times, restart chest compressions.

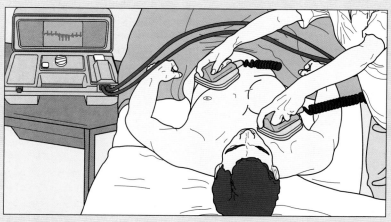

Fig. 1.69 A manual defibrillator. Apply one of the paddles over the apex of the heart and the other beneath the right clavicle.

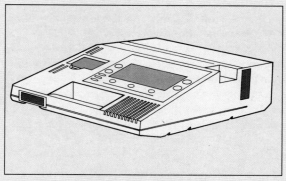

Fig. 1.70 A semi-automatic defibrillator

Semi-automatic defibrillators

2 Apply the adhesive electrodes supplied with the defibrillator to the apex and below the right clavicle, as above. Discontinue chest compressions and ventilation and order everyone to stand clear.

3 Turn on the defibrillator (Fig. 1.70) and observe the ECG trace.

4 The apparatus will display or read out the instructions which include the size of shock to be delivered.

5 If the apparatus indicates that a shock should be given, confirm that everybody is standing clear.

6 Press the defibrillate button if the machine orders it.

7 Observe the ECG trace and feel for a major pulse.

8 Follow the advice from the apparatus as to the need for further shocks.

Automatic defibrillators

2 Apply the adhesive electrodes supplied with the machine to the apex and below the right clavicle in the way described above.

3 Discontinue chest compressions and ventilation.

4 Turn on the automatic defibrillator.

5 The apparatus will issue a verbal warning if it is about to discharge a shock. Everybody should stand clear of the patient at this point, and wait for the shock to be discharged.

6 When the shock has been delivered, the machine will read the ECG again, and advise of further treatment.

7 If the patient's pulse returns, turn the defibrillator off and remove the electrodes.

Technique

Cardioversion will require general anaesthesia if the patient is conscious. The general anaesthetic should be administered by a trained anaesthetist, with the same precautions as for a surgical procedure. However, adequate starvation may be impossible if the situation is urgent, especially if haemodynamic compromise has been produced by the rhythm abnormality. Synchronous cardioversion requires an accurate ECG trace, and this should be obtained before general anaesthesia is induced. This trace needs to be analysed by the defibrillator, to allow synchrony of the DC shock.

Synchronous cardioversion

1   An ECG diagnosis of the dysrhythmia should have been made. If the patient is compromised by the dysrhythmia, cardioversion will be required urgently; otherwise, the patient should be starved of food for four hours, and clear fluids for two hours.

2   Attach the defibrillator ECG electrodes to the two arms, and the left flank. Connect the proximal end of the ECG lead to the defibrillator.

3   Switch on the defibrillator. Semi-automatic defibrillators cannot give synchronous shocks: ensure that the manual defibrillator is in the synchronous mode.

4   Ensure that the apparatus is recording the spikes of the R wave.

5   Ask the anaesthetist to induce general anaesthesia.

6   When the anaesthetist is satisfied, place defibrillator contact paddles on the apex and below the right clavicle of the patient's chest, and place the defibrillator paddles over these pads. *Do not allow the paddles to contact the ECG electrodes.* It may be more efficacious to apply the paddles over the front and back of the thorax in the midline, to increase the chance of successful cardioversion.

7   Charge the defibrillator to the selected energy.

8   Ask everybody to stand clear of the patient, and ensure that the ECG trace still picks up the R wave spikes.

9   Press the defibrillator discharge button(s).

10   Check the patient's pulse and ECG. If reversion to an acceptable rhythm has occurred, then switch off the defibrillator. If reversion has not occurred, then repeat the process up to four times, after consultation with the anaesthetist.

11   Place the patient in the recovery position, and give oxygen via a face mask.

Complications

There are very few complications from cardioversion.

- Myocardial damage may follow repeated or high energy defibrillation, but the clinical need may be so great as to make this an acceptable risk.
- R-on-T phenomenon may occur if the shock is incorrectly administered in synchronous cardioversion and if VF or VT results, it should be treated along conventional lines.
- Superficial burns to the patient's chest may occur if the paddles are not firmly applied, or if the shock arcs across the paddles or jelly.
- Accidental electrocution is a hazard to health care workers, and results from electrical contact with the patient or paddles during cardioversion.

Key points

- Understand the defibrillator, and check its function regularly.
- Apply electrode contact pads firmly, and do not allow the two pads to contact each other.
- Electrode jelly can run very easily; contact pads are a better alternative.
- Failed synchronous cardioversion may be due to an intractable structural cardiac disease or biochemical abnormalities.

Recording a 12 lead ECG

Twelve lead ECGs are used to assist the diagnosis of many cardiac and pulmonary diseases. They may also be repeated to chart the progression of such conditions as myocardial infarction, and left ventricular aneurysm. Most hospitals will have technicians skilled in obtaining good ECG records, but their services may not be available on a 24-hour basis. Thus, all medical practitioners should be familiar with the technique, to improve their diagnostic skill.

Indications

Diagnosis or exclusion of suspected myocardial infarction.

Diagnosis of pericarditis, left ventricular hypertrophy, cor pulmonale, conduction defects, pulmonary embolism and arrhythmias.

Diagnosis of myocardial ischaemia under resting and/or exercising conditions.

Diagnosis of specific conduction pathways disorders during electrophysiological testing.

Management of cardiac pacing.

Routine medical screening.

Contra-indications

Relative

Excessive muscle tremor.

Inexperience of person interpreting trace.

Arrhythmia associated with rapid deterioration; single lead rhythm strip is adequate for initial diagnosis.

Equipment

☐ ECG machine.
☐ Skin electrodes.
☐ Electrode jelly (if 'pre-gelled' electrodes not available).

Technique

The patient should be supine or semi-reclining on a bed. Encourage the patient to relax as much as possible, to reduce interference from muscle tremor. It may be necessary to shave the area over the chest, to ensure good electrical contact.

Manual ECG machines require the operator to press the chest and limb lead buttons in turn, after correct electrode placement; the fully automatic machines will move from lead to lead after correct electrode sitings by the operator.

1 Lubricate the limb and chest electrodes with electrode jelly (not water-soluble KY jelly), and wipe off any excess.

2 Attach an electrode to each limb, preferably to the hairless palmar surface. The thigh and shoulder should not be used, as muscle bulk may interfere with the signal. In amputees, the most distal part of the limb should be used, and the affected limb supported on a pillow.

3 Apply the chest leads numbered V1 to V6 as shown in Fig. 1.71. The site of the second intercostal space can be identified as that below and just lateral to the angle of Louis, or the manubrio–sternal notch.

4 Turn on the ECG machine, and wait for a signal that it is ready to record.

5 Manual ECG machines will require the operator to run in the record mode, and the 1mV signal button should be depressed briefly to calibrate the trace. Then, record the 12 leads in the order shown on the machine. At the end, return to the lead II mode, and record 20–30 seconds of this trace for a rhythm strip (Fig. 1.72).

6 Automatic machines will ask the operator if the leads are correctly applied, and then simply requires confirmation, before recording the entire ECG sequence.

7 Noisy traces should be repeated, after re-siting the appropriate electrodes. If the problem still persists, then check the wire connections and try rubbing the skin with a mild abrasive to reduce skin resistance. ▶ ▶ ▶

▶ ▶ ▶

8 At the end of the procedure, remove the electrodes, and wipe away any remaining jelly.

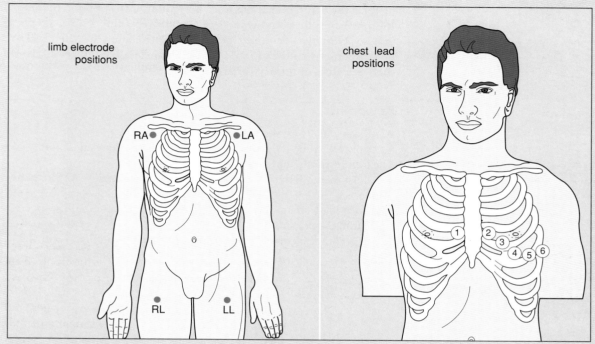

limb electrode positions

chest lead positions

Fig. 1.71 Sites of limb and chest leads for a standard ECG

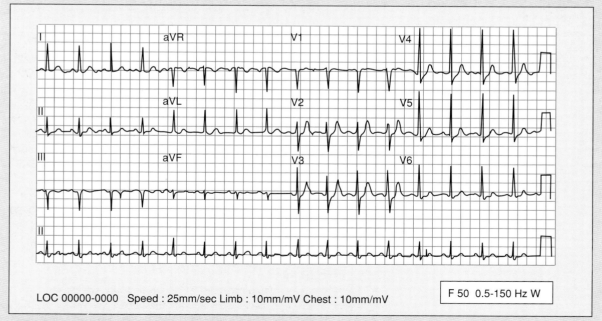

LOC 00000-0000   Speed : 25mm/sec Limb : 10mm/mV Chest : 10mm/mV

F 50 0.5-150 Hz W

Fig. 1.72 A standard 12 lead electrocardiogram (ECG/EKG)

Complications

There are no major complications of ECG recording. However, the leads may be incorrectly sited and the record may then be misinterpreted.

Automatic machines are set to provide a sensitive indication as to when medical interpretation of the trace is required ('MD opinion required'). In some cases, these indicators are actually reporting a normal variant, and so caution is required before action is based on the machines interpretation: mild right axis deviation and high ST take-off are two such examples of normal variants.

Key points

- Always make sure the patient is relaxed.
- Apply electrode jelly liberally to the limb lead electrodes, and carefully on the chest electrodes.
- Adjust the gain to produce a signal that is appropriate for the paper size.
- Run at least one to two minutes of lead II in patients with suspected rhythm disturbance.
- Always put the correct name, date and time on the final record.

Temporary and emergency cardiac pacing

Indications

Acute anterior myocardial
infarction complicated by:
- Sinus rhythm with new bifasicular block or prolonged PR
interval.
- AV node dysfunction, resulting
in either complete heart block,
shock, or sinus arrest.

Acute inferior myocardial
infarction complicated by AV
block if symptomatic or
ventricular rate <40/min.
despite atropine.

Chronic cardiac disorders listed
for pacing, associated with acute
symptoms.

Pre-operative pacing in patients
with:
- Symptomatic bifasicular block.
- Complete heart block.
- First plus second degree heart
block.
- Sinus arrest.

Contra-indications

Relative

Local sepsis demands a different
route.

Severe coagulopathy requires
careful choice of route.

The technique of cardiac pacing has advanced considerably since the time of the first generation fixed rate pacemakers. Current practices offer a wide range of facilities, to ensure that the resultant paced heart has near normal physiological function. For example, the loss of atrial activity that results from ventricular pacing, can be corrected by the use of atrial pacing, or better atrio–ventricular sequential pacing. Moreover, many pacemakers are now able to incorporate a demand function, that allows an increase in rate, and therefore cardiac output, in response to stimuli such as exercise. Further, pulmonary artery catheters are available with pacing facilities, and these may be inserted prophylactically in patients thought to be at risk of conduction disorders.

There are many indications for cardiac pacing: generally, disorders of cardiac conduction or rhythm that are likely to be recurrent or chronic necessitate a permanent pacemaker. The classification of such pacemakers is based on an international five letter system:
- The *first* letter refers to the chamber that is paced, **A**trial, **V**entricular or **D**ual.
- The *second* letter refers to the chamber that is sensed by the pacer, **A**, **V** or **D**.
- The *third* letter refers to the response of the pacemaker to the information imparted to it: **I**nhibitory, **T**riggered stimulus, **O** is zero response.
- The *fourth* letter indicates the programmability of the pacemaker: **O** is non-programmable, **P** is programmable, **M** is multi-programmable, and **C** indicates telemetry functions.
- The *fifth* letter refers to the anti-tachycardia function: **O** is none, **P** is anti-tachycardia pacing, **S** is defibrillatory shock, and **D** is dual.

In clinical practice, the critical care specialist is most likely to encounter temporary pacemakers. Therefore, this section will deal only with the technique and management of temporary pacing.

Temporary pacing is performed in patients with symptomatic ventricular bradycardia, which is likely to be short-lived. There are three methods of temporary pacing (the first is used in the majority of institutions but the second and third have found favour recently):
- A *temporary transvenous wire*, that is passed via a central vein into the ventricle. This should be done under X-ray screening, although in some situations it may be possible to obtain acceptable pacing without.
- *Temporary transcutaneous pacing* is not a new method, but recent refinements have produced a system that is useful in an emergency.
- *Temporary oesophageal pacing* is also useful in circumstances where X-ray facilities are unreliable, although it is a technique that requires some skill.

TEMPORARY TRANSVENOUS PACING

Temporary pacing is usually of the VVI type, although patients with a very low cardiac output may benefit from sequential AV pacing: special J-shaped leads are available for this procedure. This section will deal with the various methods available of providing single-chamber pacing in the emergency situation.

Equipment

☐ Central venous cannula of adequate diameter to accommodate pacing wire.
☐ Pulse generator of VVI type, with variable rate and output.
☐ Pacing wire (or other type of electrode) with connection suitable for generator.
☐ X-ray screening facilities.
☐ X-ray screening compatible tilting trolley.

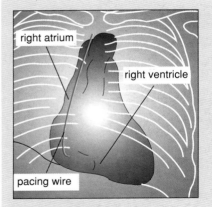

Fig. 1.73 The pacing wire passes through the tricuspid valve into the right ventricle

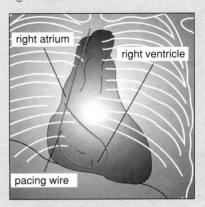

Fig. 1.74 The pacing wire is seen on the X-ray screening to cross itself as it passes into the RV outflow tract

Technique

The patient should be placed supine on a trolley that will permit X-ray screening: this may be in the X-ray department or in the coronary care unit. Attach ECG electrodes to the patient's arms, and to one leg to obtain a good ECG trace: it is important to obtain a large amplitude trace. All personnel will need to wear lead aprons, underneath the sterile gowns. Check that the selected wire has connections that will fit into the two pacing terminals of the generator when the wire is taken out of its sterile packet.

The procedure has two parts: central vein cannulation with a large bore cannula, followed by insertion of pacing wire. For the technique of central vein cannulation, see pp. 6–13. The subclavian or internal jugular veins are preferable, although the antecubital vein at the elbow and the femoral vein may be used if the situation dictates. The cannula that is inserted must be large enough to accommodate the pacing wire: the cannula may be supplied with the wire, or a 7FG pulmonary artery catheter introducer sheath may be used.

1 Ensure the cannula is correctly sited in a central vein. Secure the cannula in place with a suture.
2 Remove the pacing wire from the sterile packet, and connect the leads to the generator. Ask an assistant to check the function of the generator battery and control.
3 Insert the tip of the pacing wire into the cannula, and then advance it up to the 20cm mark.
4 Begin X-ray screening. The wire should be seen in the right atrium, which forms the right anterior part of the heart. The wire may flick straight through into the ventricle, or it may be necessary to make a loop in the right atrium, and then coax it into the right ventricle. This

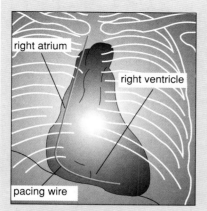

Fig. 1.75 The pacing wire is in a satisfactory position at the apex of the right ventricle

▶ ▶ ▶

will often provoke ventricular extrasystoles as the wire crosses the tricuspid valve (Fig. 1.73).

5 Advance the wire until it is seen to cross back on its own path, towards the RV outflow tract: it is now entering the pulmonary artery (Fig. 1.74).

6 Withdraw the wire at this point, until the tip lies in the apex of the right ventricle: this is represented on the screening view by the left hand side of the lower margin of the heart (Fig. 1.75).

7 Ask the assistant to turn on the generator. Set an impulse duration of 0.5ms, a voltage of 5V and a rate of 70/min (if the patient is not bradycardic, 10/min greater than the patient's heart rate should be selected). The ECG should show this new rate, followed by ventricular complexes that are different to the patient's normal QRS. waves. The pulse at the wrist should equate to the paced rate.

8 Ask the assistant to gradually turn the voltage down until the pacer no longer captures the ventricle: this is the threshold. An average threshold is around 0.5V, and it must not be more than 2V. Set the voltage at the threshold plus 2V (i.e. if the threshold is 0.8V, set the pacemaker at 2.8V).

9 Ask the patient to take a deep breath, and to move around slightly. The wire should not move from the RV on the X-ray, and the generator should continue to capture at the set voltage. If this is not the case, then re-insert the wire in the fashion described above. If the wire appears to remain in a stable position, then secure it at the point of entrance through the skin, by using special rubber clips, or sutures bound tightly around it. If the wire has been passed through a 7FG sheath, secure the latter in place.

10 Apply a sterile dressing to the wire entrance site, and take an erect chest X-ray.

11 Patients who require transvenous pacing for more than 4–5 days, should have a permanent pacing wire inserted by a cardiologist trained in the procedure.

TEMPORARY TRANSCUTANEOUS EXTERNAL CARDIAC PACING

This technique relies on the use of large surface electrodes, which reduce the resistance to current flow, and therefore the heat generated locally. The latest pacemakers function in the demand mode, through sensors placed in the electrode. The pacemaker generally drives both atria and ventricles, and the ECG is unhelpful in distinguishing the chamber that is being paced. An arterial line may be useful for patients in whom it is important to know the blood pressure.

Equipment

☐ Pacemaker of appropriate type.
☐ Large surface area electrodes with connections for pacemaker wires.
☐ Razor and mild skin abrasive.

Technique

1 Shave the area over the front of the sternum, and the mid-thoracic region posteriorly. This step may be omitted in dire emergencies.
2 Apply the first electrode underneath the right clavicle, and then turn the patient on his or her side. Apply the second electrode to the area directly behind the first, usually over the mid-thoracic region posteriorly.
3 Attach the two pacing wires to the contact plates on each electrode.
4 Set a rate of 80 beats on the pacemaker with a stimulus duration of 20–40ms. The voltage is often fixed at 100–200V, although it may be altered on some models. Slowly increase the current (to a maximum of 150mA) until pacing occurs, with a radial pulse rate of 80 beats/min. It may be necessary to observe an arterial trace display to confirm adequate ventricular response.
5 If the patient is conscious, it will be necessary to insert a temporary transvenous wire as soon as is practical. Despite the more modern large electrodes, the high voltage still results in painful muscle contractions. It will not be necessary to change the pacemaker if the patient remains unconscious and the pacing is acceptable.

This technique has value only as a temporary measure, as return of consciousness will preclude long-term use. However, it may be useful in the operating theatre in cases of ventricular or pacemaker standstill.

TEMPORARY OESOPHAGEAL CARDIAC PACING

Oesophageal pacing has not found much popularity, because of the considerable technical skill required to secure an adequate paced rhythm. However, it may be useful if the temporary transvenous route is unavailable, especially in the conscious patient.

The oesophageal pacing wire has two pacing attachments, and these should be connected to the pacemaker before electrode insertion. The pacemaker should be capable of delivering a long (10ms) duration stimulus, but voltage and sensing modes are similar to temporary transvenous values.

Equipment

☐ Suitable oesophageal pacing wire, with connections for pacing box.
☐ Pacing box capable of 5V output, and long stimulus time of at least 10ms.

Technique

1 Attach ECG electrodes to the patient.
2 Explain the procedure to the conscious patient. Lubricate the tip only of the pacing electrode, and then insert the pacing electrode into the mouth. Advance it into the oesophagus, and then turn on the pacemaker at: ► ► ►

▶ ▶ ▶
- Demand rate 80/min (or 20/min greater than the patient's own ventricular rate).
- Voltage 5V.
- Stimulus time 10ms.

3 Observe the ECG for capture of the pacing stimulus: if the heart does not capture the stimulus, advance the electrode until capture occurs. The average distance to the mid-point of the oesophagus is about 15–22cm in an adult, and markings at the lip will indicate the depth of insertion of the electrode.

4 If the ventricle captures, then gradually decrease the output until the threshold is reached. Set the output of the pacemaker at 2V above this value.

5 If the ventricle does not capture, then re-insert the electrode, and confirm oesophageal placement: this can be done by passing a large-bore nasogastric (N/G) tube, and then aspirating gastric contents. Pass the electrode down the inside of the N/G tube, and then remove the N/G tube, and cut it from around the electrode: *take care not to cut the electrode.*

6 Set the output at 10V and try to obtain atrial capture, rather than ventricular capture. This may allow a lower threshold.

Complications

Transvenous insertion

The complications of transvenous pacemaker insertion, are those of central line insertion, and in addition:
- Ventricular irritability may occur during wire insertion resulting in ventricular dysrhythmias: these should be treated symptomatically.
- Long-term complications of lead insertion include infection, pyrexia, wire perforation of myocardial wall, and loss of wire position.

Oesophageal insertion
- This method has a lower success rate, but very few complications. Oesophageal perforation may occur from traumatic insertion.

Transcutaneous external pacing
- Pain is the commonest problem, due to high voltages involved. This may be improved by the use of a lower voltage, provided the pacing threshold is reached.

Key points

- Select the technique that will have the best success rate: this should usually be the temporary transvenous route.
- Accurate radiographic screening facilities are very important .
- Aim for as low a pacemaker threshold as possible.
- Set the pacemaker box at 2V above this threshold.
- Check the position of the wire or oesophageal lead after movement or coughing: a poor position may necessitate reinsertion.

Pulse oximetry

Pulse oximetry is one of the most useful recent developments in the field of monitoring. The device utilises the differential absorption of two light frequencies by oxygenated and deoxygenated haemoglobin. The accuracy of newer versions has been improved further by the addition of a third frequency. The oximeter probe provides an accurate estimation of oxygen saturation of arterial blood, and has applications beyond the field of anaesthesia. However, certain precautions are necessary during use, to prevent inaccurate readings.

Indications

Detection of hypoxaemia in :
• Post-operative patients.
• General and regional anaesthesia.
• Sedation and sedo–analgesia.
• Controlled oxygen therapy in paediatric and adult patients.
• Critical care patients.
Analysis of limb perfusion during revascularisation.

Contra-indications

Relative
Poor regional blood flow.
Hypothermia.
Local arterio–venous fistulae
Patients receiving methylene blue.

Equipment

☐ Pulse oximeter and appropriate probe.
☐ Tape to secure probe if required.

Technique

The correct site for the oximeter is one that will indicate a value as close to arterial saturation as is possible. In most adult patients, this will be the finger. However, it may be that poor peripheral perfusion will prevent an accurate reading from a limb, and so the probe should be placed on the ear lobe or the lip. In paediatric patients, the probe site should be moved frequently, to prevent local tissue damage. Cyanotic children may require lip or ear probes.

1 Chose the correct probe, according to site and age of patient (Fig. 1.76).
2 Gently rub the chosen site, to increase local perfusion.
3 Apply the probe, and check that an appropriate reading is obtained: normal adult values are 90–100%. Check the pulse rate displayed against the patient's pulse (Fig. 1.77).
4 Secure the probe in place with some tape, although make sure that the probe site is not unduly compressed by tight application.
5 Re-assess the probe site at hourly intervals, and change the probe site if the reading is unreliable or if the site becomes painful or discoloured.

Complications

The reading from the probe may be incorrect, or it may be misinterpreted: falsely low values are the most common problem, and are usually due to poor perfusion, either globally or locally. Re-siting the probe, and warming the chosen site, may help to overcome this problem. Falsely high readings are much less common, and are usually due to inaccuracy of probe calibration.

If the probe is left *in situ* too long, tissue damage may occur, especially in paediatric patients: check the site regularly for evidence of such damage. If there is any doubt, change the probe site.

Hazards

• Check the probe site often for signs of local tissue damage.
• If the patient's apparent clinical condition and the probe value don't correlate, change the probe site.

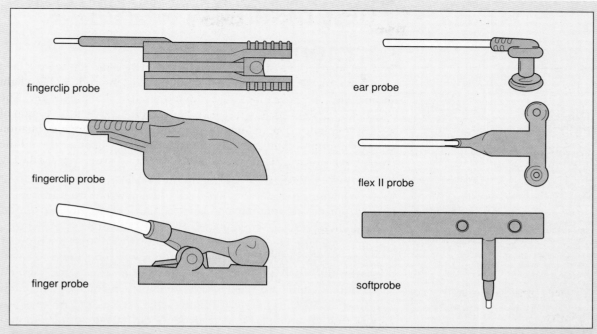

Fig. 1.76 Different types of pulse oximeter probes

fingerclip probe

fingerclip probe

finger probe

ear probe

flex II probe

softprobe

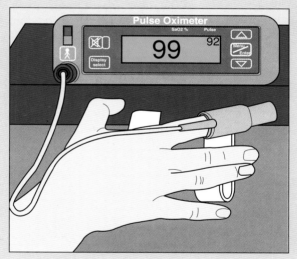

Fig. 1.77 Pulse oximeter in use with finger probe

Key points

- Make sure the probe site is well perfused.
- Make sure the probe site is not distal to a blood pressure cuff.
- If the SaO_2 value falls, check the patient's airway, ventilation and circulation: if these are satisfactory, perform an arterial blood gas analysis.
- Remember that the pulse waveform amplitude may not reflect blood pressure or perfusion. It may have been amplified electronically, and may lead to a false sense of security.

The pneumatic antishock garment

The pneumatic antishock garment (PASG), also known as military (or medical) antishock trousers (MAST), is a three-compartment, inflatable trouser suit. The device was popularised in the Vietnam War when it was used as part of the management of haemorrhagic shock. Use of the PASG is less common in the United Kingdom than in the United States, though even in the latter, its popularity is declining. Any beneficial haemodynamic effects of the PASG are brought about by: transferring blood from the peripheral venous capacitance vessels to the central circulation, increasing systemic vascular resistance, splinting fractures, and tamponade of bleeding vessels. Controversy surrounds pre-hospital use of the PASG; although external counterpressure does improve blood pressure and cardiac output in hypovolaemic patients, several comparative studies have failed to show an improvement in survival rates. Use of the PASG must not delay volume replacement or rapid transport for penetrating trauma. In some patients, such as quadriplegics and those with severe chest injuries, application of the PASG may compromise ventilatory function, and in head-injured patients the increase in central venous pressure may elevate intracranial pressure (ICP).

Indications

Pre-hospital

Hypotension due to hypovolaemia.
Hypotension from spinal cord injury.
Stabilisation of pelvic/femoral fractures.

In-hospital

Splinting pelvic fractures with continuing haemorrhage and hypotension.
Intra-abdominal bleeding from trauma (en route to definitive surgery).
Hypotension secondary to ruptured abdominal aortic aneurysm.

Contra-indications

Absolute

Congestive cardiac failure and pulmonary oedema.
Known ruptured diaphragm.
Advanced pregnancy.

Relative

Severe head injury.
Intrathoracic bleeding.
Flail chest.

Equipment

☐ Sphygmomanometer.
☐ PASG with foot pump, or automatic inflation device.
☐ Long spine board (optional).

Technique

In-hospital application of the PASG will be described. In the United States, in the pre-hospital environment, long spine boards are used routinely but would normally be carefully removed soon after the patient's admission to hospital. Spine boards are rarely used in the United Kingdom; scoop stretchers are preferred. Before application of the PASG, the patient should be supine. Initially, two attendants will be required.

1 Record the patient's blood pressure and pulse rate.
2 Unfold the PASG and open out all the Velcro fasteners. Lift up the patient's legs and slide the PASG under the patient up as far as the buttocks (Fig. 1.78a). Lift the patient's hips and slide the abdominal component into position (Fig. 1.78b). Particular care is required if spinal injury is suspected. ► ► ►

▶ ▶ ▶

3 Fold and fasten (producing a snug fit) each of the three components, starting with the left leg (Fig. 1.79a) then the right leg and finally the abdominal portion (Fig. 1.79b).

4 Attach each of the three air tubes (these may be colour coded) to the connections on the PASG. ▶ ▶ ▶

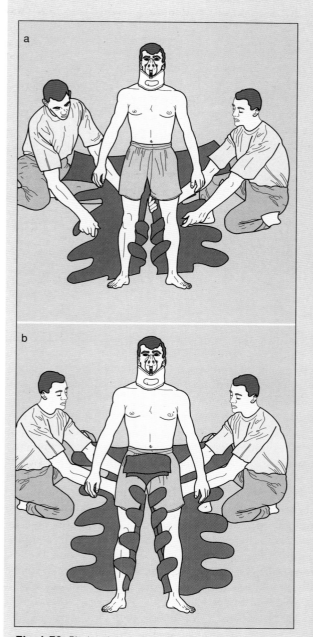

Fig. 1.78 Placing the pneumatic antishock under the patient

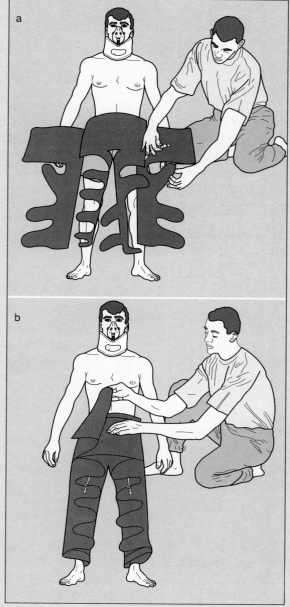

Fig. 1.79 Securing the pneumatic antishock garment

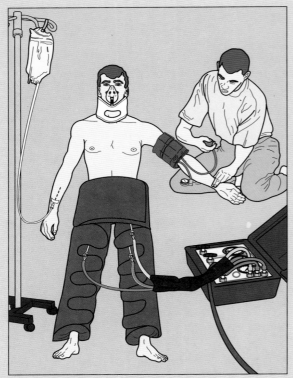

▶ ▶ ▶

5 Inflate the legs first and reassess the patient's vital signs before inflating the abdominal compartment (Fig. 1.80). Inflate the PASG to a pressure that improves the patient's blood pressure and peripheral perfusion. The maximum pressure in the PASG will be limited by pressure relief valves or slippage of the Velcro fasteners.

6 Before deflating the PASG, ensure the patient has at least two large-bore i.v. cannulae *in situ* and has received appropriate volume resuscitation. If surgery is contemplated, the patient should be taken to the operating room and anaesthetised with the surgical team at the ready. The patient should have a systolic blood pressure of at least 100mmHg before deflation is attempted.

7 Starting with the abdominal compartment, deflate the PASG slowly, while continuously monitoring the blood pressure. Stop deflation if the blood pressure falls by 5mmHg and give additional fluids to increase the blood pressure before continuing deflation. Once the abdominal compartment is successfully deflated, deflate the leg compartments slowly, one leg at a time.

8 Remove the PASG only if ongoing haemorrhage has been controlled.

Fig. 1.80 Inflation of the antishock garment

Complications

The commonest complication associated with use of the PASG is the development of severe hypotension. This may occur if it is removed prematurely before the blood volume has been re-established adequately and immediate surgical control of blood loss is not available. Increased pressure in the abdominal compartment will splint the diaphragm, increasing the work of breathing and potentially causing ventilatory failure in patients with chest injury. The increase in afterload may precipitate or worsen pulmonary oedema in patients with cardiogenic shock or congestive heart failure. Prolonged application (usually greater than two hours) of the PASG may cause skin necrosis and bullae and occasionally a compartment syndrome. Haemorrhage above the diaphragm may be exacerbated by a PASG, and in patients with severe head injuries, intracranial pressure theoretically may be increased. The PASG may limit access to the patient for examination and procedures. However, the abdominal compartment can be slowly deflated to allow access for diagnostic peritoneal lavage and intravenous access can still be obtained around the ankles, although pressure bags will be needed to provide adequate fluid infusion rates.

Hazards

- Premature and inappropriate removal of the PASG may result in severe hypotension.
- The PASG may compromise ventilation, cardiac performance, and intracranial pressure.

Upper airway control

The airway is placed in jeopardy in all supine unconscious patients, those with obtunded protective laryngeal reflexes, and those with maxillofacial or neck injury which disrupt the normal anatomy of the upper airway.

Airway patency can be established and controlled by manual and positional methods, or by using specially designed adjuncts including the oro- and nasopharyngeal airways, the laryngeal mask airway, the pharyngotracheal lumen airway and the oesophageal/tracheal Combitube airway.

Advanced techniques including endotracheal and endobronchial intubation, retrograde airway cannulation and the surgical airway will be dealt with later.

POSITIONAL AND MANUAL METHODS

The commonest cause of airway obstruction in the supine unconscious patient is the relaxed tongue falling backwards to occlude the posterior oropharynx (Fig. 2.1).

In the majority of cases, the obstruction can be overcome by appropriate manual alignment of the head, neck and mandible. These manoeuvres stretch the anterior structures of the neck and lift the base of the tongue off the posterior pharyngeal wall. The sequence of alignment should consist of backward tilt of the head, elevation of the tip of the chin (chin lift) and protrusion of the mandible (jaw thrust) (Fig. 2.2).

Indications

Complete or partial upper airway obstruction.

Contra-indications

Great care must be taken in manipulating the head and neck in patients with suspected spinal injury. In such patients in-line stabilisation of the head and neck should be maintained and the airway patency obtained primarily by jaw thrust, thus minimising head extension.

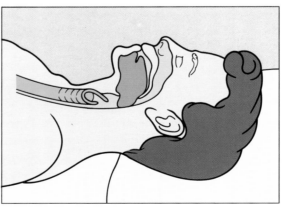

Fig. 2.1 Obstruction of the airway by the relaxed tongue

Technique

1 Ideally the supine patient's head should be placed on a small pillow or headrest.
2 Tilt the head backwards by pushing the occiput or forehead in a caudad direction to stretch the anterior tissues of the neck. ▶ ▶ ▶

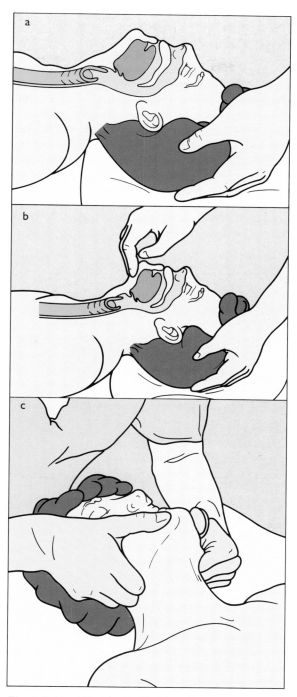

Fig. 2.2 Head tilt (**a**), chin lift (**b**) and jaw thrust (**c**) to ensure airway patency

3 Lift the chin to pull the tongue forwards.
4 Further lift the mandible upwards and forwards with the index fingers placed just proximal to the angle.
5 Reach forward with the thumbs to depress the point of the chin to open the mouth slightly.
6 Check for airway patency by observing normal chest movement and listening and feeling for exhaled air.

Complications

• Aggravation of cervical spine or maxillofacial injury.

Hazards

• Profuse bleeding may occur if chin lift or jaw thrust dislocates a fractured mandible.

Key points

• The airway is paramount to life and patency must be established without delay.

Indications

The unconscious patient at risk of airway obstruction and aspiration of foreign material who is breathing adequately and who is haemodynamically stable.

Contra-indications

Patients who require tracheal intubation or other procedures needing the supine position..

RECOVERY POSITION

Once a clear airway has been established and adequate ventilation is assured the unconscious patient should be turned into the lateral recovery position to minimise the risk of aspiration.

Even turning a large person can easily be accomplished by a single small rescuer if the correct technique is used and spinal injury is not suspected.

If a spinal injury is suspected the entire patient should be 'log-rolled' into the lateral position using a minimum of four attendants, one of whom maintains constant in-line cervical spine stabilisation.

Technique

In cases of suspected spinal injury

Log rolling into the recovery position is shown in Fig. 2.3.

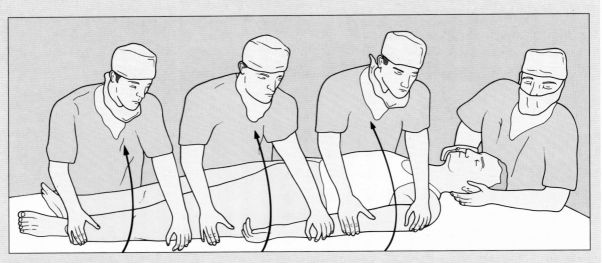

Fig. 2.3 Log rolling into recovery position

1 Three attendants stand on the same side of the supine patient. Each places one hand beneath the patient to reach to the other side – one at chest level, one at hip level and one at knee level. Their other hands are placed adjacently on the patient's opposite shoulder, hip and knee.
2 The fourth attendant maintains constant in line stabilisation of the head and neck and issues the command to turn.
3 On the command, all turn the patient towards them as one in a 'log rolling' action avoiding any rotation, flexion or extension of the spine.
4 Once the patient is in the lateral position, the arms are flexed to place the upper hand beneath the head to support it and the lower arm angled to give stability. ▶ ▶ ▶

▶ ▶ ▶

5 In-line stabilisation of the head and neck continues.
6 The upper leg is flexed to prevent the patient rolling forward.
7 The patient's airway is maintained using jaw thrust as required.

In cases where spinal injury is not suspected

A single rescuer turning the patient into the recovery position is shown in Fig. 2.4.

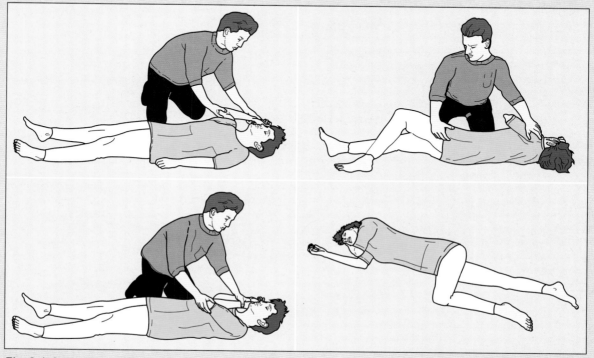

Fig. 2.4 Single rescuer turning patient into recovery position

1 Kneel beside the supine patient and pull out the nearest arm at a right angle to the body with the elbow bent and palm upwards.
2 Fold the opposite arm across the chest to place the hand against the patient's cheek on the near side.
3 Grasp the hip and shoulder furthest away maintaining the opposite hand in position near the cheek and roll the patient towards you.
4 Fix the upper leg and lower arm for stability to ensure that the head rests on the upper hand.
5 Maintain head tilt, chin lift and jaw thrust to retain a patent airway if necessary.

Hazards

- Aggravation of spinal injury by rotation or flexion of the spinal column.
- Aggravation of limb, pelvic or rib fractures.
- Disturbance of vascular lines, chest drains, urinary catheters etc.
- Pressure injury from unnoticed item in pocket or beneath patient.

Key points

- The unconscious spontaneously breathing patient is constantly in danger of airway obstruction and aspiration of foreign material. Early rotation into the lateral position minimises the risk.

CLEARANCE OF THE UPPER AIRWAY OBSTRUCTED BY FOREIGN MATERIAL

Obstruction of the upper airway by foreign material may be cleared using finger sweeps, back blows, abdominal thrusts (Heimlich manoeuvre), lateral positioning, suction, or under direct vision using a laryngoscope and forceps.

1. Finger sweeps

Technique

Finger sweeps to clear the obstructed airway are shown in Fig. 2.5.

1   Open the mouth using chin depression and jaw thrust or by prising the maxilla and mandible apart manually.
2   Using a gloved finger wrapped in a swab or handkerchief, sweep the foreign material out of the mouth.

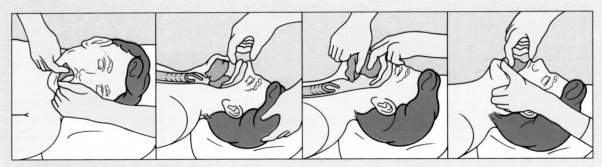

Fig. 2.5 Finger sweeps to clear the obstructed airway

Indications

A conscious patient with upper airway obstruction due to solid material not relieved by coughing.

Contra-indications

Suspected spinal or chest injury.

2. Back blows

Technique

Back blows to clear the obstructed airway are shown in Fig. 2.6.

- Ideally the patient should be placed in the lateral position with a head down tilt.
- Alternatively the patient should stand or sit and lean forward.
- Children can be placed prone and head down on the rescuer's arm or thigh.
- Apply a series of 4–6 appropriate blows to the middle of the back of the chest during expiration to enhance the expiratory flow rate and expel the impacted foreign material.

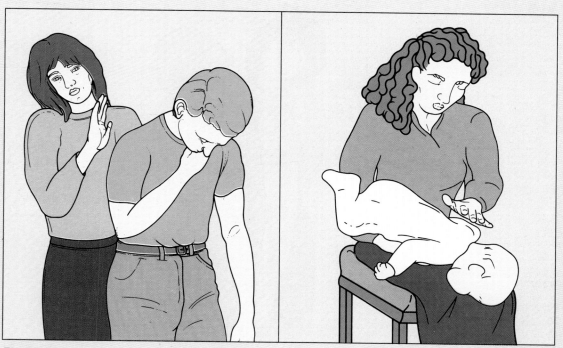

Fig. 2.6 Back blows to clear the obstructed airway

3. Abdominal thrusts (Heimlich manoeuvre)

Indications

A conscious patient with upper airway obstruction due to solid material not relieved by coughing or back blows.

Contra-indications

Children and infants.
Suspected spinal, chest or abdominal injury.
Pregnancy.
Extreme obesity.

Technique

The Heimlich manoeuvre to clear the obstructed airway is shown in Fig. 2.7.

- Stand behind the sufferer wrapping the arms around him or her at the lower margin of the rib cage.
- Clasp the hands tightly together and give a series of sharp upward thrusts timed with expiration if discernible.
- If the enhanced expiratory flow rate does not expel the foreign material be prepared for the patient to lose consciousness and attempt to remove the obstruction by finger sweeps.

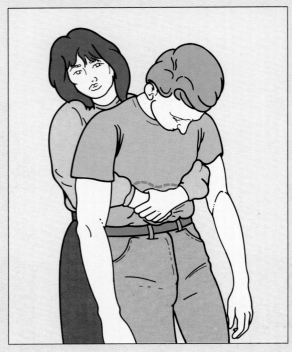

Fig. 2.7 The Heimlich manoeuvre to clear the obstructed airway

Hazards

- Abdominal visceral injury.
- Placental separation.

Lateral positioning

The lateral position with head down tilt is recommended to enhance the removal of fluid foreign material by gravity drainage in unconscious patients (for details of the procedure see p. 70).

Indications

An unconscious patient with airway obstruction due to fluid or solid material with the appropriate expertise and equipment present.

Contra-indications

None.

4. Direct laryngoscopy in combination with suction or forceps

Technique

Removal of foreign material using direct laryngoscopy and suction or forceps is shown in Fig. 2.8.

1   Place patient supine (solid material) or in the lateral position (fluid material).
2   Visualise hypopharynx directly with a laryngoscope (see p. 87).
3   Aspirate fluid material with a powerful suction apparatus using a Yankauer or wide-bore semi-stiff suction end.
4   Remove solid material under direct vision using Magill's offset forceps.

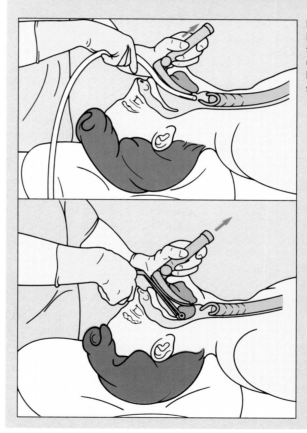

Fig. 2.8
Removal of foreign material using direct laryngoscopy and suction or forceps

Indications

An unconscious patient with upper airway obstruction or impending obstruction and absent glossopharyngeal reflexes.

To act as a protective bite block when other airways such as a tracheal tube or laryngeal mask airway are *in situ*.

Contra-indications

Clenched jaws.

At risk dentition.

Active glossopharyngeal reflexes.

Active bleeding within the hypopharynx.

Imminent danger of regurgitation or vomiting of stomach contents.

Hazards

- Trauma to lips, teeth or palate.
- Provocation of retching, vomiting or laryngeal spasm if active reflexes are present.

Remove the airway immediately at the first sign of these events occurring.

ARTIFICIAL AIRWAY ADJUNCTS

Although a clear airway may be achieved initially by manual methods in the short-term, there are occasions when airway adjuncts are helpful and necessary. Some will merely retain airway patency, others will also include airway protection from aspiration of foreign material.

The oropharyngeal (Guedel) airway

The oropharyngeal airway controls backward displacement of the tongue in the unconscious patient and provides relief for the rescuer from having to apply prolonged jaw thrust. The airway does not protect against aspiration of foreign material. A variety of sizes (000–4) are available; size 2 or 3 is suitable for the average adult.

Equipment

- ☐ Suitable sized airway(s).
- ☐ Lubrication jelly.

Technique

The oropharyngeal airway is shown in Fig. 2.9.

1 Place patient in supine or lateral position.

2a Introduce the lubricated airway into the mouth in the inverted position and rotate it through 180° as it passes over the palate.

or

2b Place a spatula in the mouth over the tongue and slide the airway over the spatula until the tip reaches the hypopharynx.

3 Check for unimpeded air entry (additional chin lift and jaw thrust may be required).

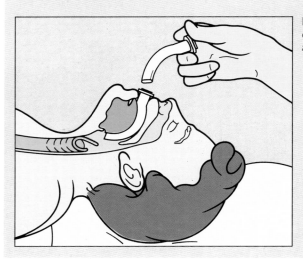

Fig. 2.9 The oropharyngeal airway

The nasopharyngeal airway

The nasopharyngeal airway is passed through the nose so that the tip lies behind the tongue in the hypopharynx just above the glottis. The specially designed airway is made of soft plastic material and has a collar flange at its proximal end to prevent it disappearing into the nose. If a purpose made device is not available, one can be made from a cut down uncuffed nasal endotracheal tube of the appropriate size with a large safety pin placed through the proximal end. Nasopharyngeal airways do not protect against aspiration of foreign material. Several sizes are available; one of 6.5–7.5mm is suitable for the average adult.

Equipment

☐ Suitable sized airway(s).
☐ Lubrication jelly.
☐ Vasoconstrictor spray (e.g. 5–10% cocaine with adrenaline) for constricting the nasal mucous membrane vasculature.

Technique

The nasopharyngeal airway is shown in Fig. 2.10.

1 In non-urgent use the nasal mucosa may be prepared by applying a vasoconstrictor spray to minimise the risk of nasal haemorrhage.
2 Introduce the well-lubricated tube of appropriate size into the right nostril directing the tip backwards, not upwards. If obstruction to advancement occurs withdraw and try the left nostril.
3 Insert the airway with rotation until the flange impinges on the nostril.
4 Check for unimpeded air entry.

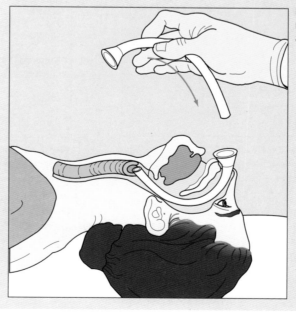

Fig. 2.10 The nasopharyngeal airway

The laryngeal mask airway (LMA)

This airway (Fig. 2.11) consists of a wide-bore tube with an elliptical inflation cuff at the distal end which is designed to seal the hypopharynx around the laryngeal opening leaving the tube orifice in close proximity to the glottic opening.

The advantage of the LMA is that it can provide a clear and secure airway without the skill required for laryngoscopy and tracheal intubation. While not guaranteeing absolute protection of the airway in every case, the LMA offers greater security and convenience than most other airways, except the endotracheal tube. Carefully applied intermittent positive pressure ventilation may be provided via the LMA which incorporates a standard connector.

The technique can be easily taught to nurses, paramedics and non-specialist doctors.

The LMA is manufactured in a range of sizes suitable for infants to large adults in both standard and reinforced materials (Fig. 2.12).

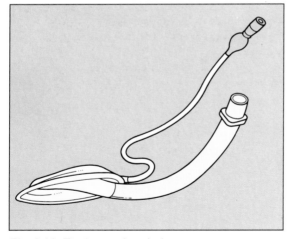

Fig. 2.11 The laryngeal mask airway

Patient	Weight	Size	Cuff volume
Neonates/ infants	up to 6.5kg	1	2-4ml
Infants/ children	6.5–15kg	2	10ml
Children	15–30kg	2.5	15ml
Small adults/ children	30–50kg	3	20ml
Adults	50–75kg	4	30ml
Large adults	>75kg	5	40ml

Fig. 2.12 Sizing and cuff inflation volumes for the laryngeal mask airway

Equipment

- ☐ LMA of appropriate size.
- ☐ Lubricating jelly.
- ☐ 50ml syringe to inflate cuff.
- ☐ Suction apparatus.
- ☐ Facility to ventilate the lungs.

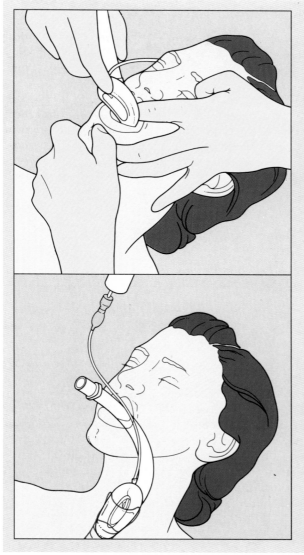

Technique

Insertion of the laryngeal mask airway is shown in Fig. 2.13.

1 Lubricate the back and sides, but not the aperture, of the completely deflated cuff.
2 Place the patient in the supine position with the head and neck aligned in the clear airway protection.
3 Ask an assistant to depress the chin to open the mouth.
4 Holding the tube like a pen, introduce the LMA into the mouth with the distal aperture facing caudad.
5 Advance the tip, applying it to the surface of the palate until it reaches the posterior pharyngeal wall.
6 Now move the operating hand to the proximal end of the tube and press the mask into position until resistance is felt as it locates in the back of the hypopharynx.
7 The black line on the tube should be aligned with the nasal septum.
8 Inflate the cuff with the appropriate amount of air. The tube rises out of the mouth 1–2cm and the larynx is pushed forward.
9 Confirm that a clear airway exists by listening for spontaneous breathing or inflate the lungs with a bag attached to the tube and note inflation pressure, chest movement, bilateral breath sounds and leakage around the cuff.
10 Insert a bite block or oropharyngeal airway alongside the tube and secure it with a tie or tape.

Fig. 2.13 Insertion of the laryngeal mask airway

Hazard

The LMA does not offer absolute protection against aspiration of gastric contents

Potential problems

Some hazards are shown in Fig. 2.14.

- Rejection, coughing, straining and laryngeal spasm in patients with active reflexes.
- Incorrect placement due to folding of the tip of the cuff during insertion. Withdraw, ensure that the tip is flat and re-insert.
- Airway obstruction due to down folding of the epiglottis. Withdraw the tube, deflate the cuff and re-insert applying the mask to the palate during introduction.
- Airway obstruction due to mask rotation. Remove and re-insert ensuring that the black line is aligned with the nasal septum.

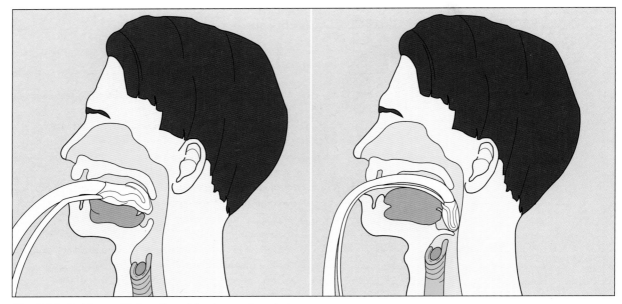

Fig. 2.14 Problems with insertion of the laryngeal mask airway

Key points

- Persistent leakage around the cuff may be due to incorrect sizing, inadequate cuff inflation, excessive inflation pressure or poor lung compliance.
- Positive inflation pressures should not exceed $20cmH_2O$. In the majority of patients adequate ventilation can be achieved within this limit by reducing the inspiratory flow rate.
- The LMA offers a method of establishing a clear airway in the profoundly unconscious patient before tracheal intubation skills and equipment are available.
- The LMA is not intended as a long-term airway in the emergency situation.

Use of the LMA to facilitate difficult tracheal intubation

The LMA may be used to help with difficult tracheal intubation by acting as an easily introduced temporary airway and a guidepath to the glottic opening through which a flexible bougie, tracheal tube or a fibre-optic intubating bronchoscope may be passed.

Indications

Difficult intubation (planned or unanticipated).

Contra-indications

Grossly distorted anatomy of the upper airway.

Equipment

- ☐ LMA of appropriate size.
- ☐ Lubricating jelly.
- ☐ 50ml syringe to inflate cuff.
- ☐ Suction apparatus.
- ☐ Flexible bougies.
- ☐ Fibre-optic bronchoscope.
- ☐ Range of endotracheal tube sizes (6.0, 8.0 and 9.0mm for adults).

Technique

In adults

1 Insert the LMA (size 3 or 4) as described above and check for a clear airway.
2 Attempt to pass a flexible lubricated bougie through the LMA and into the trachea; passage may be facilitated by cutting the bars running across the aperture of the LMA. Successful passage may be confirmed by viewing the bougie in place using a fibre-optic bronchoscope.
3 Holding the bougie in place, deflate the LMA cuff and remove it.
4 Railroad an appropriately sized, lubricated tracheal tube over the bougie until it passes into the trachea. Rotating the tube counter-clockwise will ease its passage between the vocal cords.
5 Remove the bougie.
6 Inflate the cuff of the tracheal tube; check that a clear airway is provided and that the tube is correctly positioned either by observing chest movement and listening for breath sounds or by fibre-optic bronchoscopy.

Alternative procedure

A tracheal tube may be passed directly through the LMA (size 3 or 4) into the trachea.

1 Insert the LMA as described above.
2 Pass a 6.0mm uncut tracheal tube through the LMA into the trachea. The tracheal tube can also be introduced under fibre-optic vision if the fibrescope is passed through the tracheal tube as it is inserted through the LMA.
3 Inflate the tracheal cuff; check for correct placement by observing chest movement and lung auscultation, or by fibre-optic bronchoscopy.

Hazards

- Intubation of the oesophagus. Check for correct tube placement clinically and by fibre-optic inspection.
- Further damage to soft tissues in patients with oropharyngeal injuries may occur.

Key points

- The LMA can provide an easily inserted temporary airway in emergency patients who prove difficult to intubate.

The pharyngotracheal lumen airway

The pharyngotracheal lumen airway (PTLA) (Fig. 2.15) has been introduced as a substitute for the oesophageal obturator airway which has waned in popularity. This airway consists of two tubes: a longer one with a distal cuff and a shorter one with a large cuff. The device is introduced into the mouth blindly and is designed so that the short tube lies just above the glottic opening with the large cuff inflated to obliterate the hypopharynx.

Normally the longer tube enters the oesophagus and its cuff is inflated to restrain regurgitated gastric contents and to prevent gas entering the stomach. Inflation of the short tube ventilates the lungs through the

Indications

An unconscious patient with absent glossopharyngeal and laryngeal reflexes at risk of airway obstruction and who may need artificial ventilation where endotracheal intubation is precluded by lack of available expertise or equipment.

Contra-indications

Small mouth.
Severe oropharyngeal trauma.

glottic opening. Alternatively, if the long tube enters the trachea, ventilation is applied through this route and the short tube can then act as a guide path for a separate gastric tube to remove stomach contents.

Equipment

☐ PTLA.
☐ Lubricating jelly.
☐ 50ml syringe to inflate cuff.
☐ Suction apparatus.
☐ Facility to ventilate the lungs.
☐ Capnograph.

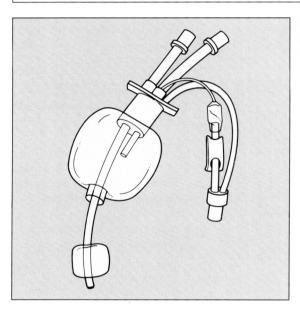

Fig. 2.15 The pharyngotracheal lumen airway

Technique

1 Place the patient in the supine position with the head and neck aligned in the clear airway position.
2 Lubricate both tubes and cuffs of the PTLA.
3 Ask an assistant to open the mouth by depressing the chin.
4 Pass the longer tube into the mouth following the line of the palate. As the shorter tube follows it will come to rest in the hypopharynx and the longer tube will enter the oesophagus or trachea.
5 Inflate both cuffs simultaneously with 100ml of air through the common self-sealing inflation port. ► ► ►

Hazards

- The device is bulky and may be difficult to introduce in patients with small mouths.
- The cuffs may be damaged by sharp teeth during insertion.
- Further damage to soft tissues in patients with oropharyngeal injuries may occur.
- Incorrect identification of the placement of the long tube may occur.
- Massive inflation of the stomach occurs if ventilation is applied to the incorrect tube.

Indications

An unconscious patient who is at risk of airway obstruction and who may need artificial ventilation where endotracheal intubation is precluded by lack of available expertise or equipment.

Contra-indications

Severe oropharyngeal trauma.

▶ ▶ ▶

6 Ventilate through the long tube.
7 If the tube has entered the trachea, breath sounds will be heard and the chest will expand on inflation. Pass a gastric tube through the short tube and continue ventilation through the long tube.
8 If the long tube has passed into the oesophagus (which is usual) gastric inflation will occur when ventilation is attempted. Ventilation should be transferred to the short tube. The long tube will allow drainage of gastric contents.

Key points

- Although relatively difficult to introduce, the PTLA does offer security of the airway.

The Combitube oesophageal/tracheal airway

The Combitube is a double lumen tube which is introduced blindly into the mouth and is designed to ventilate the patient's lungs whether the tube enters the trachea or the oesophagus (Fig. 2.16).

The 'tracheal' channel has an open distal end and the 'oesophageal' channel has a blind end with openings at supraglottic level. There is a small volume distal cuff and a high volume (100ml) cuff designed to occupy the hypopharynx.

If the tube enters the oesophagus, the patient is ventilated through the 'oesophageal' channel through the openings just above the glottic opening. The inflating gas is prevented from passing anywhere else by the distal and hypopharyngeal cuffs.

If the tube enters the trachea, ventilation should be via the 'tracheal' port. The hypopharyngeal cuff is redundant.

Equipment

- ☐ Combitube.
- ☐ Lubricating jelly.
- ☐ 50ml syringe to inflate cuff.
- ☐ Suction apparatus.
- ☐ Facility to ventilate the lungs.

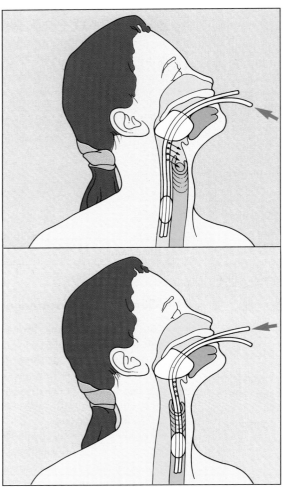

Fig. 2.16 The Combitube oesophageal/tracheal airway

Technique

1 Place the patient in the supine position with the head and neck aligned in the clear airway position.
2 Lubricate the Combitube.
3 Ask an assistant to open the mouth by depressing the chin.
4 Pass the tube to a distance of approximately 24cm.
5 Inflate the distal cuff.
6 Check for tube placement in the trachea by inflation through the 'tracheal' tube and by auscultation and observation of chest movement.
7 If the tube is placed in the trachea, continue ventilation through the 'tracheal' port.
8 If the tube is placed in the oesophagus inflate the hypopharyngeal cuff and ventilate through the 'oesophageal' port.

Key points

● The Combitube is likely to find a place as a secure airway alternative when endotracheal intubation is not possible.

Conventional tracheal intubation

Tracheal intubation provides the ultimate clear and secure airway through which positive pressure ventilation can be applied. The cuff around the distal end of the tube prevents gas leakage during ventilation and keeps the tracheobronchial airway free from aspiration of foreign material.

The tube can be passed into the trachea by a variety of means: orally or nasally using direct laryngoscopy to view the passage of the tube through the glottic opening; blind orally or nasally using a guiding light wand; or with the aid of fibre-optic laryngoscope; or by using a retrograde cannulation technique.

Fibre-optic and retrograde cannulation techniques are dealt with on pp. 98–102 and pp. 108–110, respectively.

Tracheal intubation can be performed at any age and a range of tube sizes is available to accommodate neonates to large adults. Tracheal tubes are made longer than is generally needed and usually have to be cut to the appropriate length. All should be fitted with a 15mm adapter. Conventional tracheal tubes less than 6.5mm diameter do not have cuffs. Tubes of larger size may be cuffed or uncuffed. For adult anaesthesia and critical care use, cuffed tubes are preferred as they offer protection against aspiration and allow leak-proof positive pressure ventilation.

Sizing of tubes

Adult tracheas will accommodate 7.5–9.0mm internal diameter tubes which should be cut to a length between 21–25cm (2cm longer for nasal intubation). In children the correct internal diameter and the correct length can be calculated using the formulae:
- (Age of child ÷ 4) + 4 = Correct internal diameter (mm).
- (Age of child ÷ 2) + 12 = Correct length (cm) (1–3cm longer for nasal intubation).

Indications

Airway obstruction or potential airway obstruction in the unconscious or anaesthetised patient.

Patients at risk of aspiration of foreign material.

Patients requiring positive pressure ventilation

To gain access to the lower respiratory tract for aspiration of secretions, bronchial lavage etc.

Contra-indications

Absolute

Absence of available skill and equipment.

Relative

Severe maxillofacial trauma with anatomical disruption.

Inaccessible glottis due to immobility or distorted anatomy from tumour, infection, massive pharyngeal or laryngeal oedema.

OROTRACHEAL INTUBATION UNDER DIRECT VISION USING LARYNGOSCOPY

Patients requiring orotracheal intubation for positive pressure ventilation include those with actual or impending respiratory failure. Others may require therapeutic hyperventilation, e.g. patients with head injuries.

Outline guidelines for intubation for acute respiratory failure are: $PaO_2 < 60mmHg$ (8.0kPa) while inspiring an oxygen concentration (FIO_2) of 1.0, and a $PaCO_2 > 55$–$60mmHg$ (7.5–8.0kPa). Other factors such as clouded mental state and physical exhaustion will influence the decision to intubate and ventilate.

Equipment

The necessary equipment is shown in Fig. 2.17.
- [ ] Facility to provide sedation or local or general anaesthesia if required for the procedure.
- [ ] Trolley or bed with facility for head down tilt.
- [ ] Appropriate laryngoscopes in working order.
- [ ] Appropriate range of tracheal tubes cut to correct length with connections to fit the ventilating apparatus.
- [ ] Suction apparatus.
- [ ] Lubricant jelly and swabs.
- [ ] 20ml syringe for cuff inflation.
- [ ] Clamp to secure inflated cuff.
- [ ] Flexible bougie and stylet.
- [ ] Scissors.
- [ ] Tape or tie to secure tube in place.
- [ ] Apparatus to ventilate the lungs.
- [ ] Pulse oximeter.
- [ ] Apparatus to detect correct tube placement (see p. 96).

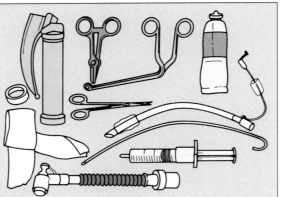

Fig. 2.17 Equipment required for tracheal intubation

Technique

This technique is shown in Fig. 2.18. ▶ ▶ ▶

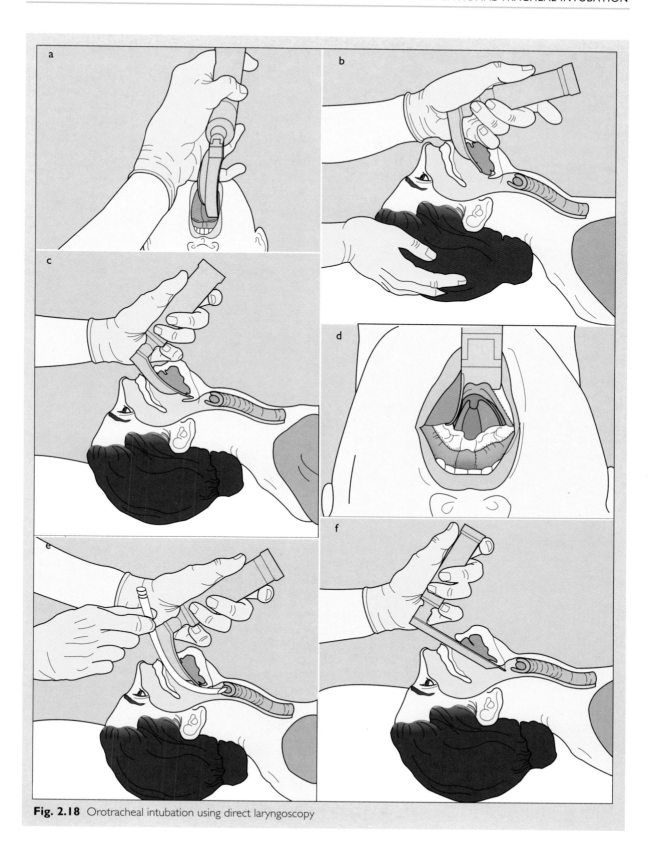

Fig. 2.18 Orotracheal intubation using direct laryngoscopy

► ► ►

1 Lubricate the tracheal tube and bougies and ensure all equipment functions correctly.

2 Place the anaesthetised or unconscious patient in the supine position with the head and neck aligned in the clear airway position using a small pillow.

3 Using the left hand to hold the laryngoscope handle, insert the *curved* laryngoscope blade into the right-hand corner of the mouth ensuring that the lower lip is not caught between the blade and the lower teeth (Fig. 2.18a). In patients with loose or absent upper teeth, a tooth guard should be placed over the upper teeth prior to introducing the laryngoscope blade.

4 Slide the laryngoscope blade towards the posterior pharyngeal wall aiming for the midline at laryngeal level and displacing the body of the tongue towards the left-hand side of the mouth (Fig. 2.18b).

5 When the laryngoscope tip reaches the laryngeal level, lift the laryngoscope handle forwards and upwards (towards the junction of the ceiling and the opposite wall) and observe the position of the tip of the laryngoscope blade (Fig. 2.18c).

6 Slide the tip of the blade between the back of the tongue and the root of the epiglottis maintaining head tilt by occipital pressure with the right hand. When using a *straight-bladed* laryngoscope, the tip of the blade should be placed beneath the epiglottis (Fig. 2.18f).

7 Visualise the larynx, adjusting the tip of the blade to get the best view of the glottic opening (Fig. 2.18d). Pressure on the cricoid cartilage is helpful and reduces the possibility of gastric regurgitation (see p. 95).

8 Pass the tracheal tube through the right-hand corner of the mouth and between the vocal cords under direct vision (Fig. 2.18e). If necessary rotate the tube 90° counter-clockwise to ease the passage through the glottic opening.

9 If a full view of the glottis is not possible, a bougie may be used. This should be well-lubricated and passed under direct vision between the cords. The tracheal tube is railroaded over the bougie into the trachea. The bougie is then withdrawn.

10 If a floppy non-precurved tracheal tube is to be used, it may be stiffened for insertion by a malleable stylet inserted through the lumen so as not to protrude, and bent to the appropriate curve. A stylet may also be used to vary the degree of curvature of a preformed tube to ease intubation.

11 Once the tube has passed between the vocal cords, it should be advanced so that the cuff lies below the glottic opening.

12 Inflate the cuff through the pilot tube until the audible leak associated with continuous positive pressure ventilation ceases; this indicates a seal between the cuff and tracheal wall. Cuff inflation volumes of more than 10–15ml should lead to a suspicion that the tube is incorrectly placed in the oesophagus, or that the cuff has burst.

13 Check that the tube is in the trachea by observing bilateral chest movement and auscultate breath sounds over both upper lung lobes. Finally, check that no sounds of air entry are heard in the epigastric area. For other methods of confirmation of correct tube placement see p. 96.

14 Secure the tube in place with a tie or tape. ► ► ►

Hazards

- Trauma to lips, teeth, tongue and structures in the pharynx or larynx.
- Exacerbation of cervical spine injury (see p. 94).
- Oesophageal intubation.
- Intubation of a single bronchus.
- Aspiration of foreign material, e.g. stomach contents, blood, etc. during the intubation attempt.
- Kinking of the tracheal tube in the pharynx or mouth.
- Over-inflation of the cuff leading to pressure necrosis of the tracheal mucous membrane or ballooning of the cuff to obstruct the lumen of the tube.

> ► ► ►
> The entire procedure of intubation should not take more than 30–40 seconds. If the attempt has failed at this time, remove the laryngoscope and tube and ventilate with oxygen by a face mask for 1–2 minutes before trying again.

Key points

- Oral tracheal intubation using direct laryngoscopy is the simplest and most reliable method in the majority of patients.

OROTRACHEAL INTUBATION USING TRANSILLUMINATION WITH A LIGHT WAND

In this method, a lighted stylet (light wand) is passed through the lumen of the tracheal tube so that the light at the end just emerges from the distal end of the tube. The principle of the technique is to pass the tube directly through the glottis into the trachea using the technique of maximal transillumination to observe the tube correctly positioned just above the larynx and to watch it pass through into the trachea.

Equipment

- ☐ Light wand.
- ☐ Lubricating jelly and swabs.
- ☐ Appropriately sized tracheal tubes cut to length.
- ☐ 20ml syringe and clip for cuff inflation.
- ☐ Suction apparatus.
- ☐ Facility to ventilate the lungs.
- ☐ Backup equipment for direct or fibre-optic laryngoscopy.

Technique

This technique is shown in Fig. 2.19.

1 Place the patient supine with the head and neck aligned in the clear airway position.
2 Pull the tongue forward wrapped in a gauze swab.
3 Pass the light wand through the lumen of the tracheal tube so that the lighted end just emerges from the distal end of the tube and bend it to a J shape (Fig. 2.19a). The base of the J should be equal in length to the thyro-mental distance.
4 Clip the distal end of the tube to the wand handle.
5 Introduce the tube or wand into the mouth aiming for the larynx (Fig. 2.19b). ► ► ►

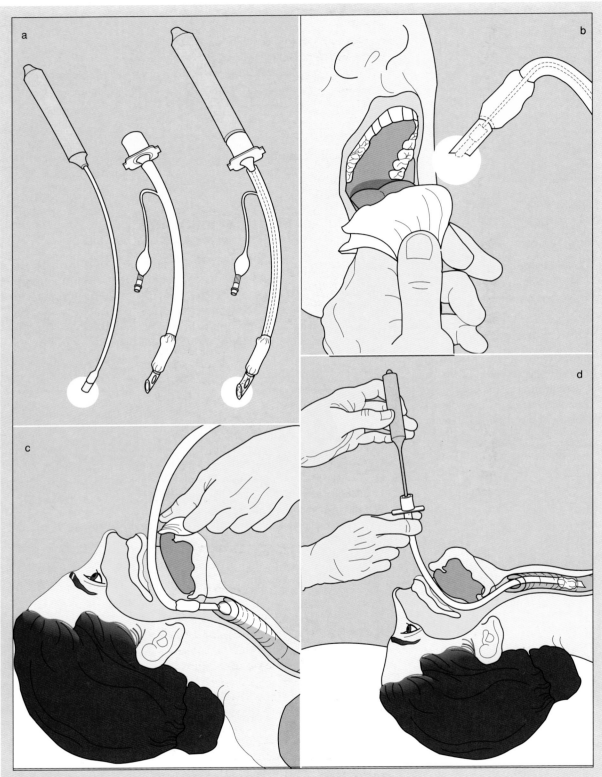

Fig. 2.19 Orotracheal intubation using a light wand

▶ ▶ ▶

6 As the tube passes behind the tongue into the hypopharynx, transillumination will be observed anteriorly (Fig. 2.19c).

7 Advance the tube further. If it passes easily and if the transillumination intensity increases in the midline, it has entered the trachea (Fig. 2.19d).

8 If the light intensity is reduced, the tube has entered the oesophagus.

9 Transillumination either side of the midline with difficulty in advancement indicates incorrect placement in the pyriform fossa.

Hazards

- Persistent lodging in the pyriform fossa or in front of the epiglottis.
- Damage to pharyngeal or laryngeal structures.

Key points

- With experience, the light wand can be successful in a substantial proportion of cases but direct laryngoscopy must always be available as an alternative technique.
- It may be useful to dim the general room lighting during trans-illumination.

NASOTRACHEAL INTUBATION

This method is used when the oral route has failed or is inappropriate, e.g. surgery is to be performed in the mouth, the jaws are to be wired together at the end of the operation, there are oral anatomical or pathological problems etc. There is some controversy as to whether the orally or nasally placed tube is more tolerable for the conscious patient. The nasal route is preferred by some authorities in patients with suspected cervical spine injury. However, it is generally agreed that the nasal route requires more technical skill. The nasal route also carries the risk of causing bleeding from the nose.

Nasotracheal tubes are available with flexible tips which allow the curve of the tube to be varied by traction on a ring pull (Fig. 2.20). This enables the tip of the tube to be adjusted to negotiate the curve from the nose into the hypopharynx and to proceed anteriorly through the glottic opening.

Three methods may be used:
- Blind nasal intubation.
- Nasal intubation assisted by direct laryngoscopy and Magill's offset forceps.
- Nasal intubation assisted by fibre-optic laryngoscopy (see p. 98).

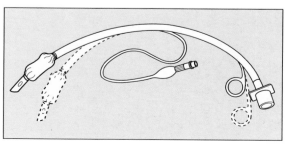

Fig. 2.20 A flexible tipped nasotracheal tube

BLIND NASOTRACHEAL INTUBATION

Technique

This technique is shown in Fig. 2.21.

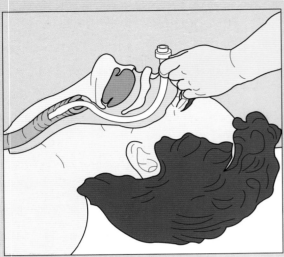

Fig. 2.21 Blind nasotracheal intubation

1 Lubricate the nasotracheal tube and ensure that all equipment functions correctly. Size 7.0–8.0mm tubes cut to 23–27cm are suitable for adults.

2 Place the patient in a supine position with the head and neck aligned in the clear airway position.

3 The patient may be unconscious, anaesthetised or awake. Awake patients require local analgesia to the nasal passages, the back of the tongue and the posterior pharynx and larynx using a local anaesthetic spray. A vasoconstrictor substance such as cocaine (up to 2ml of 10%) should be used for the nasal passages; 4% lignocaine or prilocaine is suitable for the tongue, pharynx and larynx. Additionally, the larynx should be anaesthetised by a transcricoid injection of 4% lignocaine or prilocaine or by a bilateral block of the superior laryngeal nerves using 2% lignocaine with adrenaline (see p. 100).

4 Introduce the nasotracheal tube into the right nostril directing it backwards in line with the hard palate. If resistance is encountered withdraw and try the left nostril.

5 Advance the tube through the nasopharynx.

6 Occlude the mouth and opposite nostril manually.

7 Listen at the proximal end of the tube for breath sounds in the spontaneously breathing patient.

8 Manipulating the larynx and tube, steer the tube so that breath sounds reach maximum intensity and at this point advance the tube during inspiration through the glottic opening into the trachea.

9 Generally, a cough heralds successful passage into the trachea in the awake patient.

10 Though more difficult, the technique can also be used in the apnoeic patient. With skill and practice and optimal patient positioning, the tube can often be steered blindly directly through the glottis into the trachea.

11 If the blind technique fails, resort should be made to manipulation and placement using direct or fibre-optic laryngoscopy.

NASOTRACHEAL INTUBATION ASSISTED BY DIRECT LARYNGOSCOPY AND MAGILL'S OFFSET FORCEPS

Technique

This technique is shown in Fig. 2.22.

1 Proceed as for blind nasal intubation until the tip of the tube lies just above the glottis.
2 View the larynx directly with a laryngoscope as for oral intubation.
3a Advance the tube through the glottic opening under direct vision using simple forward pressure

or

3b Grasp the tube 1–2cm from the tip with Magill's forceps and steer it through the glottic opening.
4 With either technique, if the tube appears to pass through the vocal cords but impinges anteriorly, it may be dislodged by rotation or by flexion of the head or the neck and advanced with continued downward pressure. *Flexion should not be attempted in patients with suspected spinal injuries.*
5 Secure the tube and check for correct positioning as for oral intubation.

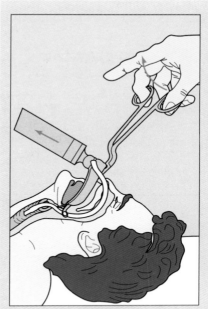

Fig. 2.22 Nasotracheal intubation using direct laryngoscopy and Magill's forceps

Hazards

- As for oral tracheal intubation.
- Trauma to the nasal passage or adenoidal tissue with associated haemorrhage.

TRACHEAL INTUBATION IN INFANTS AND CHILDREN

Tracheal intubation in infants and children follows broadly the same principles as in adults. However, there are certain important specific considerations which apply to this group of patients.

- A straight-bladed laryngoscope is generally used in infants and children under two years.
- The straight blade is passed behind the epiglottis (not in front, as with the curved blade). This is because infants have a relatively large and floppy epiglottis.
- In infants and children under six years, the narrowest diameter of the airway is just below the cricoid ring and not, as in the adult, the space between the vocal cords.

- Cuffed tubes are not used in infants and children under ten years. A slight leak during positive pressure ventilation is acceptable.
- Special care must be taken to ensure that bronchial intubation does not occur as the child's trachea is relatively short.

TRACHEAL INTUBATION IN SUSPECTED CERVICAL SPINE INJURY

Special care must be taken when intubating patients with suspected cervical spine injury. Manual in-line cervical stabilisation must be applied throughout the procedure to prevent aggravation of the injury (Fig. 2.23). Nevertheless the importance of the airway is paramount.

Certain important points should be observed in this group of patients:
- Flexion and rotation of the head and neck are the most dangerous movements.
- Many advocate awake fibre-optic nasal intubation as the method of choice.
- In the unconscious patient the fibre-optic technique may require more time than is available if the airway is obstructed.
- Oral intubation using direct laryngoscopy by a skilled operator is equally safe in the vast majority of cases and can be performed quickly.
- Cases of difficult oral intubation can be managed by the blind nasal technique, the light wand, the Combitube or with the aid of the laryngeal mask (see p. 78).
- Cases of difficult intubation with major maxillofacial injury should be managed by cricothyroidotomy (see p. 111).

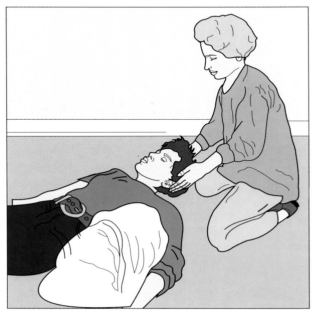

Fig. 2.23 Manual in-line cervical stabilisation

TRACHEAL INTUBATION IN PATIENTS WITH PHARYNGEAL OR LARYNGEAL OEDEMA

Patients with acute pharyngeal and laryngeal oedema due, perhaps, to inhalational thermal injury, acute epiglottis or anaphylaxis, require special care and intubation should be attempted only by a very experienced operator.

- Repeated attempts and manipulation will aggravate the oedema and may convert partial into complete airway obstruction.
- Blind techniques such as the light wand are contra-indicated.
- The use of muscle relaxants is contra-indicated.
- The technique of choice is oral intubation using direct laryngoscopy under deep inhalational general anaesthesia, although fibre-optic intubation is a reasonable alternative.
- Facilities for cricothyroidotomy should be immediately available.

CRICOID PRESSURE

Indications

Patients at risk of regurgitation and aspiration.

The majority of unconscious emergency patients are at risk of regurgitation and aspiration of gastric contents during the procedure of tracheal intubation, particularly if muscle relaxants are used. This hazard can be substantially reduced by the application of cricoid pressure by an assistant during intubation. No extra equipment is required. The application of cricoid pressure is shown in Fig. 2.24.

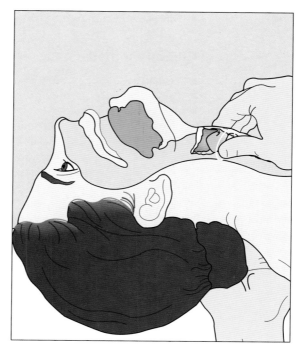

Fig. 2.24 The application of cricoid pressure

Technique

1 The patient is generally placed in the supine position but can be lying on his or her side if circumstances dictate and the intubationist is highly skilled.
2 Place the thumb, middle and index fingers astride the larynx at the level of the cricoid ring.
3 Apply firm backwards pressure to the cricoid ring to occlude the oesophagus lying behind it.
4 Counter pressure may be applied with the other hand placed behind the neck.
5 Pressure should be maintained until the trachea is safely intubated and the cuff inflated.

Hazards

- Cervical spine injury may be aggravated.
- Active vomiting against applied cricoid pressure may cause oesophageal or gastric rupture.

DETECTION OF CORRECT TUBE PLACEMENT

Nothing is more important in intubation than detection of correct placement of the tube in the trachea. Undetected tube placement in the oesophagus will have disastrous consequences and is rightly considered medically negligent.

A number of methods are available to confirm the presence of the tube in the trachea:
- Clinical methods.
- The oesophageal detector.
- Transillumination.
- Detection of carbon dioxide.
- Direct inspection using a fibre-optic laryngoscope.

Clinical methods

- Visualise the tube passing between the vocal cords.
- Palpate the tube passing into the larynx.
- Apply positive pressure ventilation and note absence of leak around the cuff, bilateral chest expansion, breath sounds heard in both axillae but not in the epigastric area.

These methods are reliable in the majority of cases.

The oesophageal detector

The oesophageal detector is shown in Fig. 2.25. A 50ml syringe or self-inflating bulb is applied to the tracheal tube connector and aspiration is attempted. Free aspiration confirms placement of the tube in the trachea. Resistance to aspiration indicates that the tube is in the oesophagus. This is a very reliable and inexpensive method.

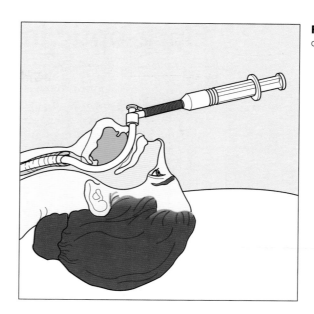

Fig. 2.25 The oesophageal detector

Transillumination

Pass a lighted stylet down the lumen of the tube (Fig. 2.19). Bright transillumination suggests that the tube is in the trachea. A dull glow suggests that it is in the oesophagus. This method is not completely reliable and depends on observed variation and background lighting.

Detection of carbon dioxide

The emergence of carbon dioxide from the tube during expiration confirms placement in the trachea. Carbon dioxide can be detected by a capnometer or by a simple inexpensive colorimetric device.

Carbon dioxide is not produced during cardiac arrest; indeed measurement of end-tidal CO_2 is a useful indication of the efficacy of CPR and may give some prediction of outcome. Values below 1.3kPa indicate a poor prognosis and above 2.0kPa may suggest a good outcome.

Fibre-optic inspection

A fibre-optic bronchoscope is passed through the lumen of the tube. Visualisation of the rings of the trachea and the carina confirms correct tube placement. This is the most reliable method.

Fibre-optic intubation

The flexible fibre-optic bronchoscope has revolutionised the approach to airway management in the patient who is expected to be difficult to intubate. The bronchoscope is a delicate instrument, comprising insulated glass fibres, a light guide cable, and a working channel for suction, oxygen insufflation, or local anaesthetic injection. Compared with diagnostic bronchoscopes, those designed for intubation tend to be of smaller diameter (4mm or less). Movement of the tip of the intubating bronchoscope, via the lever, is possible in the antero-posterior plane only. Lateral movement of the bronchoscope tip is achieved only by rotation. Fibre-optic intubation may be performed via the nasal or oral route and the patient can be awake or unconscious. Although much of the training tends to be performed on anaesthetised patients, the technique is easier in the awake patient who has more tone in the soft tissue structures of the airway. If the airway is compromised the procedure should be performed with the patient awake. Disadvantages of fibre-optic intubation are that the equipment is expensive and that considerable training is required to become adept with the technique.

Indications

Where direct laryngoscopy is expected to be difficult or impossible:
- Limited neck movement.
- Limited mouth opening.
- Short mandible.
- Over-riding upper teeth.
- Tumour, oedema, or haematoma in the airway.

Where neck extension must be avoided:
- Cervical spine injuries.
- Chronic cervical spine instability (e.g. atlanto-axial instability in rheumatoid arthritis).

Contra-indications

Where an immediate airway is required (the technique is time-consuming even in skilled hands).

Blood or other foreign material in the airway makes the procedure exceedingly difficult or impossible.

Equipment

- ☐ Flexible intubating fibre-optic bronchoscope (outer diameter 5mm).
- ☐ Light source.
- ☐ Oxygen supply.
- ☐ Intravenous cannula and infusion set primed with crystalloid.
- ☐ Cocaine solution 5% or 10%.
- ☐ Cotton buds.
- ☐ Lignocaine gel.
- ☐ Lignocaine spray 4%.
- ☐ Three 2ml syringes.
- ☐ Two 23G needles.
- ☐ Soft nasal airways (5, 6, 7, and 8mm internal diameter).
- ☐ Endotracheal tube (7mm internal diameter for nasal route; 8 or 9mm for oral route).
- ☐ Oral airway intubator (for oral route).
- ☐ Sedative drugs (for awake technique).
- ☐ Small pot containing warm water.
- ☐ Pulse oximeter.
- ☐ Anaesthesia mask with intubating port (for asleep/oral technique).

Technique

If an awake intubation is planned, reassure the patient with a comprehensive explanation of the technique, including the reasons for keeping him or her conscious. Ensure that the patient has nil by

►►►

▶ ▶ ▶

mouth for six hours beforehand to minimise the risk of vomiting and aspiration. Glycopyrrolate 0.2mg, given intramuscularly about 30 minutes before the procedure, will reduce airway secretions. If planning an awake technique, the patient may be sedated by very carefully using a combination of fentanyl (approximately 1μg/kg) and incremental doses of midazolam (0.015 mg/kg). The patient must remain rousable.

The larynx is innervated by branches of the vagus nerve, the superior and recurrent laryngeal nerves. The internal branch of the superior laryngeal nerve supplies sensory innervation to the epiglottis, aryepiglottic folds, and mucous membranes of the larynx down to the false cords. The recurrent laryngeal nerve provides sensory innervation to the larynx below the vocal cords. A combination of bilateral superior laryngeal nerve blocks and transtracheal anaesthesia will provide complete laryngeal anaesthesia for awake intubation.

Connect the bronchoscope to the light source adjusted to its maximal intensity (Fig. 2.26). Check that the optics provide a clear view, by examining some text, for example. Spray the endoscope with silicone lubricant.

Awake fibre-optic intubation can be performed with the patient in the supine or sitting position, though this may be dictated by the stability of the cervical spine. If the patient's cervical spine is stable, cervical extension tilts the larynx anteriorly and lifts the epiglottis off the posterior pharyngeal wall, thus providing the optimum position for fibre-optic laryngoscopy.

Nasotracheal route in the awake patient

1 Insert an intravenous cannula into the patient and attach an i.v. giving set primed with crystalloid. Give intravenous sedation, as required, through this cannula. ▶ ▶ ▶

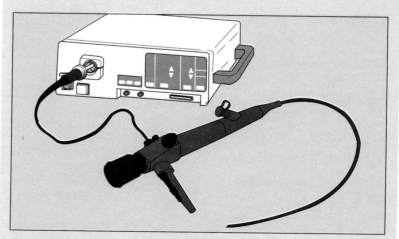

Fig. 2.26 Fibre-optic intubating bronchoscope and light source

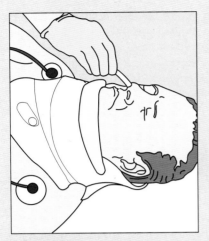

Fig. 2.27 Dilating the nasal passage

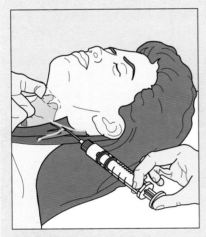

Fig. 2.28 Superior laryngeal nerve block

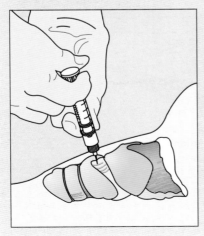

Fig. 2.29 Transtracheal anaesthesia

▶ ▶ ▶

2 Select the nostril through which the patient finds it easiest to breath. Place a cotton wool bud (nasal pledget) soaked in cocaine into the nasal passage. After a minute replace this with another, this time placing it deeper into the nasal passage.

3 Lubricate the soft nasopharyngeal airways with lignocaine gel. Remove the cotton bud and gently insert the 5mm airway into the nose (Fig. 2.27). Dilate the nasal passage progressively by using airways of increasing size, finishing with the 8mm (one size larger than the planned endotracheal tube.

4 Block the superior laryngeal nerve bilaterally: palpate the greater cornu of the hyoid bone. Using a 23G needle, and after careful aspiration (to exclude placement in the external carotid artery) inject fanwise 2ml of 1% lignocaine, 0.5cm caudad and medial to the greater cornu, 0.5cm beneath the skin surface (Fig. 2.28). Repeat on the opposite side of the neck.

5 Palpate and cleanse the skin overlying the cricothyroid membrane. Attach a 23G needle to a syringe containing 2ml of 2% lignocaine and advance through the cricothyroid membrane. Warn the patient that he or she will cough. Confirm endotracheal placement by easy aspiration of air and quickly inject the lignocaine (Fig. 2.29).

6 Spray the back of the patients tongue with 4% lignocaine.

7 Immerse the endotracheal tube in warm sterile water for a few minutes (to make it more pliable) and check the cuff for leaks. Lubricate the endotracheal tube with lignocaine gel before inserting it gently into the dilated nasal passage to a distance of 15cm (Fig. 2.30a). This will place the tip of the endotracheal tube about 1–2cm proximal to the epiglottis.

8 Attach oxygen tubing to the suction port of the fibre-optic bronchoscope. Oxygen flow increases the FIO_2, blows secretions away, and serves as a defogging mechanism. Immerse the tip of the bronchoscope in warm saline just before insertion (this also helps prevents fogging).

9 Stand behind the patient or on the right side and facing the patient (this is a matter of personal preference). Advance the fibre-optic bronchoscope through and beyond the tip of the endotracheal tube (Fig. 2.30b). The epiglottis should be visible at this stage. Advance the bronchoscope through the cords and into the trachea, noting the carina (Fig. 2.30c).

10 Advance the endotracheal tube over the bronchoscope, rotating it 90° to ease its passage through the triangular upper part of the laryngeal opening (Fig. 2.30d).

11 View the carina through the bronchoscope to confirm the correct location of the tip of the endotracheal tube in the trachea. Withdraw the bronchoscope, connect a breathing system to the endotracheal tube, and note adequate spontaneous ventilation.

12 Auscultate to confirm correct placement of the tube. ▶ ▶ ▶

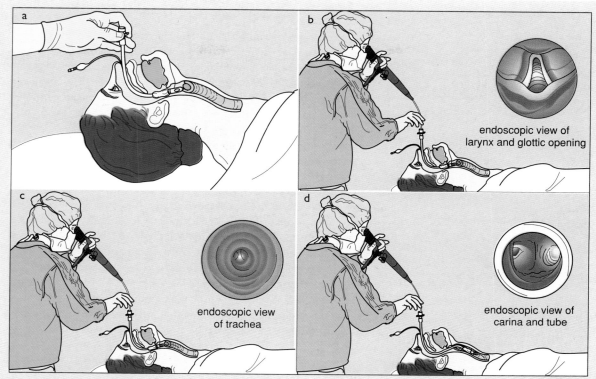

Fig. 2.30 Nasotracheal intubation in the awake patient

endoscopic view of larynx and glottic opening

endoscopic view of trachea

endoscopic view of carina and tube

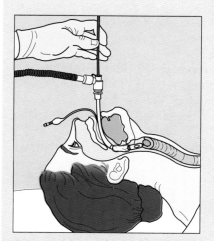

Fig. 2.31 Nasotracheal intubation in the anaesthetised patient

▶ ▶ ▶

Nasotracheal route in the anaesthetised patient

1 After securing intravenous access, induce general anaesthesia, keeping the patient breathing spontaneously. Anaesthesia can be maintained using either a volatile agent or by a continuous propofol infusion. Follow steps 1–3 above.
2 Ensure the patient is adequately anaesthetised and well oxygenated. Remove the oxygen mask and follow steps 7–12 above. Once the endotracheal tube is in the nose, attach to it a breathing system, via a catheter mount that includes a port with a diaphragm (Fig. 2.31). Oxygen and a volatile anaesthetic can then be administered during the intubation attempt. Before advancing the bronchoscope into the trachea, spray the vocal cords with 1% lignocaine via the suction port.
3 If the patient's oxygenation drops below 94% at any stage during the procedure, remove the bronchoscope and recommence mask ventilation with 100% oxygen.

Orotracheal route in the awake patient

1 Cannulate a vein and start an infusion of crystalloid.
2 Spray the patient's oropharynx with 4% lignocaine, starting with the anterior half of the tongue and progressing slowly toward the back of the oropharynx.
3 Perform superior laryngeal nerve blocks bilaterally and a transtracheal block as described in steps 4–5 above. ▶ ▶ ▶

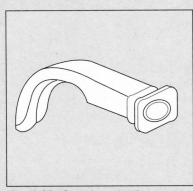

Fig. 2.32 Oral airway intubator

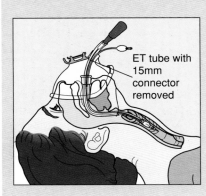

ET tube with 15mm connector removed

▶ ▶ ▶

4 Insert an oral airway intubator into the patient's mouth (Fig. 2.32).

5 Remove the 15mm connector from a 8mm internal diameter (ID) endotracheal tube and thread the well-lubricated tube over the fibre-optic bronchoscope. Advance the bronchoscope through the airway until the cords come into view. Continue to pass the bronchoscope into the trachea and thread the endotracheal tube over it, placing the tip of the tube about 2–3cm above the carina.

6 Remove the bronchoscope and oral airway intubator, replace the 15mm connector, and attach a breathing system. Auscultate to confirm adequate placement of the tube.

Orotracheal route in the anaesthetised patient

1 Obtain intravenous access and induce general anaesthesia, by inhalation if in any doubt about airway patency. If available, use an anaesthesia mask fitted with an intubating port. If not, use a nasal mask. These allow the patient to continue breathing oxygen and a volatile anaesthetic agent during the intubation attempt (Fig. 2.33).

2 Repeat steps 4–6 above, as for orotracheal intubation in the awake patient. The intubating anaesthesia mask is removed while keeping a tight grasp on the endotracheal tube close to the patient's mouth.

Fig. 2.33 Orotracheal intubation via anaesthesia mask with an intubating port

Hazards

• Take great care to ensure the patient does not become hypoxic. Insufflate oxygen down the suction port of the bronchoscope and monitor saturation with a pulse oximeter.

• Bleeding from the nasal passage will make the larynx very difficult to see. Prepare the nose thoroughly with plenty of vasoconstrictor.

Complications

• When performed by inexperienced anaesthetists or under inappropriate circumstances, attempted fibre-optic intubation is more likely to fail and can be very hazardous.

• A distorted airway or excessive secretions will make intubation more difficult.

• Hypoxia is one of the commonest complications and can occur as a result of over-sedation and/or a compromised airway (as part of the patient's pre-existing condition or as a result of bronchospasm or laryngospasm).

• The considerable doses of local anaesthetic may cause adverse reactions.

• Nasotracheal intubation often causes some bleeding which occasionally can be severe and lead to failure of the technique.

Intubation with a double-lumen endobronchial tube

Indications

Absolute

Isolation of one lung to prevent contamination from the other:
- Unilateral gross pulmonary infection.
- Unilateral massive pulmonary haemorrhage.

Control distribution of ventilation:
- Bronchopleural fistula.
- Tracheobronchial airway disruption (surgical or traumatic).
- Giant unilateral lung cyst.

Unilateral bronchopulmonary lavage.

Relative

Surgical exposure:
- Descending thoracic aortic surgery.
- Pulmonary lobectomy.
- Pneumonectomy.
- Thoracoscopy.
- Oesophageal surgery.
- Transthoracic spinal surgery.

Independent lung ventilation in asymmetrical adult respiratory distress syndrome.

Contra-indications

Children less than 10–12 years (use single lumen tube in the bronchus and/or a bronchial blocker).

A lesion in mainstem bronchus contra-indicates ipsilateral bronchial tube.

Double-lumen endobronchial tubes are used to isolate one lung from the other and were designed originally for differential lung spirometry. At present, they are used most commonly during thoracic surgery and occasionally for independent lung ventilation in patients with asymmetrical lung disease in critical care units. Several types of double-lumen tubes are available. The design of most modern tubes is based on the Robertshaw tube which has D-shaped lumina, thus providing the largest possible lumina for a given external diameter (Fig. 2.34). The original Robertshaw tube was made of red rubber, but modern tubes are manufactured from polyvinyl chloride designed for single use only. The Robertshaw-type tubes are available for both right- and left-sided endobronchial insertion and are made in five sizes (41, 39, 37, 35, and 28FG). A 41FG tube has approximately the same external diameter as an 11mm ID endotracheal tube. The distal part of the right-sided Robertshaw-type tube is slotted to allow for ventilation of the right upper lobe (the right upper lobe bronchus emerges from the mainstem only 2.5cm from the carina) and thus has an eccentrically located bronchial cuff. However, the considerable anatomical variation in the location of the right upper lobe bronchus makes it difficult to locate the bronchial slot precisely. For this reason, a left-sided tube is preferred, except where there is a proximal left mainstem bronchial lesion that could be damaged during insertion. A left-sided double-lumen tube can be used for a left pneumonectomy, and withdrawn into the trachea just before the bronchus is clamped.

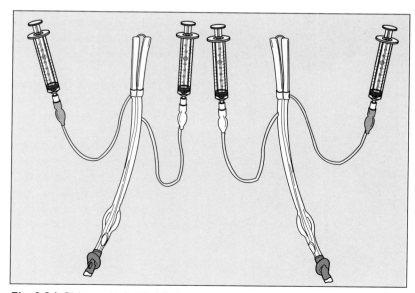

Fig. 2.34 Right- and left-sided Robertshaw-type tubes

Equipment

☐ Drugs, equipment, and monitors for induction of general anaesthesia.
☐ Sucker with Yankauer end and endobronchial catheters.
☐ Laryngoscope.
☐ Double-lumen tubes of various sizes.
☐ Single-lumen tube of suitable size.
☐ Stylet.
☐ Magill's forceps.
☐ 5ml and 10ml syringes (for cuffs of pilot tubes).
☐ Stethoscope.
☐ Flexible fibre-optic bronchoscope.
☐ Adhesive tape or tube-tie.

Technique

Assess the trachea clinically and review the chest X-ray. Select an appropriately sized double-lumen tube: typically, 37FG for a woman and 39FG for a man. Insert the stylet that comes packaged with the tube. Check both cuffs and leave a 5ml syringe on the bronchial pilot tube and a 10ml syringe on the tracheal pilot tube. Lubricate both cuffs thereby reducing the risk of tearing them on the teeth. Have a standard endotracheal tube ready in case there is a problem in placing the double-lumen tube.

Position the patient supine and in the 'sniffing' position, attach monitoring, and induce general anaesthesia and paralysis.

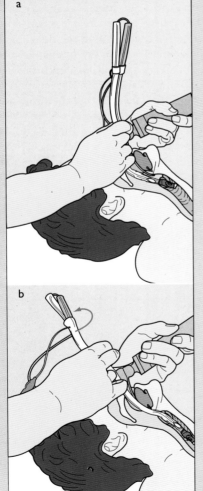

1 Ensure that the patient is well-oxygenated before proceeding to laryngoscopy.
2 Hold the double-lumen tube so that the distal end is curved anteriorly and pass it through the pharynx and between the cords (Fig. 2.35a).
3 Once the tip of the tube is through the larynx, remove the stylet, then rotate the tube 90° to the left (or to the right for a right-sided tube) (Fig. 2.35b).
4 Advance the tube until moderate resistance is encountered as it seats in the mainstem bronchus.
5 Check that the tube is in the trachea: inflate the tracheal cuff, ventilate both bronchial and tracheal sides, and auscultate both lungs to confirm breath sounds on both sides (Fig. 2.36a). *If isolating one lung to prevent contamination, inflate the bronchial cuff first, keeping it inflated to maintain isolation.* Inflate the bronchial cuff; it will require 2–3ml only (Fig. 2.36b). If the bronchial cuff requires more than 3ml it may be sitting too proximally, partly or completely within the trachea. If breath sounds are heard one side only, it is likely that both lumina have entered a mainstem bronchus. ▶ ▶ ▶

Fig. 2.35 Insertion of left-sided double-lumen tube: passing through cords, rotating the tube

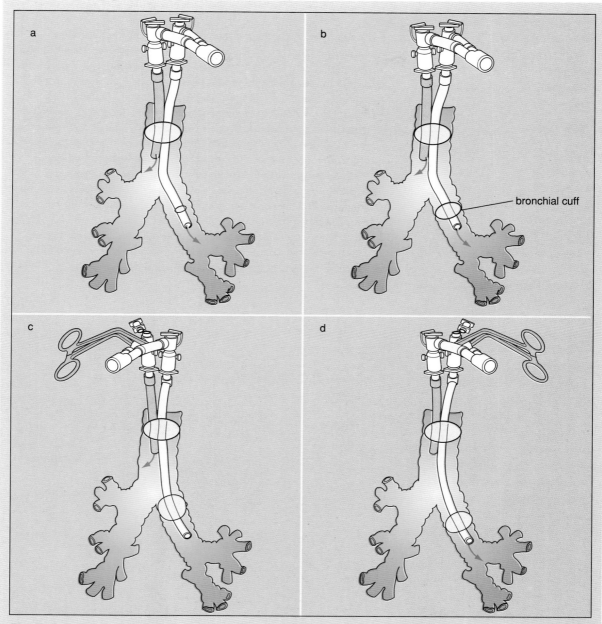

bronchial cuff

Fig. 2.36 Checking the tube position: (a) location in trachea; (b) bronchial cuff inflated; (c) checking bronchial side; (d) checking opposite side

▶ ▶ ▶

6 Check that the lung with the bronchial tube has been isolated: Clamp the tracheal lumen, squeeze the reservoir bag, and check there are breath sounds, particularly in the upper lobe, on the bronchial side only. Disconnect the catheter mount on the tracheal side and, while ventilating the bronchial side, check that there is no gas leak back up through the tracheal lumen (Fig. 2.36c). Such a gas leak suggests that the bronchial cuff is inadequately inflated or not properly seated in the bronchus. ▶ ▶ ▶

► ► ►

7 Unclamp the tracheal lumen and reconnect the catheter mount. Clamp the bronchial lumen and disconnect the catheter mount on this side (Fig. 2.36d). Squeeze the reservoir bag and check there are breath sounds on the other side only. A properly seated and sealed bronchial cuff will prevent any leakage of gas up the bronchial lumen.

8 If there is any doubt about the position of a left-sided tube, check it with a fibre-optic bronchoscope (this is the only way of confirming the exact location of the ventilation slot of right-sided tubes). A paediatric bronchoscope will pass through all sizes of double-lumen tubes.

9 Pass the bronchoscope through the tracheal lumen; this should provide a clear view of the carina. If there is excessive pressure in the endobronchial cuff, or if it is positioned too proximally, it will herniate over the carina (Fig. 2.37).

10 Remove the bronchoscope and pass it through the bronchial lumen. There should be a clear view distally and minimal compression of the lumen at the level of the bronchial cuff. ► ► ►

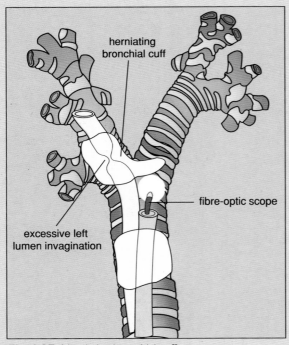

Fig. 2.37 Herniating bronchial cuff seen at bronchoscopy

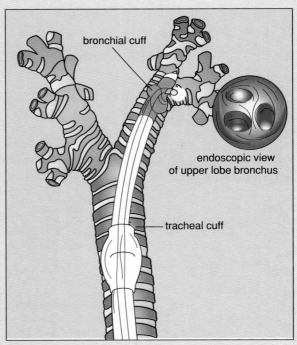

Fig. 2.38 Checking position of right upper lobe ventilation slot

▶ ▶ ▶

11 If checking a right-sided tube, pass the bronchoscope through the upper lobe ventilation slot and confirm a clear view of the characteristic trifurcating right upper lobe bronchus (Fig. 2.38). If no lumen is visible, deflate the bronchial and tracheal cuffs and slowly withdraw or advance the tube under direct vision with the bronchoscope until the right upper lobe bronchus comes into view. Re-inflate both cuffs and recheck the position.

12 The fibre-optic bronchoscope can be used to position both left and right-sided tubes initially: Once the double lumen tube is in the trachea, pass a paediatric bronchoscope through the bronchial lumen and advance it, under direct vision, into the appropriate mainstem bronchus. Railroad the double-lumen tube into the bronchus, confirm its position and remove the bronchoscope.

13 If the patient is moved (e.g. into a lateral position) the position of the double-lumen can easily change. Therefore, always recheck the location of the tube with the above tests.

14 When switching to one lung ventilation, use a tidal volume of 10ml/kg and an FIO_2 of 1.0. Increase the respiratory rate by 30% in order to maintain normocapnia. If the SaO_2 falls, recheck the tube position and apply 5–10cmH$_2$O continuous positive airway pressure (CPAP) to the lower lung.

Complications

- Double-lumen tubes are bulky, making intubation more difficult and, in comparison with single-lumen tubes, laryngeal trauma is more likely.
- In critically ill patients, difficulty with the intubation may predispose to hypoxia.
- Malposition is a common problem. The tube may be too long or too short: using too short a tube may result in herniation of the bronchial cuff over the carina and obstruction of the opposite bronchus. Malposition of a right-sided tube commonly results in collapse of the right upper lobe.
- A rare, but serious complication, is bronchial rupture. This may be caused by excessive bronchial cuff pressure, too long a double-lumen tube, or tube movement while repositioning the patient.

Hazards

- Intubation with a double-lumen tube may be difficult; take great care to avoid hypoxia.
- Excessive pressure in the bronchial cuff and/or movement of the tube may result in rupture of the bronchus.

Key points

- If there are difficulties with the airway, first place an ordinary single-lumen tracheal tube, then stabilise the patient before attempting to place the double-lumen tube.
- Nearly all surgical procedures requiring collapse of the lung can be performed adequately with a left-sided double-lumen tube.
- If a double-lumen tube cannot be positioned properly, the lungs can be separated by fibre-optic bronchoscopic placement of a single-lumen tube in a mainstem bronchus.

Retrograde tracheal intubation

A very few patients may prove impossible to intubate using the procedures described above. An alternative method for these patients can be to pass a retrograde guidewire through the cricothyroid membrane in a cephalad direction, retrieving it in the mouth or nose and railroading the tracheal tube over the guidewire, while maintaining tension at either end of the wire.

The procedure is not suitable for the unconscious emergency patient at risk from gastric regurgitation and pulmonary aspiration. Rather, it is a technique applicable to the non-urgent planned case. It is generally carried out under local anaesthesia.

Several variations of the basic technique have been reported. The commonly used ones will be described later.

Equipment

- [ ] Antiseptic solution.
- [ ] 2ml, 5ml and 20ml syringes.
- [ ] 1% lignocaine with adrenaline 1:200,000.
- [ ] 4% lignocaine.
- [ ] Scalpel blade.
- [ ] Tuohy needle 19G and epidural catheter, or 18G intravenous cannula-over-needle and Seldinger wire.
- [ ] Laryngoscope.
- [ ] Magill's offset forceps.
- [ ] Tracheal tube of appropriate size and cut to length. A tube with an additional side hole ('Murphy's eye') just below the cuff is an advantage.
- [ ] Lubricating jelly.
- [ ] Two pairs of artery forceps.
- [ ] Suction apparatus.
- [ ] Facility for lung ventilation.

Technique

The patient should be placed supine with the head and neck aligned in the clear airway position. The neck should be slightly more extended during the cricoid puncture. Spray the posterior aspect of the tongue and posterior pharyngeal wall with 4% lignocaine. The operator should now don a gown and gloves. ► ► ►

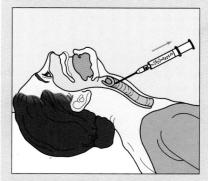

Fig. 2.39 Identification of correct needle placement in the trachea

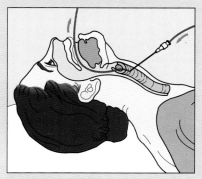

Fig. 2.40 Introduction of catheter/guideline into the oropharynx and mouth

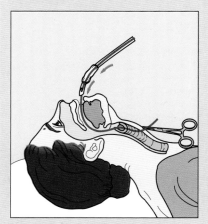

Fig. 2.41 Threading the catheter/guidewire through the side hole in the tracheal tube

▶ ▶ ▶

1　Clean and drape the skin over the anterior part of the neck.

2　Identify the cricothyroid membrane by palpation.

3　Infiltrate the skin and subcutaneous tissues over the cricothyroid membrane with 1% lignocaine and adrenaline 1:200,000.

4　Load a 5ml syringe with 2ml 4% lignocaine.

5　Pierce the cricothyroid membrane, confirm correct needle placement in the trachea by aspiration of air and then rapidly inject the 2ml lignocaine at the end of expiration. Hold the needle firmly and withdraw it quickly as injection nearly always causes coughing.

6　A bilateral superior laryngeal nerve block can also be performed for further laryngeal anaesthesia. The nerve should be infiltrated with 1% lignocaine as it lies between the greater horn of the hyoid bone and the superior horn of the thyroid cartilage (see awake fibre-optic intubation, p.100).

7　Make a small (2mm) vertical skin incision over the cricothyroid membrane.

8　Introduce a Tuohy needle (with the bevel and bend facing cephalad) or an intravenous cannula-over-needle through the cricothyroid membrane into the trachea.

9　Attach a 5ml syringe containing 2ml water and aspirate. Air bubbles entering the water confirms correct location of the needle in the trachea (Fig. 2.39).

10　Remove the syringe and direct the needle cephalad at an angle of 30° in the midline.

11　Select an epidural catheter or flexible guidewire (at least 125cm long if it is to fit later into the suction port of a fibre-optic laryngoscope). Attach an artery forceps to the proximal end of the wire to prevent it disappearing through the needle or cannula.

12　Pass the guidewire or catheter through the Tuohy needle or i.v. cannula in a retrograde direction until it emerges from the mouth or nose. It may be necessary to search for the distal end in the mouth using a laryngoscope blade and Magill's forceps. Remove the needle or cannula (Fig. 2.40).

13　Thread the wire through the 'Murphy's eye' side hole in the tracheal tube or pass it up the lumen of the tube to emerge at the proximal end. The advantage of using the 'Murphy's eye' is that the tube can be passed further through the cords before impinging on the wire as it emerges through the cricothyroid membrane (Fig. 2.41).

14　Attach a clip to the end of the wire emerging from the proximal end of the tracheal tube.

15　An assistant should hold the two ends of the wire taut; the tube is advanced over the wire until it is held up at cricoid thyroid level.

16　Correct placement of the tube can be helped by passing a flexible bougie or gastric tube down the lumen of the tracheal tube at this stage so that it lies well down the trachea and acts as a guidepath for later advancement of the tube (Fig. 2.42).

17a　Remove the proximal clip and advance the tube 1cm further so that it lies well in the trachea and then withdraw the wire from the cricothyroid end.　▶ ▶ ▶

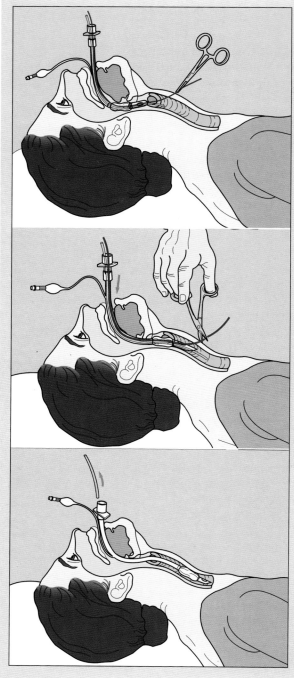

or

17b If an epidural catheter is used, cut the catheter flush with the skin, advance the tracheal tube and withdraw the catheter from the proximal end (Fig. 2.43).

18 Advance the tracheal tube to the anticipated correct level, remove the bougie or nasogastric tube (Fig. 2.44). Inflate the tracheal cuff and confirm correct placement by the usual methods described on p.96.

Fig. 2.42 Using a bougie or nasogastric tube as a guidepath for the tracheal tube

Fig. 2.43 Removal of the catheter and advancement of the tracheal tube further into the trachea

Fig. 2.44 Removal of the bougie and nasogastric tube.

Key points

- If the tube is held up at the larynx, it may usually be advanced if it is rotated through 90° counter-clockwise.
- Keep the wire taut during introduction of the tube.
- A wire is likely to be more successfully retrieved than an epidural catheter.

Surgical and percutaneous dilatational cricothyroidotomy

THE SURGICAL AIRWAY

Transtracheal intubation may be accomplished through the cricothyroid membrane or directly through the upper part of the trachea. The procedure is not without hazard and is reserved for patients in whom translaryngeal intubation is impossible, dangerous or contra-indicated.

Indications

Severe anatomical abnormality such as ankylosing spondylitis or where translaryngeal intubation has proved impossible.

Cervical spine injury where translaryngeal intubation could prove hazardous.

Extensive maxillofacial or laryngeal injury.

Upper airway obstruction which renders translaryngeal intubation impossible, for example, impacted foreign body, tumour invasion, inflammation and oedema formation. ► ► ►

▶ ▶ ▶
Where direct access to the trachea is required for aspiration of secretions for an extended period of time and prolonged translaryngeal intubation would be undesirable.
▶ ▶ ▶

▶ ▶ ▶
Where prolonged intermittent positive pressure ventilation is required and extended translaryngeal intubation is thought to be hazardous or contra-indicated.

Surgical cricothyroidotomy

Access to the trachea through the cricothyroid membrane is simpler and less hazardous than tracheostomy and is the preferred method in the emergency, except where there is severe trauma to the larynx. Tracheostomy is used in the elective situation when long-term ventilation or upper airway bypass is required.

Contra-indications

Relative

Obese bull neck with engorged veins.

Laryngeal trauma.

Recent inflammatory conditions of the larynx (tracheostomy is preferred).

Translaryngeal intubation for more than 72 hours (tracheostomy is preferred).

Children who have not yet reached puberty (tracheostomy is preferred except for an emergency short-term airway). ► ► ►

▶ ▶ ▶
In the three latter conditions, there is a danger of subglottic stenosis. If cricothyroidotomy is required as an emergency procedure, it should be replaced by a tracheostomy within 48 hours should the indication for a surgical airway remain.

Equipment

- ☐ Antiseptic solution.
- ☐ 5ml and 10ml syringes and needles.
- ☐ 10ml 1% lignocaine with 1:200,000 adrenaline.
- ☐ Drapes.
- ☐ Scalpel handle with no. 10 blades.
- ☐ Small and medium artery forceps.
- ☐ Self-retaining retractor.
- ☐ Tracheal dilators.
- ☐ Sterile lubricant.
- ☐ 6.0mm or 6.5mm tracheostomy tube for an adult (if not immediately available a similar size cut-down endotracheal tube will suffice in the emergency situation).
- ☐ Suction apparatus and catheters.
- ☐ 20ml syringe for inflation of tracheal tube cuff.
- ☐ Appropriate connection to ventilation device.
- ☐ Cotton ties.
- ☐ Sutures, needle holder and scissors.
- ☐ Optional: electrodiathermy; headlight.

Hazards

- Access may be restricted in patients with cervical spine injury. Some cervical collars permit the procedure to be done through an anterior window in the collar. If the collar has to be removed to gain access, in-line cervical stabilisation should be meticulously maintained by an assistant.
- Care should be taken not to pierce the posterior aspect of the airway.
- Bleeding may occur restricting visual access to the membrane, especially in patients with airway obstruction.
- Air embolism may occur in the head up position, particularly in the gasping patient with engorged neck veins.

Technique

The technique is shown in Fig. 2.45. Place the patient supine with the head hyperextended on the neck by inserting a sandbag or rolled sheet beneath the shoulders. The occiput should be placed on a soft ring to stabilise the head. The table or trolley should be tilted 15° head up to reduce venous bleeding. Hyperextension of the head and neck should be avoided in suspected cervical spine injury.

1 Clean and drape the skin over the anterior and lateral aspects of the neck from chin to sternum.
2 Identify the cricothyroid membrane by palpation of the dimple just below the thyroid cartilage (Figs. 2.45a–c).
3 In conscious patients infiltrate the skin and subcutaneous tissue with 1% lignocaine with adrenaline.
4 Make a 2–3cm transverse skin incision over the cricothyroid membrane (Fig. 2.45d).
5 Dissect the subcutaneous tissues down to the membrane using artery forceps.
6 Insert the self-retaining retractor to expose the membrane.
7 Incise the membrane 1cm transversely, insert the scalpel handle through the incision and rotate it 90° to achieve an airway (Fig. 2.45e).
8 Insert the lubricated tracheal tube through the incision alongside the scalpel handle directing it caudally into the trachea. Remove the scalpel handle as the tube enters the airway (Fig. 2.45f).
9 Inflate the cuff of the tube through the pilot tube. ▶ ▶ ▶

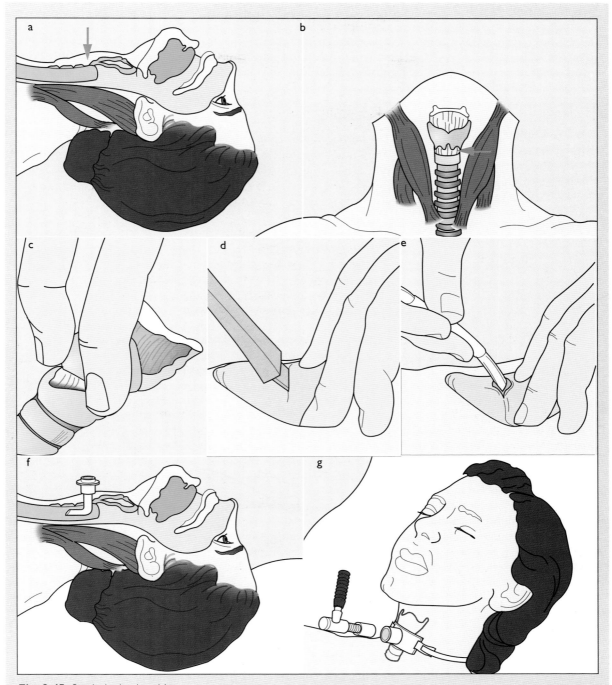

Fig. 2.45 Surgical cricothyroidotomy

▶ ▶ ▶

10 Connect the tube to the ventilating apparatus and check for correct tube placement by observing chest movement and CO_2 content of the exhaled air.

11 Suture the edges of the skin around the tube.

12 Fix the tube in position using tape or sutures (Fig. 2.45g).

Blind stab cricothyroidotomy

Purpose-designed cricothyroidotomy sets have been produced which are based on the 'blind stab' principle. Examples include the Portex Minitrach II and the NuTrach.

Hazards

- It may be difficult to locate the stab incision in the membrane with the bougie especially in the gasping patient whose larynx is moving up and down in relation to the skin. This problem can be minimised by transfixing the skin and membrane by two needles placed laterally to the proposed incision and asking an assistant to hold them so that the original alignment of larynx and skin is maintained.
- Bleeding may be a hazard in the asphyxiating patient.
- The 4.0mm tube provided is too narrow for anything but a very short-term emergency airway. To achieve a better airway the bougie can be re-inserted and tracheal tubes of increasing diameter can be introduced until a 6.0 or 6.5mm tube is accommodated in the trachea.

Technique

The Portex Minitrach II

The set is shown in Fig. 2.46. It includes a scalpel, bougie, 4.0mm tube and connector and suction catheter. It was originally designed for tracheal access for suction in the intensive care setting but has also been used to achieve an emergency airway.

1 Position and prepare the patient as for surgical cricothyroidotomy.
2 Ask an assistant to hold the larynx steady throughout the procedure.
3 Make a 2–3mm incision in the skin over the cricothyroid membrane and continue the incision to pierce the anterior aspect of the membrane.
4 Pass the bougie through the incision in the membrane and direct it caudally.
5 Railroad the 4.0mm lubricated tube over the bougie into the trachea. Remove the bougie.
6 Connect the tube to the ventilatory device and check for correct placement before securing with a tie or sutures.

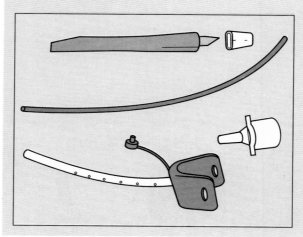

Fig. 2.46 The Portex Minitrach II kit

The NuTrach

The NuTrach consists of a patent expandable trochar system which pierces the membrane through a skin incision. A series of dilators of increasing size are passed through the expandable trochar until a tube of 6.0 or 6.5mm is accommodated in the trachea.

PERCUTANEOUS DILATATIONAL CRICOTHYROIDOTOMY

A kit for this technique is shown in Fig. 2.47. This method uses the Seldinger principle of passing a guidewire through a needle placed in the trachea via the cricothyroid membrane. A dilator is passed over the wire to enlarge the hole in the membrane sufficiently to admit a 6.0–6.5mm tracheal tube. The technique can also be applied for tracheostomy using a guiding catheter and a number of serial dilators.

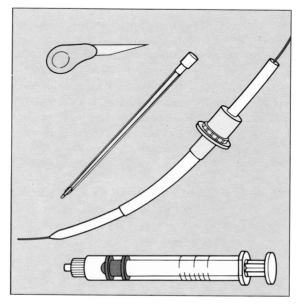

Fig. 2.47 The Melker percutaneous dilatational cricothyroidotomy kit

Technique

1 Position and prepare the patient as for surgical cricothyroidotomy.
2 Make a transverse skin incision through the skin and subcutaneous tissues across the intended guidewire entry point and extend it to make a small incision in the cricothyroid membrane beneath.
3 Insert an 18G cannula-over-needle into the trachea through the cricothyroid membrane and direct it caudally.
4 Confirm correct placement of the needle in the trachea by the aspiration of air into a syringe partly filled with sterile water.
5 Remove the aspirating syringe and needle and pass the guidewire through the cannula well down into the trachea.
6 Remove the cannula leaving the guidewire *in situ*.
7 Pass the dilator over the guidewire to enter the trachea. Move the dilator up and down a few times to ensure a hole of sufficient size in the membrane. ▶ ▶ ▶

Hazards

- Care must be taken not to pierce the posterior aspect of the trachea with the cannula-over-needle. Confirmation of correct placement by aspiration of air is essential.
- The procedure takes some minutes to complete and is therefore less suitable for the asphyxiating patient *in extremis*.
- The procedure may be difficult in the gasping patient.

▶ ▶ ▶

8   Railroad a lubricated 6.0–6.5mm tube over the dilator into the trachea. Remove the dilator.
9   Inflate the tube cuff, attach to the ventilation equipment and check for correct placement.
10   Secure the tube with a tie or sutures.

Key points

- The surgical technique has proved to be the most reliable in the majority of hands.
- Blind cricothyrotomy using a prepacked kit requires practice and experience. The 4.0mm tube is only suitable for very short-term use as an emergency airway but can be used for several days if the upper airway is clear and the tube is merely being used for aspiration of secretions.
- The percutaneous dilatational method is relatively simple to perform but does take some minutes to complete.

Surgical and percutaneous tracheostomy

Indications

To provide:
- A reduction in dead space to facilitate weaning from a ventilator or for those with borderline respiratory function.
- A secure long-term airway for those with permanently absent protective laryngeal reflexes.
- A secure long-term airway for those requiring permanent or prolonged artificial ventilation.
- An airway in patients who require laryngectomy or who have long-term unrelievable upper airway obstruction.
- A secure airway temporarily after head and neck surgery.

Contra-indications

Absolute
The emergency situation with asphyxia or apnoea.
Patients in whom the indication is likely to be short-lived and alternative methods such as cricothyroidotomy or tracheal intubation would be suitable.
Local infection.

Relative
Coagulation defects.
Anatomical deformities.

SURGICAL TRACHEOSTOMY

Surgical tracheostomy is an operation which is not without hazard. There are effective alternatives for obtaining an airway in emergency conditions such as tracheal intubation or cricothyroidotomy. Therefore, surgical tracheostomy should not be contemplated as a procedure for the hurried relief of an obstructed airway. It is an operation which can be fraught with technical difficulty, particularly in the obese patient and in those with congested veins in the neck, arising from the futile and exaggerated respiratory efforts associated with asphyxia.

Nevertheless, tracheal intubation and cricothyroidotomy are but temporary measures to secure a bypass of the upper airway and if the indications for this continue for more than a week or two, surgical tracheostomy offers the most satisfactory long-term option.

The operation is usually performed in an operating room in patients whose airway has already been secured. Occasionally, surgical tracheostomy is performed in a critical care unit. It may be performed under local or general anaesthesia, according to the patient's individual circumstances.

Relevant anatomy

The trachea lies in the neck, normally in the midline. It is overlain by skin, fat, the platysma, the strap muscles of the neck, partly (covering the second to fourth rings of the trachea) by the isthmus of the thyroid gland, and finally by the pretracheal fascia (Fig. 2.48).

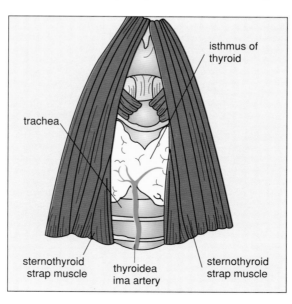

Fig. 2.48 The anatomy of the trachea

isthmus of thyroid

trachea

sternothyroid strap muscle

thyroidea ima artery

sternothyroid strap muscle

The strap muscles lie in two layers bordering either side of the trachea. The more superficial layer consists of the sternohyoid muscles and the deeper layer consists of sternothyroid muscles which run from the relevant cartilage to the back of the sternum and medial ends of the clavicles. Both sets of strap muscles can be parted in the midline and the thyroid isthmus can, in most patients, be retracted cephalad to reveal the second ring of the trachea and below. Rarely, the thyroidea ima artery runs from below arising from the aortic arch and supplying the thyroid isthmus. This vessel must be divided before cephalad retraction is possible.

Equipment

- ☐ Antiseptic solution.
- ☐ Sterile surgical drapes.
- ☐ 5ml and 20ml sterile syringes.
- ☐ 23G and 20G needles.
- ☐ Lignocaine 1% with 1:200,000 adrenaline.
- ☐ Scalpel with no.15 blades.
- ☐ Haemostat forceps x10.
- ☐ Retractors, e.g. Langenbeck and self-retaining.
- ☐ Scissors.
- ☐ Preferred sutures, ties and needle holder.
- ☐ Tracheal dilators.
- ☐ Cuffed tracheostomy tubes sizes 7.0, 7.5, 8.0 and 8.5mm diameter with obturator.
- ☐ Lubricating jelly.
- ☐ 20ml syringe to inflate tube cuff.
- ☐ Tape to secure tracheostomy tube.
- ☐ Catheter mount to connect to ventilator system.

Check that the tube sizes are correct, that the obturator can be easily removed from the tube, the cuffs on the tubes are intact and the connections fit the ventilating system.

Technique

Fully extend the patient's neck by placing a rolled towel or sandbag under the shoulders. Ask an assistant to help with the operation.

1 Don sterile gown and gloves.
2 Clean the neck and upper chest with antiseptic solution and apply drapes to the area.
3 If local anaesthesia is to be used, infiltrate the skin and underlying tissues in front of the trachea with local anaesthetic solution.
4 Make a 5cm transverse skin incision, 2cm above the sternal notch extending the incision through the platysma to expose the strap muscles. Identify and tie the anterior jugular veins. ► ► ►

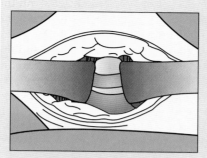

Fig. 2.49 Separation of the strap muscles

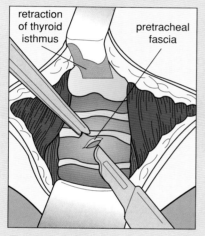

Fig. 2.50 Exposure of the pretracheal fascia

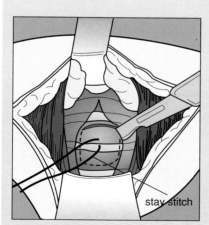

Fig. 2.51 Excision of a window to form the tracheostomy

▶ ▶ ▶

5   Incise the fascia joining the strap muscles in the midline and separate the muscles to either side of the trachea holding them apart with a self-retaining retractor (Fig. 2.49).

6   Retract the thyroid isthmus in a cephalad direction securing any bleeding points which may arise. In many patients the isthmus of the thyroid will need to be divided and transfixed to gain access to the upper part of the trachea.

7   Incise and dissect away the pretracheal fascia overlying the second and third tracheal rings (Fig. 2.50). Ensure haemostasis.

8   Warn the anaesthetist that an incision is about to be made in the trachea so that he may begin to withdraw the endotracheal tube.

9   Pass a stay stitch through the lower border of the second ring.

10 Cut a circular window on the front of the trachea through the second and third rings (Fig. 2.51). Some surgeons prefer to create an inverted U shaped flap sewing the lower edge to the skin to allow for easier tube changing. Others believe that this procedure is associated with delayed healing when the tracheostomy is eventually closed.

11 Remove the window by pulling gently on the stay stitch.

12 Ask the anaesthetist to withdraw the endotracheal tube sufficiently to admit the tracheostomy tube as it is passed through the window into the tracheal lumen (Fig. 2.52).

13 Remove the obturator, inflate the cuff to obtain an airtight seal, attach the catheter mount to the tracheostomy tube and pass the other end to the anaesthetist to connect to the ventilation system.

14 Aspirate the trachea to clear away any blood or secretions.

15 Secure the tracheostomy tube in place with a tape.

16 Place two skin sutures in the incision on either side of the tube. Ensure that the wound is sufficiently open to prevent surgical emphysema developing in case of an air leak occurring around the tracheostome.

17 Apply a dry dressing.

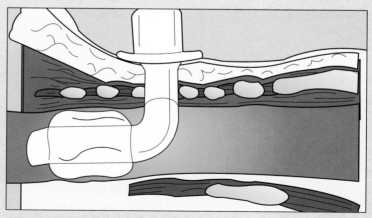

Fig. 2.52 The tracheostomy tube in place

Hazards

- Haemorrhage during dissection to expose the trachea.
- Poor visual access to the trachea in the obese patients.
- Failure to intubate the trachea associated with premature withdrawal of the endotracheal tube through the vocal cords.
- Contamination of the airway by blood.
- Displaced tracheostomy tube.

Indications

The indications for percutaneous tracheostomy are the same as for the surgical technique with the exception of those patients undergoing laryngectomy.

Contra-indications

As for the surgical approach plus:
- Whenever the cricoid cartilage is impalpable.
- Patients with an enlarged thyroid gland.
- Children.
- Anatomically difficult patients.

Key points

- Ensure that all equipment is satisfactory and compatible before beginning.
- Do not incise the first tracheal ring as this may lead to tracheal stenosis after the tracheostome has closed.
- A vertical incision rather than a window is mandatory in small children. Tracheal dilators are required to assist with the tube insertion.
- Make sure that the anaesthetist does not withdraw the endotracheal tube through the vocal cords until the tracheostomy tube is correctly in place.

PERCUTANEOUS DILATATIONAL TRACHEOSTOMY

Percutaneous dilatational tracheostomy was described first by Ciaglia in 1985. The potential advantages over formal surgical tracheostomy are that the percutaneous technique results in the smallest possible stoma and reduced bleeding, and can be performed by non-surgeons on the critical care unit. Thus, there is no need to arrange for a full theatre team or to transport the patient to the operating theatre. A prepacked kit is used to place a standard tracheostomy tube of up to 9.0mm ID.

Equipment

- ☐ Ciaglia percutaneous dilatational tracheostomy set.
- ☐ Indelible skin marker.
- ☐ 4 packets of gauze swabs.
- ☐ Suction apparatus.
- ☐ Antiseptic solution.
- ☐ Scalpel with no. 23 blade.
- ☐ Artery forceps x3.
- ☐ 5ml, 10ml and 20ml syringes.
- ☐ 23G and 25G needles.
- ☐ 20ml 1% lignocaine with 1:200,000 adrenaline.
- ☐ Small diathermy (e.g. battery powered disposable).
- ☐ Lubricating jelly.
- ☐ Silicone lubricant.
- ☐ Tracheostomy tube (8.0mm ID in most cases).
- ☐ Tracheostomy tube tie.
- ☐ Suitable dressing and sutures.
- ☐ Reserve endotracheal intubation set.
- ☐ Reserve surgical tracheostomy set.

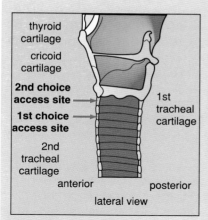

Fig. 2.53 Access site for percutaneous dilatational tracheostomy

Technique

Position the patient supine. Place a pillow under the shoulders and extend the head and neck. An anaesthetist should attend to the ventilator and endotracheal tube throughout the procedure. The endotracheal tube should be withdrawn until the top of the cuff is across the cords. Some adjustment may need to be made to the ventilator to maintain adequate tidal volumes.

It is helpful to have a second person scrubbed. This person can support the guidewire and, with a gauze swab, control the leak from the hole during change of the dilator.

The recommended access site is between the first and second tracheal rings. Alternatively, the space between the cricoid and first tracheal rings can be used. Identify the cricoid cartilage (Fig. 2.53) and mark the skin. Do not proceed if the cricoid cartilage cannot be identified clearly. Arrange the contents of the percutaneous tracheostomy set (Fig. 2.54) on a trolley. An 8.0mm ID tracheostomy tube is adequate for most adult patients and this should fit over the 24FG dilator.

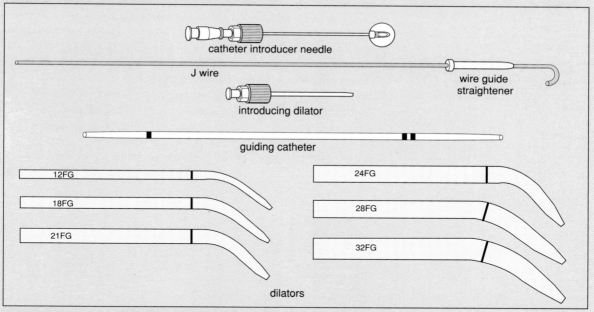

Fig. 2.54 Ciaglia percutaneous tracheostomy introducer set

1 Clean the anterior neck with antiseptic solution and drape the area.
2 Infiltrate the skin and subcutaneous tissues over the upper trachea and cricoid cartilage with 1% lignocaine and adrenaline. Additionally, soak a swab with some of this solution. ▶ ▶ ▶

▶ ▶ ▶

3 Make a 1.5cm vertical incision through the skin from the lower edge of the cricoid downwards and strictly in the midline. Some clinicians prefer a horizontal incision. This may make definition of the midline clearer, but the risk of bleeding is slightly higher.

4 Using an artery clip, gently dissect down between the strap muscles until the cricoid cartilage and first and second tracheal ring can be palpated clearly. Be particularly careful to avoid veins which may cross the midline. Stop minor bleeding by applying pressure with the swab soaked in lignocaine and adrenaline or use the portable diathermy. Apply an artery clip and tie obvious bleeding vessels.

5 Mount the catheter introducer needle and sheath on a 10ml syringe containing 3ml 1% lignocaine and 1:200,000 adrenaline. While gently aspirating, insert this between the first and second tracheal ring, aiming caudad (Fig. 2.55). Once air is aspirated into the syringe (indicating entry into the trachea), inject the lignocaine and, in a caudad direction, slide the sheath off the needle and into the trachea.

6 Ask the anaesthetist looking after the airway to gently move the endotracheal tube. If the sheath moves, it has impaled the endotracheal tube. In this event, remove the sheath, withdraw the endotracheal tube 1cm, and reintroduce the needle and sheath into the trachea.

7 Insert the J wire through the sheath and feed 5–8 cm into the trachea.

8 Remove the sheath, leaving the wire in the trachea (Fig. 2.56).

9 Advance the introducing dilator over the wire and into the access site. Remove the dilator, leaving the wire in position.

10 Advance the translucent guiding catheter over the wire and into the trachea (Fig. 2.57). The two positioning marks (to be aligned at skin level) are toward the leading or distal end. In more recent kits, the guiding catheter is shouldered at the position of the skin marker. Align the proximal end of the guiding catheter with the solder mark on the wire.

▶ ▶ ▶

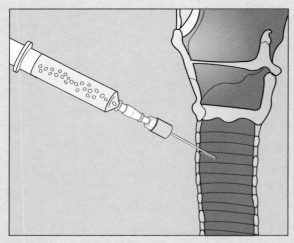

Fig. 2.55 Aspiration of air into syringe confirms entry into the trachea

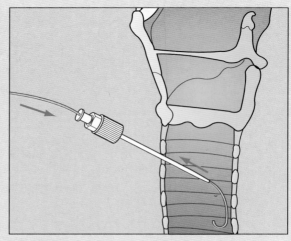

Fig. 2.56 Remove the sheath, leaving the 'J' wire in the trachea

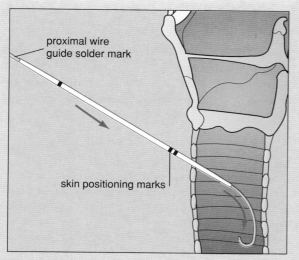

Fig. 2.57 The correct position of the guiding catheter on the wire

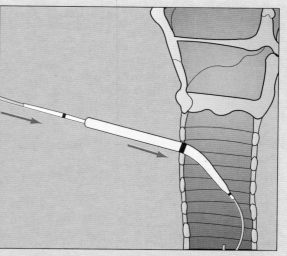

Fig. 2.58 Dilate the access site by advancing the dilator, wire and guiding catheter as a single unit

▶ ▶ ▶

11 Place the smallest dilator (12FG) over the guiding catheter and wire and dilate the access site. Align the proximal end of the dilator with the single mark on the guiding catheter. Advance the dilator, guiding catheter and wire as a single unit into the trachea, as far as the skin level mark on the blue dilator (Fig. 2.58). Advance and pull back the dilating assembly several times.

12 Exchange the dilator for the next largest size and repeat step 11 for each dilator.

13 While exchanging dilators, ask an assistant to hold a swab over the hole. This will reduce the loss of tidal volume.

14 Having dilated with the bougie that introduces the tracheostomy tube, lubricate the dilator with lubricating jelly or silicone spray and mount the tracheostomy tube with the balloon fully deflated. This will minimise the time between removing the last dilator (when the leak will be large) and locating the tracheostomy tube. Position the tracheostomy tube onto the dilator so that its tip is approximately 2cm back from the tip of the dilator.

15 If inserting a 8.0mm or 9.0mm tracheostomy tube, dilate the access site with the largest dilator (32FG).

16 Advance the preloaded tracheostomy tube into the trachea (Fig. 2.59). Remove the dilator, guiding catheter, and wire. Inflate the cuff and connect the catheter mount and ventilator. Confirm adequate ventilation.

17 Place a dressing on the site and secure the tracheostomy tube with tapes.

18 Arrange for a check chest X-ray.

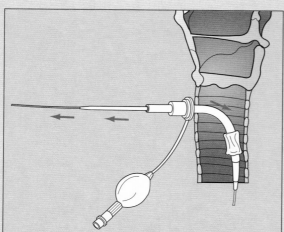

Fig. 2.59 Advance the preloaded tracheostomy tube into the trachea

Hazards

- Profuse bleeding may result if this procedure is undertaken in patients with an enlarged thyroid gland.

Complications

Significant bleeding is rare, but if it occurs it may require attention by a surgeon with possible conversion to an open tracheostomy. It is possible to misplace the tube, particularly if the cricoid is not identified clearly. The posterior tracheal wall can be penetrated with the needle, sheath, J wire or dilators.

Key points

- Do not proceed if the cricoid cartilage cannot be identified clearly.
- Control minor bleeding with a swab soaked in 1:200,000 adrenaline.
- Be careful not to get lubricant jelly on the dilators (except when loading the tracheostomy tube) or on your hands.
- There are few, if any, indications to use a tracheostomy tube larger than 8.0mm ID.
- In patients with short necks, it may be preferable to use the space between the cricoid and the first tracheal rings.

Basic ventilation techniques

This chapter will cover basic ventilation techniques ranging from expired air methods to the use of the self-inflating bag/valve device and automatic resuscitators.

EXPIRED AIR RESPIRATION

Expired air respiration (EAR) can be provided by the direct mouth-to-mouth (Fig. 2.60), mouth-to-nose (Fig. 2.61) and mouth-to-mouth-and-nose in infants (Fig. 2.62) methods. The mouth-to-mouth method is recommended for adults by the majority of authorities.

Alternatively, a protective device such as a mask, tube airway or foil may be interposed between the patient and the rescuer to avoid direct contact. With some protective devices, a nipple is fitted to allow for oxygen enrichment of the inspired air.

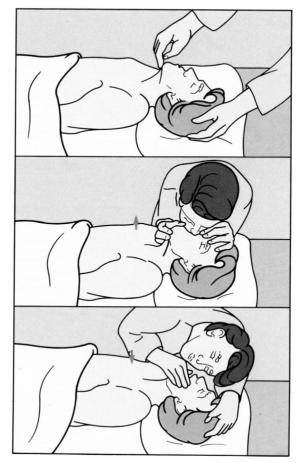

Fig. 2.60 The mouth-to-mouth method for EAR

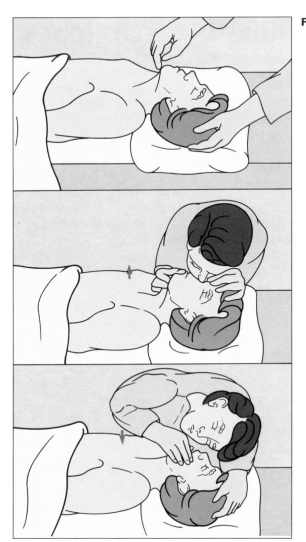

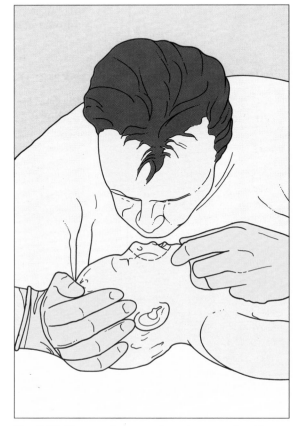

Fig. 2.61 The mouth-to-nose method for EAR

Fig. 2.62 The mouth-to-mouth-and-nose method for EAR

'Naked' EAR carries with it the advantage that no equipment whatsoever is required and so artificial ventilation can be carried out immediately anywhere provided there is a respirable atmosphere.

However, there are aesthetic drawbacks to the direct methods, and there is also a fear of cross infection between the patient and rescuer which is not currently justified by scientific data.

Rates, volumes, flow rates and pressures with EAR

Respiratory rates should equate to normal physiological values related to the patient's age and weight. A rate of 10–12 breaths/min is recommended for adults, 20 breaths/min for children over 1 year and 25–30 breaths/min for infants under one year.

Tidal volumes should be slightly greater than normal, values ranging from 25–50ml in infants, up to 800ml in adults.

Inspiratory flow rates should mimic normal values of 20–30 litres/min in adults. Inspiration should take 1.5–2.0 seconds with twice that time for exhalation.

Excessive inflation pressures can occur with high flow rates, large tidal volumes and respiratory rates which do not allow enough time for complete exhalation. Excessive inflation pressures (>20cmH$_2$O) are associated with gastric distension, regurgitation and pulmonary aspiration and pneumothorax, particularly in paediatric patients.

Cricoid pressure (see p. 95) should be applied by an assistant during EAR to minimise the risk of regurgitation.

Direct methods of EAR

Indications

An apnoeic patient without serious maxillofacial injury in a situation where no equipment is immediately available.

Contra-indications

A major maxillofacial injury producing facial distortion and serious intra-oral haemorrhage.
Obvious mortal injury.
Patient's express wish not to be resuscitated is known to the rescuer.

Technique

The mouth-to-mouth method

1 The patient is placed supine with the head and neck aligned in the clear airway position. The airway is cleared of any foreign material.
2 The rescuer kneels at one side of the patient's head.
3 The nostrils are pinched closed with the finger and thumb of one hand. The heel of that hand produces downward pressure on the forehead to maintain correct head and neck alignment.
4 The other hand supports the chin holding the mouth 1cm open.
5 The rescuer inhales deeply, opens his own mouth widely and seals it over the patient's mouth and blows until the patient's chest rises as with a normal breath.
6 If inflation is difficult, tilt the head further back and check that the airway is not obstructed by foreign material and try again.
7 Once inflation has occurred, the rescuer removes his mouth allowing complete passive exhalation to occur.
8 The process is repeated at a rate of 10–12 times per minute in adults.

The mouth-to-nose method

1 The patient and rescuer are placed as for the mouth-to-mouth method.
2 The rescuer maintains head tilt by downward pressure on the patient's forehead with one hand and seals the patient's lips with the thumb of the other hand which is supporting the chin.
3 Inflation of the patient's lungs is provided by the rescuer forming a seal with his lips around the patient's nostrils and blowing until normal inspiratory chest expansion is achieved.
4 Passive exhalation is assisted by opening the patient's mouth in case there is a degree of nasal obstruction.

The mouth-to-mouth-and-nose method

This method is used in resuscitation of infants and small children.

1 The patient and rescuer are positioned as before. The relatively large infant's head should be placed in the neutral rather than extended position.
2 The rescuer applies his mouth over the infant's mouth and nose and blows to achieve normal chest expansion for that child.
3 The process should be repeated 20–30 times per minute.

Hazards

- In patients with suspected cervical spine injury only the minimum head extension and neck movement required to achieve a clear airway should be applied.

Key points

- Direct EAR has saved many lives and health care professionals faced with an apnoeic patient in a situation without immediate access to equipment should not hesitate to apply it.
- The concentration of inspired oxygen can be increased (if oxygen and tubing are available) by placing the end of the tube in the rescuer's mouth and turning on the oxygen at a flow rate of 3–5 litres/min.

EXPIRED AIR RESPIRATION USING SIMPLE PROTECTIVE APPLIANCES

Simple inexpensive protective devices are available which are designed to prevent direct contact between patient and rescuer during EAR. These devices are of three types:
- The mask type.
- The tube/flange type.
- The foil type.

Their use has a number of advantages:
- They avoid aesthetic concern about direct patient/rescuer contact especially in the presence of blood, vomit or nasal secretions.
- They may reduce the possibility of cross infection.
- With certain models oxygen can be added.
- With certain types airway patency may be improved by an oropharyngeal tube extension.

The mask type

This device consists of a moulded face mask similar to that used in anaesthesia. Better models incorporate a unidirectional valve which diverts the patient's expired air away from the rescuer and traps any macroscopic particles emerging from the patient. It is unlikely that this valve acts as an effective barrier to airborne bacteria and viruses.

Technique

This technique is shown in Fig. 2.63.

1 Place the patient supine with head and neck aligned in the clear airway position.
2 Apply the mask to the face to cover the patient's mouth and nose.
3 Using both hands, apply bilateral jaw thrust with the fingers and press the mask tightly onto the face with the outstretched thumbs and thenar eminences.
4 Blow into the port of the mask to inflate the patient's chest as in the mouth-to-mouth method.
5 Some adjustment of the mask and hand position may be necessary to prevent leaks at the mask/patient interface. ► ► ►

▶ ▶ ▶

6 If an oxygen nipple is fitted, give oxygen at 8 litres/min to increase the FIO$_2$

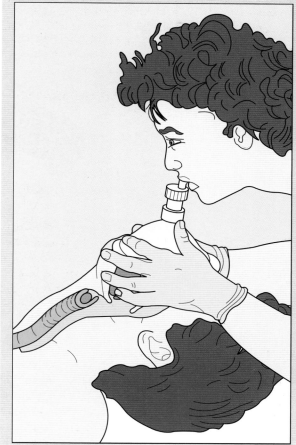

Fig. 2.63 EAR using the mouth to mask technique

The tube/flange type

This device consists of a flange to seal the lips and a tube resembling a short oropharyngeal airway. Certain models incorporate an unidirectional valve and some have a nose clip provided.

Technique

This technique is shown in Fig. 2.64.

1 Place the patient supine with the head and neck aligned in the clear airway position.

2 Introduce the distal end of the tube into the mouth taking care not to displace the patient's tongue backwards. ▶ ▶ ▶

▶ ▶ ▶

3 Apply the flange firmly to the face around the patient's mouth using both hands to provide jaw thrust and maintain an airtight seal between the patient's face and the flange.
4 Occlude the nostrils by the tip of the thumbs or by a nose clip.
5 Inflate the patient's lungs by blowing into the proximal end of the tube as in the mouth-to-mouth method.
6 The patient's expired air is diverted away from the rescuer, through a unidirectional valve.

Hazards

- Damage may occur to the teeth or lips during insertion of the tube.
- It may be difficult to achieve an airtight seal between the flange and the patient's face.
- Introduction of the tube into the patient's mouth may induce retching and vomiting.
- The rescuer may experience damage to his own mouth and teeth during a bumpy ride in ambulance or helicopter.
- Certain devices have a relatively high resistance to airflow.

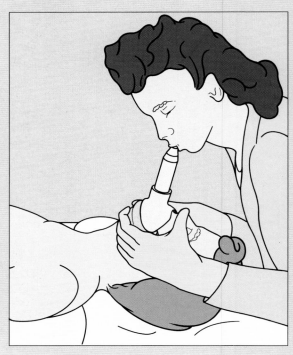

Fig. 2.64 EAR using the mouth to tube/flange airway

The foil types

The foil types consist of a small area of plastic film which can be applied to the oronasal region. An orifice with a one way valve or textile filter is provided to be aligned with the patient's mouth. These devices are very inexpensive, compact and lightweight and are designed for use by members of the public.

Technique

The technique is shown in Fig. 2.65.

1 Place the patient supine with head and neck aligned in the clear airway position.
2 Place the foil over the patient's mouth and nose locating the orifice over the mouth. ▶ ▶ ▶

▶ ▶ ▶

Hazards

- On occasion the foil may tear due to contact with the patient's or rescuer's teeth.

3 Stand or kneel at the side of the patient's head as with the mouth-to-mouth method.
4 Use fingers and thumbs to apply chin lift, occlude the nostrils and seal the foil to the face.
5 Inflate the patient's lungs by blowing over the valve or filtered orifice as with the mouth-to-mouth method.
6 Some adjustment of the hand position may be required to provide an effective seal between the foil and the face.

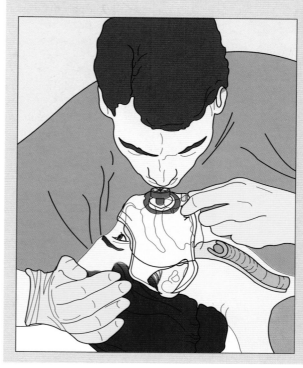

Fig. 2.65 EAR using a foil device

THE SELF-INFLATING BAG/VALVE DEVICE

The self-inflating bag/valve device is capable of inflating the patient's lungs with air or an air–oxygen mixture entrained through an inlet valve. Inflation of the lungs occurs through the patient valve when the bag is compressed and the patient's exhaled air is directed to the atmosphere during the relaxation and bag re-expansion phase.

The bag may be used with a face mask or may be attached to any standard 15mm connector on an endotracheal tube, laryngeal mask, etc. Use of the bag and mask by a single operator requires a particular skill to achieve airway alignment and a seal between the mask and the patient's face with one hand. Many authorities advocate using two rescuers (if available) – one using both hands to align the airway and apply the mask to the face and one to squeeze the bag.

Oxygen enrichment is best provided using a reservoir bag attached to the inflating bag. Inspired oxygen concentrations of 90% are possible with flow rates of 8–10 litres/min using this system. The addition of oxygen

Indications

Apnoeic patient.

Contra-indications

None other than lack of skill in the technique.

through a nipple directly attached to the inflating bag without a reservoir is much less efficient as the high flow rates necessary to achieve a high FIO_2 (25 litres/min) jam the patient valve in the inspiratory mode.

Technique

This technique is shown in Fig. 2.66.

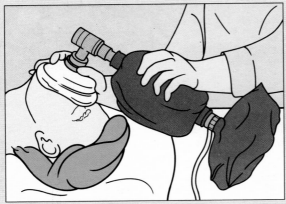

Fig. 2.66 Artificial ventilation using a self-inflating bag/valve mask (single rescuer)

1 Place the patient supine with the head and neck aligned in the correct airway position.
2 Apply the mask firmly to the patient's face using the thumb and forefinger to form a collar around the mask near the port attached to the patient valve.
3 The other fingers support the jaw to maintain a clear airway.
4 The airtight seal is achieved by opposing the thumb and forefinger towards the other fingers.
5 Compression of the bag with the other hand inflates the patient's lungs.
6 Greater inflation volumes may be achieved using the open palm method and compressing the bag against a part of the rescuer's anatomy, e.g. thigh or chest (Fig. 2.67).
7 Positive end expiratory pressure may be applied using a special patient valve and a filter may be attached to the inlet valve for use when the atmospheric air is contaminated by noxious gases.

Hazards

- The technique is not easy to acquire and requires continued practice to maintain a patent airway and an airtight seal between the mask and the face throughout.
- An inadequate seal results in hypoventilation.
- High inspiratory flow rates or volumes, particularly in the presence of an imperfectly aligned airway, result in gastric inflation and regurgitation and pulmonary aspiration. Cricoid pressure (see p. 95) by an assistant reduces the chances of this occurring.
- The valves should be easy to take apart for cleaning. Incorrect assembly should be impossible.

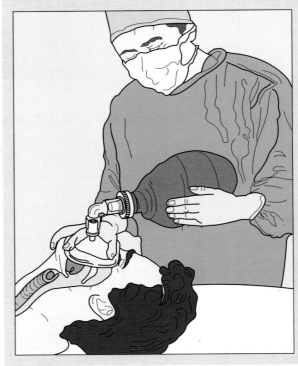

Fig. 2.67 Use of the open palm method for compression of the self-inflating bag

Key points

- Use of the self-inflating bag with a mask should be confined to those expert and experienced in its use. Others will achieve better artificial ventilation by using the mouth-to-mask method with oxygen enrichment (see p. 129).
- As soon as an endotracheal tube or laryngeal mask or other sophisticated airway has been introduced, the self inflating bag/valve with oxygen reservoir should be attached.

MANUALLY-TRIGGERED OXYGEN POWERED RESUSCITATORS

These devices are powered by a high pressure (300–400 kPa) oxygen source. Triggering of the inspiratory and expiratory phase is done by manually compressing and releasing a lever or button at the patient valve which is attached to a face mask, endotracheal tube or laryngeal mask.

Both hands are free to ensure an airtight fit between the mask and the face and control airway alignment.

Some models have a triggering device to provide assisted ventilation in time with the patient's own respiratory efforts.

Indications

As for the self-inflating bag/valve device.

Contra-indications

As for the self-inflating bag/valve device.

Hazards

- Lack of direct contact ('feel') during the inspiratory phase may lead to gastric inflation and regurgitation in an airway which is slightly less than perfectly controlled.
- The equipment should be designed to restrict the inspiratory flow rates to less than 40litres/min and a blow-off valve with audible warning should operate if the inflation pressure reaches 60cmH$_2$O in adults.

Technique

Use of the device with a face mask is shown in Fig. 2.68.

1 Place the patient supine, with the head and neck aligned in the clear airway position.
2 Turn on the oxygen supply.
3 Using both hands, apply the mask over the mouth and nose to form an airtight seal as with mouth-to-mask EAR (see p. 129).
4 Inflate the chest by depressing the lever or button trigger on the patient valve.
5 Release the trigger to allow passive exhalation.
6 Continue to ensure airway patency on a breath by breath basis.

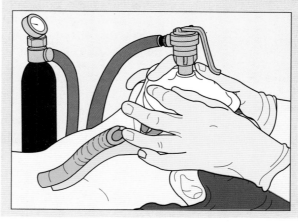

Fig. 2.68 Use of a manually triggered oxygen powered device with a mask

AUTOMATIC RESUSCITATORS

These devices are small portable ventilators powered by a high pressure (300–400 kPa) oxygen source. They cycle between inspiration and expiration using a fluid logic arrangement or by electronic control. Cycling should be triggered by volume, not pressure.

The versatility of control of the inspiratory and expiratory phase varies from model to model. Some models have the facility to ventilate with an air/oxygen mixture and/or a demand valve triggered by the patient's inspiratory efforts.

They can be used with a face mask or may be attached to an endotracheal tube, laryngeal mask or other sophisticated airway adjunct.

Indications

As for the self-inflating bag valve device.

Contra-indications

As for the self-inflating bag/valve device.

Technique

The technique for an automatic resuscitator used with a mask is shown in Fig. 2.69.

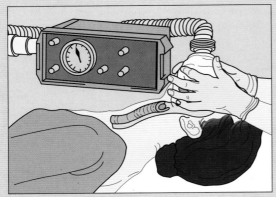

1 Place the patient supine with the head and neck aligned in the clear airway position.
2 Turn on the oxygen supply.
3 Apply the mask to the mouth and nose to form an airtight seal as with mouth-to-mask ventilation (see p. 129).
4 Adjust the controls for tidal volumes and respiratory rate to achieve normal chest expansion at a suitable rate. Some models have additional controls to adjust the inspiratory and expiratory times and flow rates and to introduce a triggering mode.
5 Adjust the air–oxygen mixture as appropriate (generally 100% oxygen or 60% oxygen).
6 Ensure airway patency with each breath.
7 As soon as possible, connect the device to an endotracheal tube or laryngeal mask.

Fig. 2.69 Use of an automatic resuscitator with a mask

Hazards

- As with manual triggered devices, there is a loss of 'feel' during inflation with the attendant danger of gastric inflation and regurgitation. However, experience with models which have a low inspiratory flow rate and a blow-off valve with audible warning, has shown that the danger of gastric inflation is less than with the self-inflating bag or mouth-to-mask method.

Key points

- Automatic resuscitators provide consistent automatic ventilation at the preset tidal volume, rate, and respiratory pattern. Manual methods are, perforce, subject to continual variation. Once the automatic resuscitator is connected to an endotracheal tube, the rescuer is free to undertake other tasks, e.g. venous cannulation.

Ventilatory modes

Patients undergoing general anaesthesia or being managed in critical care units will often require some ventilatory assistance. This ranges from a small level of support in the spontaneously breathing patient who has poorly compliant lungs, to full mechanical ventilation in the paralysed and heavily sedated patient. As ventilator technology has progressed, new and often more complex modes of ventilation have been developed. Using the equipment available, and in the light of current knowledge, the clinician must attempt to select the safest and most appropriate mode of ventilation for any given patient.

Although mechanical ventilation often produces improvement in oxygenation and carbon dioxide removal, it has a number of adverse effects. The increase in intrathoracic pressure can have potentially adverse effects on the lungs and on the cardiovascular system. High airway pressures, particularly when transmitted to the distal airways, can cause alveolar hyperinflation and subsequent disruption. The high intrathoracic pressure will impede venous return and compromise cardiac output. The net result may be a fall in tissue oxygen delivery despite an increase in red cell oxygen content. Recent trends in ventilatory techniques have emphasised the importance of reducing distal airway pressure by encouraging the patient to maintain some spontaneous respiratory effort while gaining a degree of assistance from the ventilator. Keeping the alveoli open and eliminating large swings in alveolar pressure may reduce shear forces, thus limiting parenchymal damage.

CONTINUOUS POSITIVE AIRWAY PRESSURE (CPAP)

CPAP raises the baseline airway pressure of the spontaneously breathing patient (Fig. 2.70a) and can be provided through a tight-fitting face mask or endotracheal tube. The increase in expiratory pressure provided by CPAP increases end expiratory lung volume and recruits collapsed alveoli. The improved ventilation–perfusion matching increases oxygenation. Tidal ventilation is moved up to a more advantageous part of the respiratory system's compliance curve and, when using an efficient CPAP circuit, this should reduce work of breathing.

Originally, CPAP was provided by continuous flow systems. As a result of the high gas flows, these systems are very noisy, but they do provide a stable airway pressure. Modern ventilators provide CPAP by means of a demand valve. There tends to be some delay in the opening of even the most sensitive of these valves, and this results in a short phase of zero flow and a momentary drop in airway pressure. However, ventilators permit better monitoring of the respiratory system during CPAP.

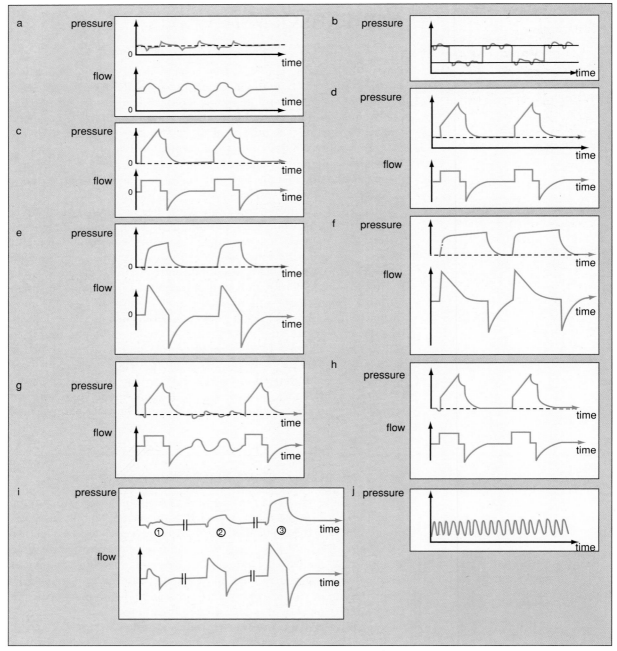

Fig. 2.70 a Pressure and flow curves for continuous positive airway pressure (CPAP). **b** Pressure curve for airway pressure release ventilation. **c** Pressure and flow curves for controlled mechanical ventilation. **d** Pressure and flow curves for positive end expiratory pressure. **e** Pressure and flow curves for pressure-controlled ventilation.

f Pressure and flow curves for inverse ratio ventilation. **g** Pressure and flow curves for synchronised intermittent mandatory ventilation. **h** Pressure and flow curves for assist-controlled ventilation. **i** Pressure and flow curves for pressure support ventilation. **j** Pressure curve for high-frequency ventilation

Indications

Hypoxaemia in the presence of adequate ventilatory drive:
• Atelectasis e.g. post-operative.
• Adult respiratory distress syndrome (ARDS).
• Pulmonary oedema.
• Thoracic trauma.

Contra-indications

Lack of patient co-operation.
Inadequate ventilatory drive (retaining carbon dioxide).
Mask CPAP contra-indicated:
• Immediately after gastric and pulmonary surgery (distension may rupture suture lines).
• Basal skull fractures (risk of pneumocephalus).

Equipment

☐ Ventilator with facility for CPAP or continuous flow CPAP system with valve and with or without a reservoir bag.
☐ Face mask with restraining strap, or endotracheal tube.
☐ Pulse oximeter.
☐ Facilities for blood gas analysis.

Technique

Before connecting a conscious patient to a CPAP system, provide an explanation of what you plan to do. The tight-fitting mask makes CPAP very uncomfortable and it requires considerable patient co-operation. If possible, place the patient in a sitting position; this will improve functional residual capacity. Review the patient's chest radiograph and make certain there is no pneumothorax. CPAP is likely to convert a simple pneumothorax into a life-threatening, tension pneumothorax.

1 Check the patient's blood gases before attaching the CPAP system and attach a pulse oximeter probe to the patient's finger.
2 If using some form of continuous flow system, assemble the components (as in Fig. 2.71) and add a bacterial filter to prevent contamination of the system and a CPAP valve. The valve can be an adjustable pressure device or one of a number of fixed pressure valves (e.g. 5, 10, 15, and 20cmH$_2$O). If the patient has not been receiving any form of respiratory assistance, start with a 5cmH$_2$O valve. If the patient is being weaned from mechanical ventilation, set the valve to the same level as any PEEP already being used.
3 Turn on the gas supply (oxygen–air mix) and select an appropriate FIO$_2$. Depending whether or not a reservoir is present, fresh gas flows will need to be of the order of 60 litres/min. Check the manufacturer's instructions to confirm the gas flow requirement of the particular system. If using a ventilator, turn the selector knob to the CPAP position and select an appropriate CPAP pressure.
4 In the unintubated patient, apply the mask to the patient's face, pass the straps around the back of the head and attach them to the mask. The mask must be applied tightly and must make a good seal with the face.
5 Attach the tubing from the CPAP system or ventilator to the mask, or to the catheter mount of the endotracheal tube.
6 Carefully observe the patient's ventilatory effort and note the respiratory rate. After approximately 30 minutes repeat these observations and check the blood gases. Aim for an arterial oxygen saturation of at least 90%, while keeping the FIO$_2$ below 0.6.

▶ ▶ ▶

Attain this goal by adjusting the level of CPAP in increments of 5cmH$_2$O, while repeating the respiratory observations. Find the level of CPAP at which the patient is most comfortable, as this is likely to represent the optimum position of the respiratory system's compliance curve. Use the pulse oximeter for continuous monitoring of arterial oxygen saturation.

7 As the patient's condition improves reduce the level of CPAP, while monitoring all the observations above.

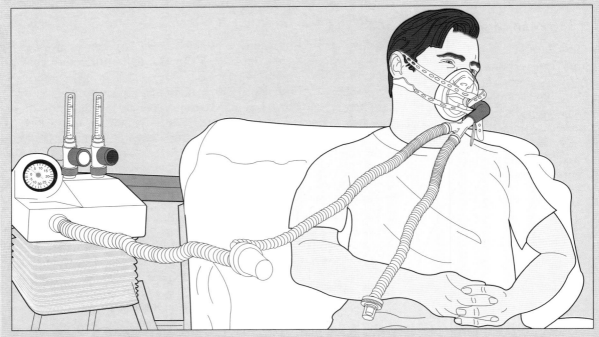

Fig. 2.71 Patient breathing through a mask CPAP system

Hazards

- In the presence of rib fractures, CPAP will increase the risk of pneumothorax, therefore consider prophylactic placement of a chest drainage tube.
- The demand–flow mechanism on many ventilators, particularly some of the older models, is very inefficient, increasing considerably the work of breathing in the CPAP mode.

Complications

- If the level of CPAP is inappropriately high, alveolar over-distension will increase the work of breathing.
- Excessive CPAP will reduce venous return and cardiac output, and can cause barotrauma in the form of pneumothorax and pneumomediastinum.
- Mask CPAP can cause significant gastric distension with the accompanying risk of regurgitation and aspiration. Few patients will tolerate very prolonged periods of mask CPAP and removal of the mask results in episodes of hypoxia.

AIRWAY PRESSURE RELEASE VENTILATION

While CPAP will often improve oxygenation, in patients with respiratory muscle weakness or ventilatory failure from other causes, carbon dioxide retention will force the clinician to find another mode of ventilatory support. Airway pressure release ventilation (APRV) has been designed especially for patients suffering from both lung failure and ventilatory pump failure. The main benefits of APRV are reduced mean airway pressure and peak inflation pressure. One form of APRV, known as BIPAP, comprises a CPAP system with an additional APRV valve placed in the respiratory limb, which drops the airway pressure intermittently. The pressure can be dropped either to ambient levels or to a second level of CPAP (Fig. 2.70b). The release of pressure allows lung volume to decrease and in so doing, clear CO_2. As soon as the APRV valve is closed, CPAP returns rapidly to its higher level. The two pressure levels and the frequency and duty cycles of the APRV valve can be altered to suit individual patients. As originally described, by setting an appropriate frequency of pressure release, APRV can provide the entire alveolar ventilation in the patient making no spontaneous respiratory effort. Until recently, APRV has been regarded as an experimental technique, but there are now available a number of ventilators equipped with some form of APRV mode.

Indications

Similar to those for CPAP plus:
• Moderate ARDS.
• Ventilatory failure.

Contra-indications

Similar to CPAP, with the exception of ventilatory failure.

Technique

• The technique for setting up APRV will vary greatly between specific systems. Follow manufacturers instructions, while applying the same monitoring principles as for CPAP.

CONTROLLED MECHANICAL VENTILATION

In many ways standard controlled mechanical ventilation (CMV) is the most unsophisticated of today's ventilatory modes. It was developed in the 1950s and can be considered the prototype of positive pressure ventilation. CMV involves delivery of breaths at a preselected rate and volume, thus guaranteeing a set minute volume (Fig. 2.70c). In both the intensive care and operating theatre environments, a wide range of ventilators are available with a CMV mode. The main limitation of this mode is that it does not allow any contribution from the patient and it may be difficult to 'settle' the patient without resorting to deep sedation and paralysis. However, when patients cannot or are not permitted to breath spontaneously, CMV is the mode of choice.

Indications

During general anaesthesia.
Drug overdose.
Other causes of respiratory muscle paralysis.
Head injury.

Contra-indications

There are no absolute contra-indications to CMV, but in many circumstances other modes of ventilation are more appropriate.

Equipment

☐ Appropriate mechanical ventilator.

Technique

Check the ventilator has an effective power and gas supply. To initiate CMV safely, the conscious patient must be first anaesthetised, and then is usually paralysed before intubation. A patient who is already unconscious, as a result of a head injury for example, may still benefit from an intravenous anaesthetic agent, in addition to neuromuscular blockade. Intubation techniques have been described elsewhere (p. 85). Once intubated, the patient is sedated with a respiratory depressant agent (opioid and often a benzodiazepine) which usually eliminates the need for continuous neuromuscular blockade.

1 Precise ventilator controls vary from one machine to the next, but in general select the following settings:
   - Tidal volume, 10–12ml/kg body weight.
   - Respiratory rate, 8–12 breaths/min.
   - FIO_2, 0.3–0.6.
   - I:E ratio, 1:2–1:3.
   - PEEP, zero.
   - Inspiratory waveform, square.
2 Connect the ventilator breathing system to the catheter mount of the patient's tracheal tube. After 15 minutes of ventilation, recheck the patient's blood gases or note the end-tidal CO_2 and SaO_2.
3 Aim for a $PaCO_2$, or end-tidal CO_2, of 35–40mmHg and an SaO_2 of at least 95%. If the $PaCO_2$ is low, reduce the respiratory rate and/or tidal volume. Increase these for hypercapnoea. If the SaO_2 is low, increase the FIO_2 or, if this is already >0.5, consider adding PEEP (see below).

Hazards

- If not properly monitored, patients can be grossly under- or over-ventilated during CMV.

Complications

- CMV may result in significant cardiovascular depression, particularly if peak airway pressures are high.
- If the patient attempts to breath spontaneously and 'fights' the ventilator, oxygenation may deteriorate while demand increases, and the accompanying pressure peaks may cause pulmonary barotrauma.

POSITIVE END EXPIRATORY PRESSURE (PEEP)

The effects of adding PEEP to the patient undergoing mechanical ventilation are much the same as the effects of CPAP in the spontaneously breathing patient. A pressure limiting valve is placed in the expiratory limb of the ventilator system so that expiratory flow is stopped before airway pressure falls to atmospheric (Fig. 2.70d). PEEP improves oxygenation by opening more alveoli and increasing functional residual capacity (FRC). Many clinicians add at least 5cmH$_2$O of PEEP to all ventilator systems in order to counteract the loss of physiologic PEEP (resulting from intubation and sedation). Others add PEEP only when an $FIO_2>0.5$ is required for adequate oxygenation. However, the potential adverse affects of PEEP must be taken into account.

Indications

ARDS.
Pneumonia.
Atelectasis during prolonged general anaesthesia.

Contra-indications

Bronchopleural fistula.
High PEEP contra-indicated in head-injured patients.
Uncorrected hypovolaemia (severe hypotension may result).

Technique

1 Check the patient's blood gases and if a pulmonary artery flotation catheter (PAFC) is *in situ*, calculate the oxygen delivery (DO_2).
2 Set the PEEP valve to 5cmH$_2$O and after 15 minutes recheck the blood gases and DO_2. Increase the PEEP in increments of 2.5cmH$_2$O, reassessing blood gases and, if possible, DO_2 after each change. 'Best PEEP' equates to that providing the highest DO_2. If not *in situ* initially, insert a PAFC if contemplating PEEP>15cmH$_2$O.

Complications

- Barotrauma (pulmonary hyper-inflation, pneumothorax).
- Cardiac output depression represents the major adverse effect of PEEP.

Any improvement in oxygenation is, to some extent, opposed by reduced venous return and stroke volume, with the result that DO_2 is not necessarily improved.

Indications

Moderate to severe ARDS.

Contra-indications

Lack of adequate respiratory monitoring (sudden reduction in compliance will drop the minute volume).

PRESSURE-CONTROLLED VENTILATION

The pressure-controlled ventilation (PCV) mode is now available on a number of ventilators designed for the critical care unit. Inspiratory pressure is limited to a level selected by the clinician, while inspiratory flow will vary with the resistance and compliance of the patient's respiratory system. Tidal volume depends on the inspiratory flow rate and inspiratory time. In the relaxed patient the decelerating flow pattern that occurs (Fig. 2.70e) results in a reduction of peak airway pressure. Mean airway pressure, however, is likely to be raised. Initially, PCV was used in conjunction with inverse I:E ratios and was reserved for severe acute lung injuries, but it is becoming increasingly popular as a first choice ventilation mode, and is often used with conventional I:E ratios.

Technique

1 Note the peak inspiratory pressure and tidal volume while in CMV mode. Set the pressure limit to 5cmH$_2$O below that value.
2 Select pressure-control mode on the ventilator. Select the appropriate breath rate. An I:E ratio of 1:1 or 1:2 will provide more time for an adequate tidal volume at any given pressure. ► ► ►

141

> ▶ ▶ ▶
> **3** Adjust the pressure limit to provide a tidal volume similar to that given during CMV. The peak airway pressure should be significantly lower than that during CMV.
> **4** After 15 minutes, recheck the blood gases and, if available, DO_2, and make appropriate adjustments.

Complications

- The higher mean airway pressure associated with PCV may reduce the cardiac output.
- Tidal volume and minute volume are not guaranteed, therefore careful respiratory monitoring must be used.

INVERSE RATIO VENTILATION

Inverse ratio ventilation (IRV) is defined by an I:E ratio greater than 1:1 and can be performed in conjunction with volume-controlled or pressure-controlled modes (Fig. 2.70f). I:E ratios as high as 4:1 have been used. The longer inspiratory time reduces peak airway pressures. The short expiratory time may not allow for complete lung deflation, and there may be a significant increase in end-expiratory alveolar pressure (so called auto-PEEP or intrinsic-PEEP) even when external PEEP is zero. This is the likely mechanism for any increase in oxygenation.

Indications Severe ARDS. **Contra-indications** Severe obstructive pulmonary disease (dangerous hyperinflation may occur).

> **Technique**
>
> **1** Make a baseline set of respiratory and cardiovascular observations at the current I:E ratio.
> **2** Increase the I:E ratio one notch on the control knob (e.g. from 1:2 to 1:1). Reduce the inspiratory flow to provide an appropriate tidal volume.
> **3** Recheck blood gases after 15 minutes.

Complications

- IRV is unphysiological and very uncomfortable for a conscious patient. Heavy sedation and often paralysis is required. Pulmonary hyperinflation may reduce cardiac output dramatically and cause pulmonary barotrauma.

INTERMITTENT MANDATORY VENTILATION (IMV) AND SYNCHRONISED IMV (SIMV)

IMV and SIMV assist the patient's ventilation while allowing a variable amount of spontaneous respiratory activity and were designed originally as weaning modes. In IMV mode, volume-controlled time-cycled

Indications

Any patient requiring mechanical ventilation.
To aid weaning from mechanical ventilation.

Contra-indications

Paralysed or apnoeic patients.

mechanical breaths are delivered according to a frequency selected by the clinician. Between mechanical breaths, the patient is free to breath spontaneously. IMV was refined with the development of SIMV which synchronised the mechanical breaths to the patient's spontaneous inspiratory effort and thereby eliminated inspiratory volume stacking which could occur if a mechanical breath was delivered at the end of a spontaneous inspiration (Fig. 2.70g). More recently, SIMV has become popular as a basic mode of ventilation in the critical care unit. In comparison with CMV, SIMV is associated with lower intrathoracic pressure, less barotrauma, and less adverse effects on cardiac output.

Technique

1 Obtain a baseline set of respiratory and cardiovascular observations.
2 Select the IMV or SIMV (preferable) mode on the ventilator. Set the tidal volume to 10–12ml/kg and start with a mandatory rate of 8 breaths/min. If available, set extrinsic PEEP to 5cmH$_2$O.
3 Recheck respiratory observations, including blood gases, after 15 minutes. An appropriate ventilator rate should maintain normocapnoea and a normal pH coupled with a spontaneous respiratory rate of less than 30/min.
4 If attempting to wean the patient, make small reductions in the mandatory rate (1 breath/min changes) and recheck the arterial blood gases after 1–2 hours.

Complications

- If the mandatory rate is set too low, the patient's spontaneous rate may rise leading to fatigue and hypoventilation. A sudden drop in the patient's spontaneous respiratory activity will cause severe hypoventilation.

Indications

Patients requiring considerable ventilatory assistance but who retain some spontaneous respiratory effort.

Contra-indications

Apnoeic patients.

ASSIST-CONTROLLED VENTILATION

Like SIMV, assist-controlled ventilation (ACV) assures the delivery of a pre-set volume while preserving some patient ventilatory activity. Volume-controlled time-cycled breaths are synchronised with the patients inspiratory efforts and, in the absence of spontaneous activity, set to deliver a minimal frequency (Fig. 2.70h). The sensitivity of the triggering mechanism varies between ventilators, but many machines demand significant respiratory muscle activity. On the other hand, if the ventilator trigger is too sensitive, hyperventilation may result.

Technique

- The principles involved in setting up ACV are much the same as for CMV.

PRESSURE SUPPORT VENTILATION

Pressure support ventilation (PSV) synchronises the patient's inspiratory effort with a mechanical breath, delivered to a pre-set pressure limit (Fig. 2.70i). The very high flow rate associated with this mode reduces significantly the work of breathing. The pressure support continues until the inspiratory flow rate drops below a predetermined level (e.g. 25% of peak flow), when the ventilator cycles to the expiratory phase. This method of cycling is said to be one of the most comfortable for the patient. Low levels of pressure support ($5-10cmH_2O$) can be used to counteract the extra work of breathing imposed on spontaneously breathing patients by ventilator circuits, valves, and endotracheal tubes. PSV can be used on its own or in combination with SIMV.

<table>
<tr><td>

Indications

To reduce work of breathing in the spontaneously breathing patient.

Contra-indications

Apnoea.

</td></tr>
</table>

Technique

1 Determine whether PSV is to be used alone or in association with SIMV.
2 If there is any impairment to oxygenation set the PEEP valve to $5cmH_2O$.
3 The appropriate level of pressure support will depend on the patient's respiratory system compliance. The goal is normocapnoea and a respiratory rate of less than 30 breaths/min.

INDEPENDENT LUNG VENTILATION

The lungs of patients with severe asymmetric lung disease will have marked differences in compliance, resulting in unevenly distributed ventilation. By placing a double-lumen endobronchial tube and attaching two ventilators, one to each lumen, it is possible to optimise the ventilatory parameters for each lung individually. Some ventilators can be connected electronically, enabling full synchronisation between the two sides. However, it has been shown that ventilation of each lung may be out of phase by as much as $90°$ without adverse effect.

<table>
<tr><td>

Indications

Severe unilateral lung disease e.g. contusion, aspiration, pneumonia.
Bronchopleural fistula.

Contra-indications

Inability to place double-lumen endobronchial tube.
Absence of PAFC

</td></tr>
</table>

Technique

1 Place a left-sided double-lumen endobronchial tube (see p. 103).
2 Ensure the patient has a PAFC *in situ*.
3 Set up the ventilators as directed by the manufacturer. Increase the level of PEEP to the affected lung and titrate to maximise DO_2. The rationale for the remaining ventilator settings is complex and outside the scope of this book.

Complications

- The endobronchial tube can be difficult to position initially, and later can migrate out of position. The relatively narrow lumina of the double-lumen tube can make aspiration or suction difficult.

HIGH-FREQUENCY VENTILATION

Three slightly different modes of ventilation may all be termed high-frequency ventilation: high-frequency positive pressure ventilation (HFPPV, 60–100 breaths/min); high-frequency jet ventilation (HFJV, 60–150 breaths/min); and high-frequency oscillation (HFO, 180–3000 breaths/min). All modes of HFV are able to maintain adequate gas exchange with low tidal volumes, thereby reducing peak airway pressures (Fig. 2.70j). The initial promise shown by these techniques has not been realised and, with certain exceptions, they are not commonly used in clinical practice. Current indications are listed below. HFPPV and HFJV involve the use of a flow-interrupting device coupled to a high-pressure flow generator and distally to a small diameter cannula. These modes can be used to ventilate through a rigid bronchoscope or transcricothyroid cannula. HFO remains largely experimental.

Indications

Ventilation during rigid bronchoscopy and laryngeal procedures.

Transtracheal or transcricothyroid ventilation in patients who are difficult to intubate.

Bronchopleural fistula.

Technique

- The precise technique for setting up HFV varies from one device to another and should be performed under the supervision of a person experienced in the use of that specific equipment.

LOW-FREQUENCY POSITIVE-PRESSURE VENTILATION WITH EXTRACORPOREAL CO_2 REMOVAL

Low-frequency positive-pressure ventilation with extracorporeal CO_2 removal (LFPPV–$ECCO_2R$) was developed by Gattinoni in Milan and should be considered experimental; it is practised in a few centres only. It is outside the scope of this book but, in summary, the technique comprises CO_2 removal and partial oxygenation by an extracorporeal membrane lung and venovenous bypass at 20%–30% of the cardiac output. Additional oxygenation is achieved by LFPPV at 3–5 breaths/min. LFPPV–$ECCO_2R$ is used to manage very severe respiratory failure.

Key points

- Successful use of mask CPAP will prevent the need for a more invasive technique employing intubation and mechanical ventilation.
- For patients requiring some form of mechanical ventilation, select a mode that minimises airway pressures and thus reduces barotrauma. Modes that preserve some degree of spontaneous respiratory activity will best achieve this goal.
- If possible, try to maintain the FIO_2 below 0.6.
- Monitor continuously any patient receiving ventilatory assistance.

Transtracheal jet ventilation

Indications

The emergency situation

To achieve pulmonary ventilation in patients with upper airway inspiratory obstruction who cannot be ventilated with a self-inflating bag/valve/mask even with the aid of an oro- or nasopharyngeal airway, a laryngeal mask or other airway, and who cannot be intubated immediately using the translaryngeal route.

To 'buy time' in such patients with upper airway obstruction while more time-consuming methods of translaryngeal intubation, such as the fibre-optic or retrograde techniques, are accomplished.

The elective situation

To provide ventilation during surgical or diagnostic procedures requiring 'the shared airway' such as laryngeal microsurgery, surgery for the correction of laryngeal stenosis, laryngoscopy and bronchoscopy. Jet ventilation may be provided using either the direct transtracheal route or through a bronchoscope or small bore translaryngeal tube as dictated by the circumstances.

To provide ventilation with oxygen or lavage for patients with severe dyspnoea due to cystic fibrosis, etc.

Contra-indications

Lower airway obstruction.
Obstruction to exhalation.
Laryngeal injury.
Distorted anatomy of the neck.
Trachea-oesophageal fistula.

Ventilation of the lungs may be achieved rapidly using a high pressure oxygen source delivered through a cannula placed in the trachea through the cricothyroid membrane. The technique may be used in the emergency situation when other methods are impossible or hazardous, in elective surgery or diagnostic procedures to achieve optimal operating conditions and, in certain situations requiring lavage of the lower respiratory tract.

The efficiency and safety of the technique are dependant on a clear route for exhalation and a reliable system for controlling the inspiratory time and the inspiratory and expiratory ration.

The procedure is relatively simple to perform, but is not without hazard.

Equipment

☐ Antiseptic solution.
☐ 5ml and 10ml syringes and needles.
☐ Drapes.
☐ 10ml 1% lignocaine with 1:200,000 adrenaline.
☐ 5ml sterile water.
☐ 12 or 14G cannula-over-needle.
☐ Suitable apparatus for lung ventilation (see below).
☐ High pressure oxygen source (414kPa).

Ventilation apparatus

Three methods may be used to ventilate the lungs through a trans-tracheal cannula.

• A purpose-designed jet injector control system (Sanders) connected to a high pressure (414kPa) oxygen source (Fig. 2.72). The Sanders system may also be modified to incorporate a needle injector attached by a clip to a bronchoscope or small bore tracheal tube.

The high-pressure oxygen source may be derived from a designated outlet on the anaesthetic machine.

Alternatively, the oxygen source may be produced from the wall outlet point of the piped oxygen supply or from an oxygen cylinder (tank) fitted with a step-down regulator to reduce the pressure to 414kPa.

• The high pressure oxygen source may also be connected via non-compliant narrow bore tubing (e.g. i.v. giving set or oxygen bubble) to the transtracheal cannula with a hole in the tubing allowing intermittent pulmonary inflation by occlusion with a finger.

• A self-inflating bag or anaesthetic circuit may be attached to the tracheal cannula via a 3mm endotracheal tube connector or via a

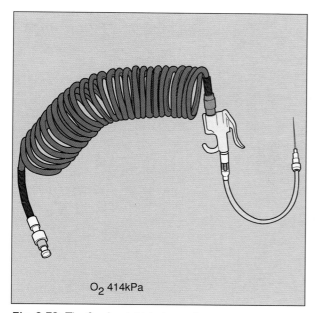

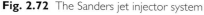

Fig. 2.72 The Sanders jet injector system

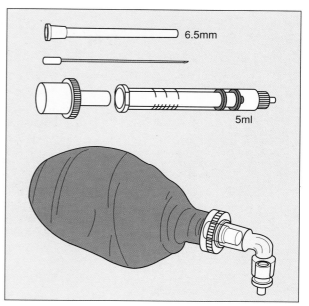

Fig. 2.73 Jet ventilation using a self-inflating bag or anaesthetic circuit

cuffed endotracheal tube plugged into the barrel of a syringe (Fig. 2.73). A 6.5mm tube will fit into a 5ml syringe and an 8.5mm tube will fit a 10ml syringe. Ventilation of the lungs by this system is inefficient and much of the effort is dissipated in overcoming the compliance of the system. Nevertheless the technique can be life-saving over a short period of time.

Technique

1 Place the patient supine with the head hyperextended by inserting a sandbag or rolled sheet beneath the patient's shoulders. Head and neck hyperextension should be avoided in patients with suspected cervical injury.
2 Don sterile gloves.
3 Clean and drape the skin over the anterior and lateral aspects of the neck (if time permits).
4 Identify the cricothyroid membrane by palpation of the dimple just below the thyroid cartilage.
5 Infiltrate the skin and subcutaneous tissues with 1% lignocaine with adrenaline in conscious patients.
6 Insert a 12–14G cannula over needle percutaneously through the cricothyroid membrane into the trachea directing it 30° caudally (Fig. 2.74).
7 Confirm correct placement in the trachea by free aspiration of air into a syringe partly filled with sterile water.
8 Remove the needle and syringe from the cannula.
9 Connect the ventilation apparatus to the cannula. ► ► ►

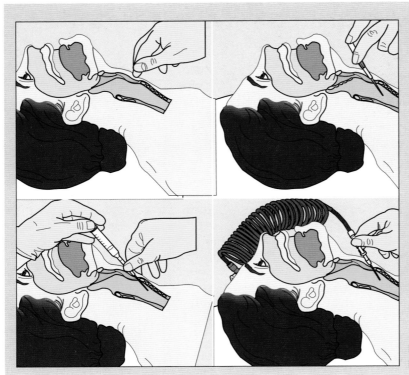

► ► ►

10 Using the Sanders jet injector system apply intermittent positive pressure to the lungs by manual compression of the injector trigger control. Each inflation must be carefully observed and the trigger released immediately normal chest expansion occurs. Ample time must be left for passive lung deflation.

Fig. 2.74 Transtracheal cannula placement

Hazards

Transtracheal jet ventilation is not without hazard. Incorrect needle placement leading to massive emphysema and pulmonary barotrauma are the most dangerous consequences.

Complications

- Needle placement in the subcutaneous tissues.
- Needle placement in the oesophagus.
- Needle placement only partly in the trachea.
- Puncture of the posterior aspect of the airway.
- Puncture of the great vessels in the neck leading to massive haemothorax.
- Local bleeding.
- Puncture of lymphatic chain.

Key points

- Correct needle and cannula placement must be absolutely assured.
- An inadequate escape route for exhaled gases through the upper airway will rapidly cause pulmonary barotrauma.
- Prolonged inflation times cause pulmonary barotrauma.

Arterial blood gases and end-tidal CO_2 measurement

Measurement of arterial blood gas values is one of the more common clinical procedures. Direct analysis of arterial PaO_2 and $PaCO_2$ is essential in the assessment of all types of ventilatory failure, and is used to follow the progress of acute and chronic disease of the cardio–respiratory system. Arterial pH and bicarbonate (HCO_3) analysis is useful in most types of metabolic disorders.

End-tidal $P\acute{E}CO_2$ is used in intensive care units and operating rooms, to provide a value of the partial pressure of carbon dioxide in the expired gas mixture. It provides an approximation of arterial $PaCO_2$, and can be measured in patients with either spontaneous or mechanical ventilation. It can also act as a disconnection alarm, for patient breathing circuits, and may detect air or fat embolism.

ARTERIAL BLOOD GASES

Indications

Analysis of respiratory or metabolic disorder.

Contra-indications

Absolute
Local sepsis.
Relative
Analysis device more than 30 minutes away.
Known severe coagulation disorder.

Equipment

☐ Alcohol swab (e.g. 70% w/v isopropyl alcohol).
☐ Local anaesthetic: lignocaine 1% without adrenaline.
☐ Heparinised 2ml or 5ml syringe.
☐ Ice for transportation.
☐ Assistant to provide pressure on puncture site.

Technique

It is not possible to provide an absolute guide on the best artery for reliable sampling: however, a distal artery should be chosen first. The radial or brachial artery are popular; the femoral or axillary are second choices. An assistant will be required to help immobilise the limb chosen, and to provide pressure on the puncture site after the procedure.

The description of the sampling technique will be for the radial artery, although it is similar for the other puncture sites. Choose the non-dominant hand in a conscious patient, and a perform a modified Allen's test (see p. 30). However, the clinical condition of the patient may be such that the test is not performed, and anyway there is doubt over the value of the test. ► ► ►

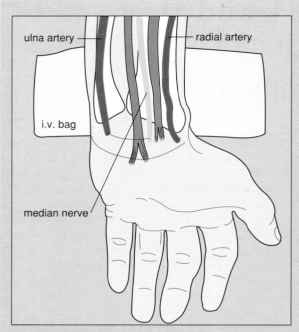

Fig. 2.75 The position of the hand for radial arterial puncture

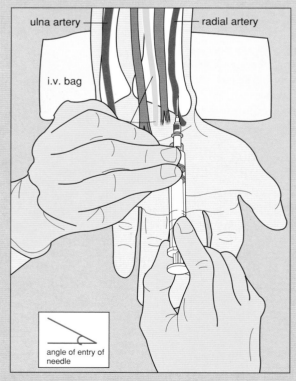

Fig. 2.76 The needle is inserted at an angle of about 30°

▶ ▶ ▶

1 Place the arm on an arm-board over a suitable rest such as a 500ml bag of i.v. fluid, and tape the forearm gently to arm-board (Fig. 2.75).

2 Don sterile gloves.

3 Clean and drape the area over the radial artery with an antiseptic solution, and infiltrate the area with 1–2ml. of local anaesthetic (without adrenaline).

4 Attach a 22G or 25G needle to the syringe and ensure that it is heparinised with a tiny amount of 1000U/ml heparin.

5 Advance the syringe at 30° to the horizontal, along the long axis of the artery, gently aspirating continually (Fig. 2.76).

6 Arterial blood should appear bright red and will sometimes push the plunger back. If there is any doubt, remove the syringe, and arterial blood should pulse out the needle.

7 Collect 2ml of blood, and then remove the syringe and needle.

8 Ask the assistant to apply firm pressure to the puncture site for five minutes. Expel all the air from the syringe after removing the needle, and then cap the syringe (Fig. 2.77).

9 Introduce the blood gas sample into an analysis machine: if this is more than three minutes away, the sample should be packed in ice for transportation.

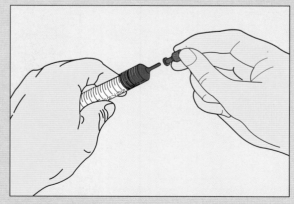

Fig. 2.77 Cap off the syringe with a sterile bung

Hazards

- Patients with bleeding disorders may require more than five minutes of pressure to prevent haematoma formation.

Complications

- Local haematoma and sepsis are the two most common complications, and can be avoided by strict attention to the details given above.
- More serious damage to the artery may result in thrombosis or embolism and resultant distal ischaemia.

Key points

- Always check that the syringe is adequately heparinised.
- Secure the arm firmly, and with the hand fully extended.
- Always use local anaesthetic.
- If arterial blood does not appear, withdraw the needle gently, as the artery may have been already punctured.

END-TIDAL CO_2 MONITORING

Indications

Assessment of adequacy of ventilation.
Confirmation of endotracheal tube placement.
Detection of air or blood embolism.

Contra-indications

Relative
Failure of machine to calibrate accurately.
Excessive secretions/ vomit in airway.

Equipment

☐ Suitable sampling site.
☐ Sampling tube with water trap or absorber.
☐ Capnometer.
☐ Reference gas for calibration.

Technique

The end-tidal sample can be taken from any source of expired gas. However, to give an accurate reading, it should be sampled from the exhaled limb of a breathing system, connected to a cuffed endotracheal tube, tracheostomy or laryngeal mask airway. Patients breathing via a face mask will produce a qualitative (but not quantitative) signal of exhaled CO_2.

It is essential that the sampling tube has a means of either trapping or filtering moisture, as excessive water droplets will cause an inaccurate signal.

1 Turn on the CO_2 analyser, and perform any calibration checks that are required: the machine may perform these automatically, but it may be necessary to provide gas sample(s) of known CO_2 concentration. These will be supplied with the machine.
2 When the calibration checks are complete, attach the sampling tube to the patient breathing circuit (Fig. 2.78).
3 The CO_2 pattern should appear as in Fig. 2.79; variations of this pattern can occur in pathological conditions, and these have also been indicated. ► ► ►

▶ ▶ ▶

4 Periodically empty any droplets of water that may have accumulated from the sampling tube in the water trap.

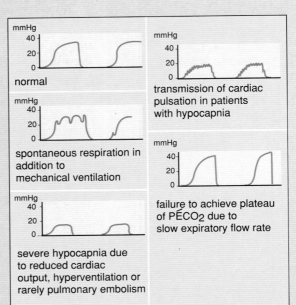

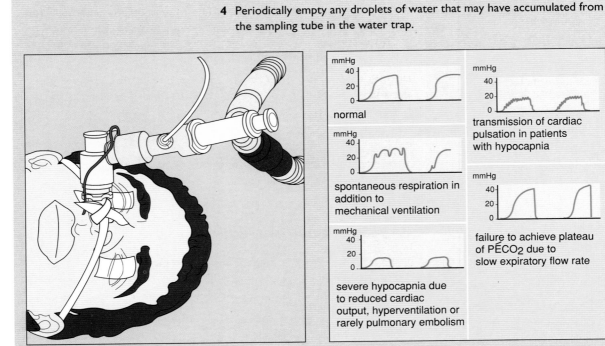

mmHg
40
20
0
normal

mmHg
40
20
0
spontaneous respiration in addition to mechanical ventilation

mmHg
40
20
0
severe hypocapnia due to reduced cardiac output, hyperventilation or rarely pulmonary embolism

mmHg
40
20
0
transmission of cardiac pulsation in patients with hypocapnia

mmHg
40
20
0
failure to achieve plateau of $P\bar{E}CO_2$ due to slow expiratory flow rate

Fig. 2.78 The gas sampling tube is inserted in the breathing system

Fig. 2.79 Normal and abnormal end-tidal CO_2 traces

Complications

- There are very few complications of this technique: false negative readings and poor calibration are the most common problems in clinical practice. False negative readings can be caused by foreign material in the sampling tube or the airway, and can be corrected by clearing such material. Disconnection and sampling tube kinking may also produce an absent trace.
- Rarely, oesophageal intubation may produce a CO_2 trace, especially if the patient has recently ingested carbonated drinks. However, oesophageal intubation should always be excluded by other methods, if there is an absent or abnormal CO_2 trace.

Key points

- Accurately calibrate the machine.
- Regularly clean the sampling tube.
- Changes in the CO_2 waveform or value are much more significant than absolute values.

Needle thoracostomy and chest drainage

Decompression and drainage of the normally only potential pleural space is required when air, other gases, blood, serous fluid, lymph or gastro–oesophageal contents enter the space in significant amounts. Major, and potentially rapid, accumulations in the space cause pulmonary collapse with ventilation perfusion disruption and mediastinal shift with reduction in cardiac output, sometimes to the point of cardiac arrest.

A pneumothorax may arise as a result of chest wall perforation (open pneumothorax), commonly caused by a stab wound or missile injury. A closed pneumothorax arises from a lung or bronchial leak. This may occur apparently spontaneously from rupture of an emphysematous bulla (often brought on by a rise in intrathoracic pressure associated with coughing or sneezing). More frequently, however, a pneumothorax occurs in association with barotrauma related to blast injury, injury with rib fracture or a penetrating wound or after cardiothoracic surgery or high positive pressure lung inflation.

A pneumothorax can come under increasing tension if a valvular leak in the lung occurs which allows gas to escape from the respiratory tract into the pleural space but does not permit its return. A simple closed pneumothorax can be converted to a tension pneumothorax when intermittent positive pressure ventilation is used. A tension pneumothorax is the commonest life-threatening result of chest injury and barotrauma.

Haemothorax commonly arises as a result of blunt or penetrating chest injury and occasionally after cardiothoracic surgery. Frequently a pneumothorax is also present.

The presence of gastric contents in the pleural space heralds injury or rupture of the oesophagus or a leak after oesophageal surgery. Rupture of the oesophagus associated with trauma is related to penetrating injury or to sudden severe abdominal compression or restrained rapid deceleration by a seat belt.

Speedy decompression of the pleural space is required as a life-saving procedure in patients with tension pneumothorax. Early chest drainage is needed for rapidly accumulating blood, air or other foreign material in the pleural space.

Temporary decompression of a pneumothorax can be achieved using simple needle thoracostomy. Formal chest tube drainage is required for fluid removal and longer term relief of a pneumothorax.

NEEDLE THORACOSTOMY (THORACOCENTESIS)

Needle thoracostomy rapidly but temporarily decompresses the pleural space using a wide-bore intravenous cannula-over-needle placed through an intercostal space.

Indications

Decompression of a rapidly accumulating pneumothorax (which is usually under tension).

To diagnose if a pneumothorax or haemothorax is present.

Removal of a serious pleural effusion associated with cardiac, renal or hepatic failure or neoplasm.

Analysis of a pleural effusion for diagnostic purposes.

Equipment

☐ Antiseptic solution.
☐ 5ml and 20ml syringes, 22G needle and 16G cannula-over-needle.
☐ 5ml 1% lignocaine with adrenaline.
☐ 3-way tap.
☐ 50ml aspirating syringe.
☐ Gauze and tape.

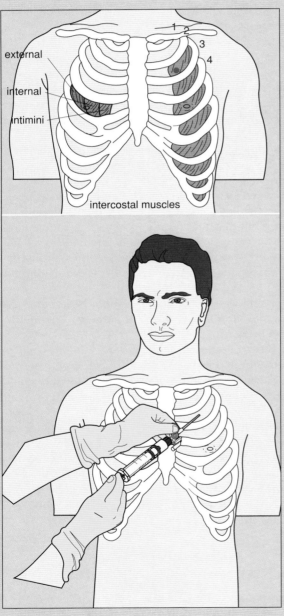

Technique

The position of the patient will be determined by the intercostal space to be used. For the decompression or diagnosis of a pneumothorax the patient should be placed supine and slightly head up and the cannula placed in the second intercostal space in the mid clavicular line on the appropriate side (Fig. 2.80).

For removal of serous fluid, the patient should be sitting up with elbows on a table and the cannula placed posteriorly in the eighth intercostal space in the mid scapular line (Fig. 2.81).

For diagnosis of a haemothorax the patient should lie supine and the cannula is inserted in the seventh intercostal space in the mid axillary line.

1 Place the patient in the appropriate position.
2 Don gloves.
3 Clean the area with antiseptic solution.
4 Infiltrate the skin and subcutaneous tissues with 1% lignocaine with adrenaline (if time permits in the conscious patient).
5 Insert a 16G i.v. cannula-over-needle through the skin and subcutaneous tissues advancing it slowly over the upper rib margin until a 'pop' is felt, heralding penetration of the parietal pleura. Prevent excessive penetration by placing a finger 2.5cm from the distal end along the cannula. ► ► ►

Fig. 2.80 Needle thoracostomy for the relief or diagnosis of a pneumothorax

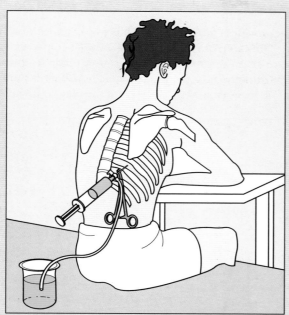

Fig. 2.81 Needle thoracocentesis for the drainage of a pleural effusion

► ► ►

Pneumothorax

6 Listen for escaping air.

7 Remove the needle.

8 Attempt to aspirate air with the syringe through the cannula.

9 Leave the cannula *in situ* if air is aspirated, placing sterile gauze loosely over the end and taping the cannula securely in place.

10 If air is aspirated proceed to formal chest tube drainage (see below).

11 If air is not aspirated remove the cannula.

Serous fluid drainage

6 Remove the needle leaving the cannula *in situ*.

7 Attach the 50ml syringe with a 3-way tap to the cannula.

8 Aspirate the pleural fluid into the syringe and expel it through the open port of the 3-way tap into a suitable receptacle after saving a sample for laboratory analysis.

9 Continue aspiration of 50ml aliquots until all available fluid is removed. The procedure should not be hurried and up to an hour may be required for removal of large pleural effusions of 1.0–1.5 litres. Excessively rapid removal of large volumes may result in unilateral pulmonary oedema.

Diagnosis of haemothorax:

6 Remove the needle leaving the cannula *in situ*.

7 Attach a 20ml syringe with 3-way tap to the cannula.

8 Aspirate with the syringe.

9 If blood is aspirated proceed to formal chest tube drainage (see below).

Hazards

- A pneumothorax may occur as a result of the needle puncturing the lung, particularly if previous pneumothorax, haemothorax or pleural effusion are absent. Puncture of the lung is most likely if the patient coughs during penetration of the pleura.

Complications

- Haemorrhage may occur if an intercostal or other vessel is punctured. The cannula-over-needle should be introduced above rather than below the rib margin to avoid the intercostal neurovascular bundle.
- Unilateral pulmonary oedema (see above).
- Infection and empyema.
- Previous intrapleural adhesions may cause loculation of the pleural space which will reduce the efficacy of the procedure.

CHEST TUBE DRAINAGE

Chest tube drainage provides continuing decompression and drainage of the pleural space. The external end of the tube must be connected to an underwater seal or flap valve to prevent aspiration of air from the atmosphere through the tube into the pleural space. A suction pump may be attached to enhance removal of blood from the pleural cavity.

Indications

Pneumothorax (post traumatic or postoperative).

Haemothorax (post traumatic or postoperative).

Chyle or gastric contents in the pleural space.

Long-term drainage of empyema.

Equipment

☐ Antiseptic solution.
☐ 5ml and 10ml syringes with 22G and 25G needles.
☐ 10ml lignocaine 1% with adrenaline.
☐ Scalpel handle with no. 10 blade.
☐ Medium artery forceps.
☐ Kelly's blunt forceps.
☐ Chest drainage tubes 30–36FG.
☐ Skin sutures.
☐ Needle holders.
☐ Gauze swabs and a dressing.

Technique

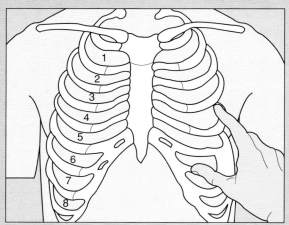

Fig. 2.82 Site for chest tube drainage

Theoretically the tube should be introduced high in the thorax for removal of air and low in the thorax for removal of fluid. However, anterior tube placement in the second or third intercostal space is difficult because of the close apposition of the ribs at that point and the presence of the overlying pectoralis muscle. It is also a particularly painful site and breathing and coughing may be impeded.

It is generally agreed that the most suitable all round site for introduction of the chest tube is in the fifth or sixth interspace in the mid axillary line. A tube placed in this space will generally drain both air and fluid (Fig. 2.82).

With a penetrating injury, the chest tube should be sited away from the original injury.

1 Place the patient supine with the ipsilateral arm at right angles to the chest.
2 Don gloves.
3 Clean the skin over the area with antiseptic solution.
4 Drape the area.
5 Infiltrate the skin and subcutaneous tissues over the proposed site with 1% lignocaine with adrenaline in the conscious patient (Fig. 2.83a).
6 Continue infiltration until the needle is felt to penetrate the parietal pleura. ▶ ▶ ▶

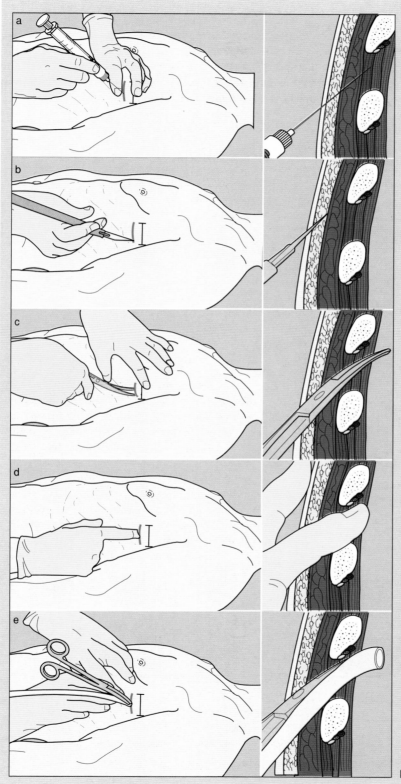

▶ ▶ ▶

7 Make a 3cm incision in the skin over the upper border of the rib at the proposed level (normally the sixth rib) (Fig. 2.83b).

8 Place a skin suture as a purse string around either end of the incision and wrap the ends around the gauze swab taped to the chest wall.

9 Bluntly dissect the subcutaneous tissues with Kelly's forceps seeking a path into the pleural cavity over the upper border of the 6th rib (Fig. 2.83c).

10 Introduce a finger into the pleural cavity and sweep around to ensure that the lung is not adherent to the chest wall at that point (Fig. 2.83d).

11 Grasp the chest tube with the Kelly's forceps and introduce it cephalad into the pleural cavity ensuring that all side drainage holes are well within the chest cavity (Fig. 2.83e). ▶ ▶ ▶

Fig. 2.83 Insertion of chest tube

▶ ▶ ▶

12 Connect the tube to an underwater seal system or to a chest drainage bag with built in flap valve. (Figs. 2.84, 2.85).

13 Secure the tube firmly in place with a second suture placed alongside, wrapping the ends of the suture around the tube again and again in a garter fashion before tying securely in a surgeon's bow knot (Fig. 2.86).

14 Observe initial flow of air and or blood or other pleural cavity contents through the tube.

15 Observe a 'swing' of the fluid level in the underwater seal system with respiration.

16 Drainage of more than 1.5–2.0 litres of blood or a continuing loss of more than 200ml/hour should suggest the need for an exploratory thoracotomy.

17 Continuing massive air leak suggests serious lung laceration or a bronchial rupture which may require confirmatory bronchoscopy, or thoracoscopy and surgical repair.

18 Check the position of the tube and lung expansion by chest X-ray.

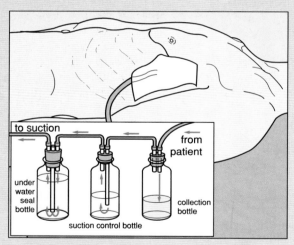

Fig. 2.84 Chest tube drainage using an underwater seal system

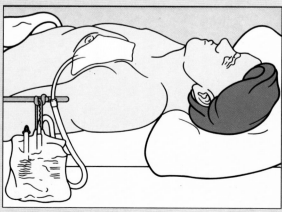

Fig. 2.85 Chest tube drainage using a drainage bag with built in flap valve

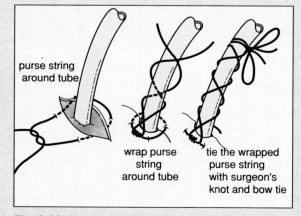

Fig. 2.86 Securing a chest tube *in situ*.

Hazard

- Serious damage to the lung, great vessels or heart can occur if a trochar is used to position the chest drain.

Complications

- Haemorrhage, generally due to an injury to an intercostal vessel, or erosion of an intrathoracic vessel.
- Injury to the lung or other structures inside the thorax.
- Misplacement of the tube outside the pleura.
- Placement of the tube in a loculated area confined by adhesions.
- Subcutaneous emphysema occurring from leakage of air around the tube if too big a hole is made or if one of the side holes lies within the chest wall.
- Pneumothorax occurring during removal of the tube.

REMOVAL OF THE CHEST TUBE

Indications

Cessation of drainage of fluid and air.

No detectable air leak during coughing or a Valsalva manoeuvre.

Full expansion of the lung on X-ray.

Technique

1 Clamp the tube for 12–24 hours to ensure that there is no build up of pneumothorax or intra pleural fluid.
2 Undo the surgeon's bow knot and unwind and remove the suture from around the tube.
3 Remove the purse string from around the gauze swab, pull the ends together and place a single throw knot loosely between them.
4 Ask the patient to breathe in deeply and then breathe out deeply.
5 Sharply remove the tube at the end of expiration and pull the knotted purse string tight.
6 Place a gauze swab firmly over the tube tract and complete the knot in the purse string.
7 Apply a waterproof airtight dressing to the site.

Key points

- Analgesia for this procedure may be provided by inhaled 50% O_2 50% N_2O mixture (Entonox).

Bronchoscopy

Indications

Fibre-optic

Awake or asleep tracheal
intubation.
Diagnosis and management of
bronchial or pulmonary
pathology.
Focal bronchial lavage.
Removal of foreign bodies.

Rigid bronchoscopy

Removal of tracheal or first
division bronchial foreign
bodies.
Diagnosis of tracheal pathology.

Contra-indications

Inexperience with the particular
technique.
Severe hypoxaemia occurring
during the procedure.
Copious blood or viscid
secretions in the airway.

Anaesthetists and critical care physicians may be required to perform bronchoscopy for diagnostic or therapeutic purposes. In the critical care setting, fibre-optic bronchoscopy is used to assess lobar or segmental collapse, and to perform focal bronchial lavage. It is also used to assist in endotracheal or endobronchial intubation, in either awake or asleep patients, see p. 98.

Rigid bronchoscopy can be used to remove inhaled foreign material or foreign bodies; this method should not be used by the inexperienced operator.

Equipment

☐ Rigid or flexible bronchoscope (Fig. 2.87).

Fibre-optic bronchoscopy

☐ Appropriate size bronchoscope.
☐ Right angle connector with valve port to admit the bronchoscope.
☐ Suction equipment with sputum trap.
☐ Bronchial brushing and biopsy equipment.
☐ Topical anaesthesia for awake intubation.
☐ Oxygen via bubble tubing.
☐ Pot of warm water to 'de-mist' the bronchoscope tip.
☐ Facilities and qualified personnel to monitor the patient's vital signs during sedation or general anaesthesia.

Rigid fibre-optic bronchoscopy

☐ Topical anaesthesia for awake intubation.
☐ Rigid bronchoscope of appropriate size.
☐ Facility and qualified personnel to ventilate patient via the bronchoscope (e.g. Sanders injector).
☐ Bronchial biopsy and brushing equipment.
☐ Forceps to remove foreign bodies.
☐ Facilities for total intravenous anaesthesia.

Technique

Awake fibre-optic bronchoscopy is performed via the nose or the mouth, using topical anaesthesia of the airway, together with intravenous sedation. The technique of topical anaesthesia will not be described here, as it has been described previously (p. 100). Awake bronchoscopy is most conveniently performed with the patient sitting at 45°, to aid tracheal intubation.

Asleep fibre-optic bronchoscopy can be performed through a nasal or oral airway during spontaneous inhalational anaesthesia. ► ► ►

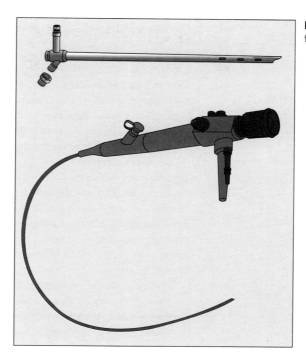

Fig. 2.87 Rigid and flexible bronchoscopes

▶ ▶ ▶

However, it is usually carried out via an endotracheal tube, with the patient ventilated using a flow generator ventilator. In this case, total intravenous anaesthesia is required using a muscle relaxant and an intravenous anaesthetic, such as propofol or midazolam.

Rigid bronchoscopy is usually performed under general anaesthesia. The bronchoscope is introduced instead of an endotracheal tube. There are several possible ways of ventilating the patient at this point: using either a Sanders jet injector, or apnoeic oxygen insufflation. In the former technique, the patient is ventilated by high-pressure oxygen source that flows into the side of the bronchoscope. In apnoeic oxygenation, the patient is oxygenated by a continuous flow of oxygen that is passed via a fine catheter or tube, inside the bronchoscope. This technique relies on mass diffusion of gases, and does not adequately remove carbon dioxide. It is therefore limited to about 10–15 minutes of bronchoscopy, to prevent excessive hypercapnia.

Fibre-optic bronchoscopy

1 Attach the bronchoscope to the light source, and check that the view through the bronchoscope is clear: attempt to read some small print through the bronchoscope.
2 Attach suction to the suction port of the bronchoscope, and check that adequate pressure is generated: draw some water through the bronchoscope. (If the patient is hypoxic, or if there are unlikely to be secretions, insufflate 100% oxygen via bubble tubing instead of suction through the suction port). ▶ ▶ ▶

▶ ▶ ▶

3 Look through the bronchoscope, and identify the indented line in the view; this is used to orientate the bronchoscope. Decide whether you wish to stand at the foot or the head of the patient. The former position will mean that the left-sided pulmonary structures will appear on the right of the viewer; the latter position will mean that left-sided structures appear on the left of the viewer (Fig. 2.88).

4 Advance the bronchoscope through the valve on the endotracheal tube connector, or through the nostril/mouth (Fig. 2.89). If the bronchoscope is being passed through an endotracheal tube, the first structure that will be seen is the carina and trachea. If the bronchoscope is passing through the nose/mouth, identify the larynx, and pass the bronchoscope through the vocal cords, and then down into the trachea. The presence of tracheal rings should confirm entry into the trachea.

5 Identify the carina, as the bifurcation of the trachea.

6 Identify the left and right main bronchus; the following rules will help:
   • If standing at the patients head, the left main bronchus will be to the left for the viewer, if the bronchoscope has not been rotated.
   • The left main bronchus arises at a more acute angle than the right main bronchus, so the right bronchus will be seen more clearly when passing down the trachea.
   • The right main bronchus gives off a branch to the upper lobe bronchus, which is directed in a supero-posterior direction some 2.5–5cm beyond the carina. The left upper lobe bronchus is 5–7.5 cm along from the carina. (Fig. 2.90). ▶ ▶ ▶

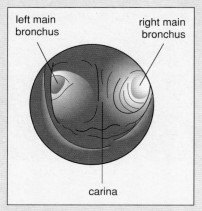

Fig. 2.88 The carina as seen through a bronchoscope

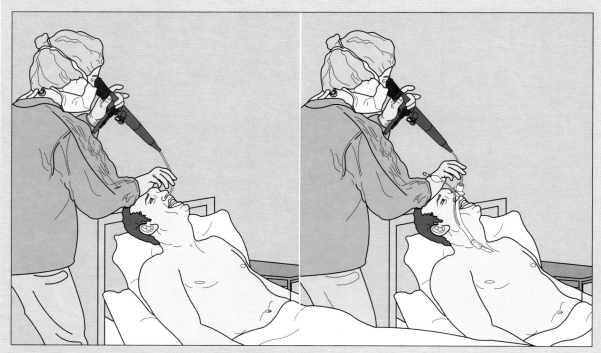

Fig. 2.89 The bronchoscope can be introduced through the mouth, nose or an endotracheal tube

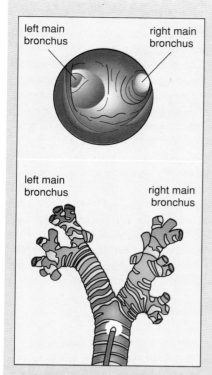

Fig. 2.90 Anatomy of the main bronchi

▶ ▶ ▶

7　Perform the appropriate biopsies and/or lavage, and then inspect the opposite lung.

8　Withdraw the bronchoscope slowly, and check for any bleeding points as the bronchoscope ascends the trachea.

9　In ventilated patients, reconfirm that the patient is ventilating adequately on both sides. In spontaneously breathing patients, administer oxygen via face mask until any sedation has worn off.

Rigid bronchoscopy

1　Ensure that the patient is adequately anaesthetised with stable vital signs.

2　Check that there is a suitable and functioning means of ventilation available. Usually, this will be a Sanders injector attached to the side port of the bronchoscope. There should be a switching device to control inspiration, that is either electrically, manually or mechanically driven. Ensure that you understand how the device functions (Fig. 2.91).

3　Ask the anaesthetist to place the patient's head as flat as possible. Remove the endotracheal tube (if present) and fit a gum shield to the patient's upper teeth.

4　Introduce the bronchoscope into the mouth and identify the larynx. Pass the bronchoscope through the vocal cords and identify the tracheal rings (Fig. 2.92).

5　Begin ventilation of the patient's lungs.

6　Identify the carina and then the right main bronchus. The bronchoscope will usually pass to the proximal portions of the segmental bronchi and will allow identification, foreign body removal and biopsy of lesions to this point.

7　The anaesthetist will indicate if the time limit of the procedure has been reached: this may occur because of a rising $P\acute{E}CO_2$ or a falling SaO_2.

8　Withdraw the bronchoscope carefully and then remove the gum shield. Replace the endotracheal tube in the trachea and re-commence ventilation.

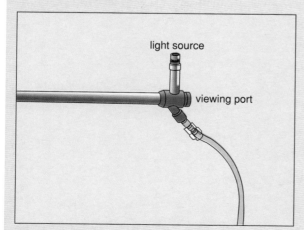

Fig. 2.91 The Sanders injector is used to provide jet ventilation during rigid bronchoscopy

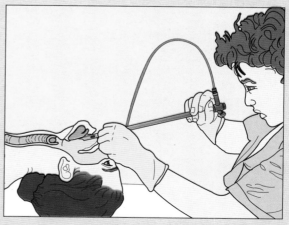

Fig. 2.92 The rigid bronchoscope is introduced via the mouth (note the extension of the head)

Complications

- The complications of bronchoscopy are related to the sedation/anaesthesia required, and the procedure itself.
- Local trauma to the lips, teeth, mouth, nose or pharyngeal structures may occur during introduction of the bronchoscope.
- Major complications of fibre-optic bronchoscopy are due to over-sedation. It is essential that the patient is monitored for signs of respiratory depression, or airway obstruction. A decrease in SaO_2 should be promptly treated.
- Rigid bronchoscopy may result in hypoxia or hypercapnia, and it is essential to have an anaesthetist supervising the patient's general condition.
- Bronchial or lung biopsy may be followed by pulmonary haemorrhage, sepsis, pneumothorax, and pneumomediastinum. These complications are rarer these days, because of the high yield of histological specimens from bronchial brushings, and lavage. However, a chest radiograph is mandatory where the patient has developed symptoms or signs suggestive of such a complication.

Hazards

- Check the degree of neck movement, mouth opening and dentition before anaesthesia is induced; this is essential for safe conduct of the procedure.
- Rigid bronchoscopy should not be attempted in patients who are likely to be difficult intubations.

Key points

Fibre-optic bronchoscopy

- Use local anaesthetics with vasoconstrictor to reduce coughing and have a qualified assistant to provide additional intravenous sedation.
- In awake patients, the nasal route is preferable to the oral route.
- Paediatric bronchoscopy requires special size bronchoscopes, which cannot normally be used for bronchial lavage or suction.
- Oxygen may be insufflated via the suction port in patients who are hypoxaemic.

Rigid bronchoscopy

- Make sure that the method of oxygen ventilation or insufflation works, and that you understand how to use it.
- The procedure is only of value in patients with lesions down to the major bronchi.

Broncho-alveolar lavage

Indications

Diagnosis and management of pneumonia.
Alveolar proteinosis.
Pulmonary aspiration of particulate and liquid material.
Bronchial obstruction due to viscid secretions.

Contra-indications

Bronchial carcinoma.
Lung abscess.
Broncho-pleural fistula.

Therapeutic broncho-alveolar lavage is less commonly used today and is reserved for the management of certain conditions. It is not first-line therapy in any of the conditions mentioned, but can be used as an adjunct to other treatment. It is generally performed in the critical care setting, although it may occasionally be performed in the operating room.

There are two types of bronchial lavage: focal lavage is performed in patients with disease confined to one lobe or segment, whilst lung lavage is performed for bilateral widespread disease, such as alveolar proteinosis. Focal lavage is performed through a flexible bronchoscope, and involves injection of small volumes of fluid under direct vision via the injection port. Lung lavage is performed without the aid of a bronchoscope, and is not aimed at one focal area. Both techniques are performed under controlled ventilation and general anaesthesia, via a cuffed endotracheal tube.

Equipment

The equipment necessary for this technique is shown in Fig. 2.93.
☐ 1.6% (one-fifth molar) sodium bicarbonate or 0.9% normal saline.
☐ Flexible bronchoscope for focal lavage.
☐ Biopsy forceps and sputum trap.
☐ Fine sterile suction catheters and high volume suction device.
☐ Facilities and qualified personnel for ventilating and monitoring the patient's vital signs during general anaesthesia.

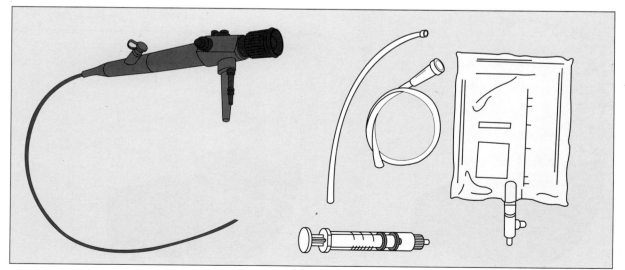

Fig. 2.93 Equipment for broncho–alveolar lavage

Technique

General anaesthesia is required for the procedure. A cuffed endotracheal tube is inserted in the trachea, and a special right angle connector is fitted, to allow the passage of a flexible bronchoscope. The anaesthetist should then ventilate the patient with 100% oxygen, and monitor the SaO_2 with a pulse oximeter.

Bilateral lung lavage

1 Disconnect the patient from the ventilator, and instill 50–100ml of lavage fluid into the endotracheal tube. The fluid may flow out of the end of the tube, which is of no concern (Fig. 2.94).

2 Wait for 30–60 seconds, provided the SaO_2 remains satisfactory.

3 Insert the suction catheter into the tracheal tube to a depth of 25cm. Apply maximum suction to remove all the fluid from the endotracheal tube. Do not continue this suction for more than 20 seconds (Fig. 2.95).

4 Ventilate the patient for at least two minutes with 100% oxygen.

5 Repeat the process twice more: on each occasion, the fluid aspirated should become clearer and less viscid. ▶ ▶ ▶

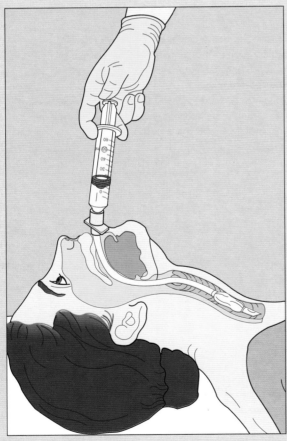

Fig. 2.94 Lavage fluid is instilled down the endotracheal tube

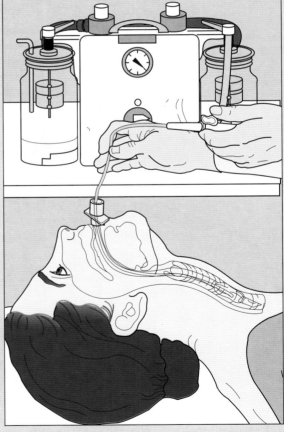

Fig. 2.95 The lavage fluid is sucked out of the lungs via the endotracheal tube

► ► ►

6 If the patient becomes increasingly difficult to ventilate, the suction catheter should be briefly re-inserted. If the patient remains hard to ventilate, it will be necessary to perform flexible bronchoscopy, to remove any plugs of mucus etc.

Focal bronchial lavage

1 Continue to ventilate the patient with 100% oxygen. Resistance to gas flow will be increased during bronchoscopy, and the ventilator may require adjustment.

2 Insert the flexible bronchoscope through the special right angle connector, and pass it to the affected bronchial segment (for anatomical identification, see p. 162 on bronchoscopy).

3 Aspirate any pus or foreign material into the suction trap, and send this for culture and microscopy.

4 Inject 10–20ml. of normal saline through the injection port of the bronchoscope while occluding the suction tubing (Fig. 2.96).

5 Wait 30 seconds, and then aspirate the fluid completely into the suction trap. Send this fluid for culture and microscopy.

6 Repeat the process up to five times, until the fluid aspirated is clear.

7 Remove the bronchoscope and recap the right angle connector on the endotracheal tube.

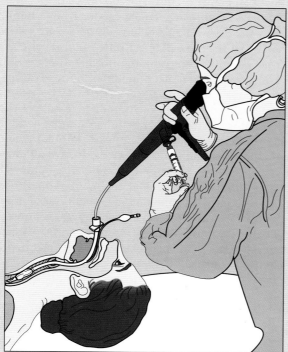

Fig. 2.96 Focal lavage can be performed via a flexible bronchoscope

Complications

- Dissemination of infection or tumour is possible during lung lavage, although it is difficult to quantify.
- Hypoxaemia, hypertension and bradycardia are all recognised complications of both types of bronchoscopy and will require intervention by the anaesthetist.

Key points

- General anaesthesia with muscular relaxation is essential to prevent coughing.
- Hypoxaemic patients will require a rapid procedure.

Hazards

- If hypoxaemia worsens, abandon the procedure unless the lavage is thought to be life-saving.

How to set-up and use a nebuliser

Nebulisers and humidifiers are often considered under the same heading in descriptions of equipment. The major difference between the two types of device is that humidifiers produce vapour from a liquid, while nebulisers produce droplets of liquid of any size. There are several uses for these devices. Patients on mechanical ventilation receive dry medical gases via a tracheal tube by-passing the normal upper airway humidification mechanisms. Inclusion of a humidifier in the breathing system will prevent excessive drying of the airways.

Nebulisers can also be used to administer medication to the upper and lower airway. Bronchodilators are the most common example because this route reduces many of their systemic side effects. Antibiotics and anti-viral agents, particularly pentamidine and ribovirin, are administered preferentially via this route. Nebulised racemic adrenaline will reduce stridor in patients with laryngo-tracheo-bronchiolitis. This section will deal only with the technique of nebulisation of liquid forms of drugs and water although humidification has many similar physical features.

The purpose of the nebuliser is to produce droplets of liquid of a size that will allow their passage to the distal bronchial tree. A droplet size of less than five micrometres is required to ensure delivery to the alveoli although in practice many gas driven nebulisers do not achieve this small droplet size. Larger size droplets will condense out in the more proximal bronchial tree, which may be adequate for drugs such as bronchodilators. All nebulisers may be used to humidify inspired air with water and in this respect they possess the same function as humidifiers. Three main types of nebuliser will be described.

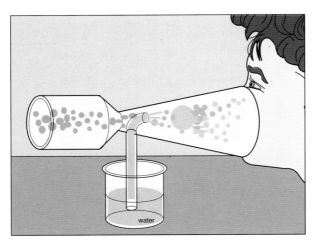

Fig. 2.97 Gas driven nebulisers work according to Bernoulli's principle. Droplets of liquid are drawn up the tube, because of·a pressure drop across the gas stream coming out of the nozzle

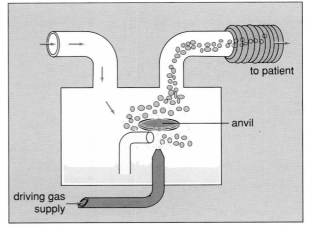

Fig. 2.98 Smaller droplets may be produced if the gas flow from the first stage of the nebuliser falls onto an anvil

THE GAS DRIVEN NEBULISER

This device (Fig. 2.97) works on the Bernoulli principle, which is an application of the Venturi effect. Gas is passed through a nozzle where there is an area of low pressure. Liquid is drawn up into the air stream as droplets which are then carried forward by the gas stream. The gas stream may then strike an anvil which has the effect of breaking the droplets up into yet smaller droplets (Fig. 2.98). These are then passed to the patient via a face mask or into the inspiratory tubing of a ventilator. The gas driven type of nebuliser produces droplets of size 5–20 micrometres although multiple anvils will result in smaller droplets.

THE ULTRASONIC NEBULISER

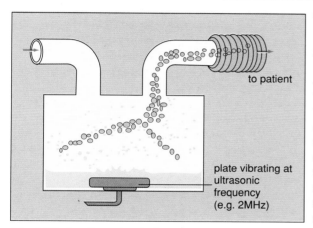

to patient

plate vibrating at ultrasonic frequency (e.g. 2MHz)

Fig. 2.99 An ultrasonic nebuliser

This device generates fine droplets by the action of a continuous sonic bombardment from a high frequency generator (Fig. 2.99). The sonic transducer may be in the air and droplets of liquid are allowed to fall onto it. Alternatively, the transducer may be submerged and the droplets will rise up from the surface of the transducer as the energy beam increases their kinetic energy. Both types of nebuliser may be damaged if the supply of liquid dries up so many machines incorporate design features to prevent this happening. It is claimed that these nebulisers can produce liquid droplets of a constant size (1–2 micrometres). Ultrasonic nebulisers are expensive and are not generally used for routine nebuliser therapy.

THE SPINNING DISC NEBULISER

This device works on the principle of liquid impinging on a rotating disc. The liquid is then broken up into droplets of widely varying sizes. This type of nebuliser is less popular as it does not allow for accurate prediction of droplet size and therefore the effect of the administered drug is variable.

The gas driven nebuliser will be described as this is the type that is most commonly used for drug administration in clinical practice.

Indications

Administration of drugs into the bronchial tree, e.g. antibiotics, bronchodilators, and adrenaline. Humidification of airway with water.

Contra-indications

Known sensitivity to selected agent.

Equipment

☐ Gas supply (air or oxygen) at 4 bar pressure with flow meter.
☐ Nebuliser.
☐ Liquid form of drug to be administered.
☐ Face mask or ventilator tubing for administration of gas carrying droplets.

Technique

The choice of driving gas depends on the general condition of the patient. Patients who are hypoxic will require oxygen as the driving gas; otherwise air or air/oxygen mixtures will be acceptable. The gas flow required by the nebuliser will be stated in the manufacturer's instructions and this should be adhered to closely: low flows will produce liquid droplets that are too small. The choice of face mask depends on the condition of the patient and the connections from the nebuliser to the mask. Generally, most gas powered nebulisers are incorporated within a face mask and the mask will be of the fixed performance type. This ensures that the patient receives a known FIO_2.

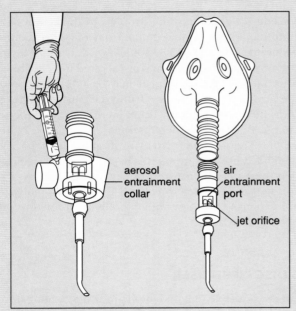

aerosol entrainment collar

air entrainment port

jet orifice

1 Draw up the dose of drug prescribed and dilute it with sterile saline or water to a volume of 2.5–5ml.
2 Inject this liquid into the chamber of the nebuliser, and replace the top of the nebuliser (Fig. 2.100).
3 Attach the fresh gas tubing to the nebuliser and start the gas flow at the stated rate.
4 Check that a mist of droplets is produced and then attach the nebuliser outflow to the patient via a mask or the inspiratory tubing of the breathing circuit.
5 When the liquid chamber of the nebuliser is empty and no mist is seen, stop the fresh gas flow and either repeat the dose or replace the mask with a conventional mask to deliver the required FIO_2 to the patient.

Fig. 2.100 Put the liquid in the chamber of the gas-driven nebuliser and close firmly

Complications

- Inadequate gas flow may result in a failure to deliver the drug far enough distally in the bronchial tree. Some patients find the mist distressing and it may be useful to reduce the flow briefly to lower the hissing noise that accompanies such nebulisers. The flow should be returned to normal values later.

Key points

- Ensure that the drug can be given via the nebulised route.
- Systemic side effects are rare but can occur if stated dosage is exceeded.
- Do not allow the ultrasonic type of nebuliser to run dry.

SECTION 3
Gastro-Intestinal System

Insertion of a nasogastric tube

There are a wide variety of tubes available for nasogastric insertion. These include single lumen tubes for general purposes, double lumen, sump tubes for easy drainage and fine-bore feeding tubes.

Complex multi-channel tubes designed for tamponading bleeding oesophageal varices are described on p. 178.

Indications

Decompression of the stomach:
• After trauma or major surgery.
• Sepsis.
• Bowel obstruction or ileus.
Nutrition.
Evacuation of toxic substances, e.g. drug overdose.
Active warming or cooling by lavage with fluid of the appropriate temperature.
Contrast studies of the upper gastrointestinal tract.

Contra-indications

Fractures of the base of skull and/or midface.

Equipment

☐ A nasogastric tube of the appropriate size (for general gastric decompression a 14FG is adequate).
☐ Lubricating jelly or 2% lignocaine gel.
☐ Glass of drinking water and a straw.
☐ 60ml syringe.
☐ Stethoscope.
☐ Blue litmus paper.
☐ Laryngoscope.
☐ Magill's forceps.
☐ Adhesive tape.

Technique

Place awake patients in the sitting position; unconscious patients will have to be supine. Select the most patent nasal passage by getting the patient to sniff through each nostril in turn, or by examining the nares to detect obstruction or asymmetry. A sterile technique is not required, although simple hygiene should be observed.

1 The distance from the nares to the stomach can be approximated by placing the tube tip at the patient's earlobe and extending the tube via the bridge of the nose to the tip of xiphoid process. Place a piece of sticky tape on the tube to mark this distance.
2 Lubricate the tube with 2% lignocaine gel (conscious patients) or water soluble jelly (unconscious patients).
3 Pass the tube gently along the floor of the nasal cavity in a directly posterior (not superior) direction (Fig. 3.1). ▶ ▶ ▶

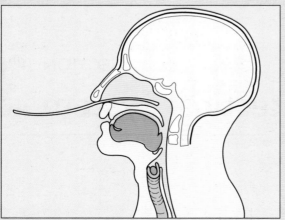

Fig. 3.1 Passage of the nasogastric tube along the floor of the nose

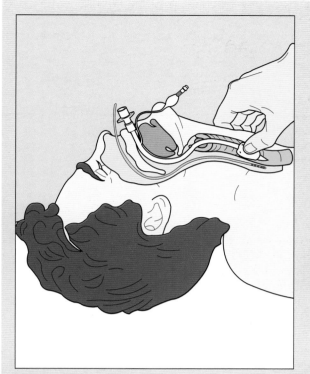

Fig. 3.2 Thyroid traction to aid nasogastric tube placement

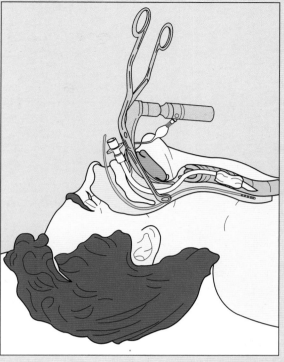

Fig. 3.3 Use of a laryngoscope and Magill's forceps to aid nasogastric tube placement

► ► ►

4   Use firm but gentle pressure to overcome the slight resistance encountered as the tip reaches the nasopharynx. Get the patient to swallow sips of water from the drinking straw, while continuing to pass the tube to the predetermined distance.

5   In patients who are unconscious or who have endotracheal tubes in place, passage of the nasogastric tube is aided by grasping the thyroid cartilage and pulling it anteriorly (Fig. 3.2). If this fails, insert a laryngoscope into the oropharynx and under direct vision pass the nasogastric tube into the oesophagus using Magill's forceps (Fig. 3.3). Alternatively, cut a nasotracheal tube longitudinally, pass it through the nose and into the oesophagus (Fig. 3.4a), insert the nasogastric tube (Fig. 3.4b) and finally peel away the outer split tube (Fig. 3.4c).

6   Attempt to aspirate gastric contents into the 60ml syringe. Test any aspirate with the blue litmus paper: it should turn red immediately.

7   If there is no aspirate, connect the tube to the 60ml syringe filled with air and auscultate the stomach while injecting air (Fig. 3.5). An obvious gurgling is heard if the tube is correctly positioned.

8   Secure the nasogastric tube to the nose with adhesive tape.

9   Check the position of the tube with an X-ray if:
    • The patient is unconscious.
    • The patient has a chest or abdominal injury.
    • A fine-bore tube has been used.
    • There is any doubt about the position of the tube.   ► ► ►

▶ ▶ ▶

10 If the tube is to be used for feeding purposes, the first feed should be water.

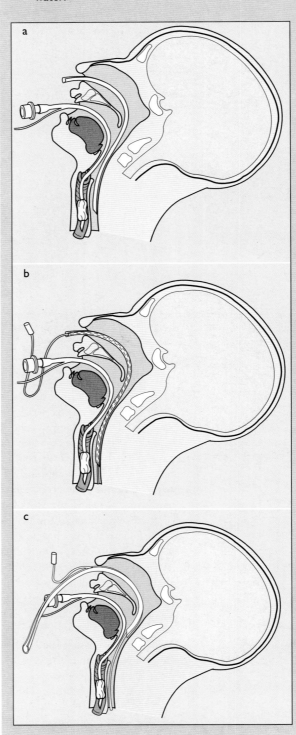

Fig. 3.4 Use of a split naso-oesophageal tube to aid nasogastric tube placement

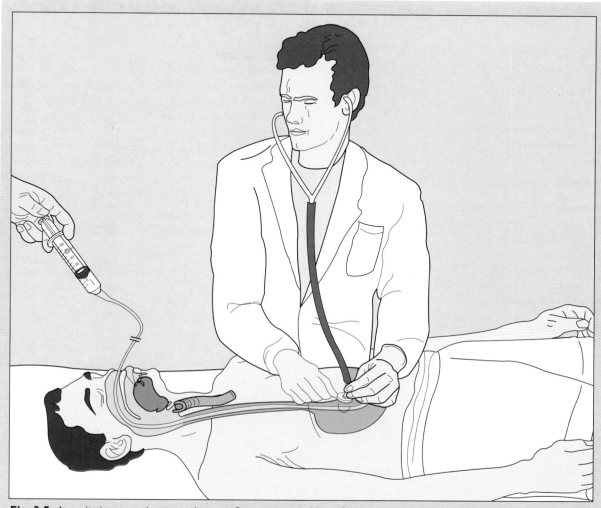

Fig. 3.5 Auscultation over the stomach to confirm correct position of the nasogastric tube

Hazards

- Do not place a nasogastric tube in any patient who may have a fractured base of skull; use the orogastric route instead.
- Do not feed the patient through a nasogastric tube until correct placement has been confirmed.

Complications

- A difficult insertion may cause bleeding, particularly in the presence of coagulopathy.
- Other problems relating to trauma include ulceration of the nose, oesophagus, stomach and (rarely) cranial placement through a basal skull fracture.
- Obstruction of nasal sinus drainage may result in sinusitis and secondary sepsis.
- The tube may migrate back into the oesophagus or into the trachea, resulting in pulmonary soiling with gastric contents or feed.

Key points

- In the conscious patient, lubricate the tube with a liberal quantity of 2% lignocaine gel. This can be supplemented by 10% lignocaine spray to the oropharynx.

175

Gastric lavage

Gastric lavage is most commonly performed in the accident and emergency department to remove toxic substances after an intentional or accidental overdose. It is most effective if performed within an hour of ingestion of the poison, but some drugs will delay gastric emptying and it may be effective up to four hours later. In the critical care unit, gastric lavage is more likely to be used as a method of temperature control in the hypothermic or hyperthermic patient. In this situation, where very large fluid volumes are required, use saline or Hartmann's solution, as water may cause electrolyte disturbances.

Indications

Following drug overdose.
Correction of hypothermia or hyperthermia.

Contra-indications

Any patient with obtunded airway reflexes must first have a cuffed endotracheal tube inserted.
Caustic chemicals and petroleum will cause severe pneumonitis if aspirated, thus lavage is absolutely contra-indicated in the absence of a cuffed endotracheal tube.

Equipment

- ☐ Large-bore (1cm diameter) orogastric stomach washout tube.
- ☐ Water-soluble lubricant (KY jelly).
- ☐ Bite-block.
- ☐ Funnel.
- ☐ Lukewarm water.
- ☐ Bucket.

Technique

The patient should be in the lateral position on a tipping trolley. Check for the presence of good laryngeal reflexes (strong gag reflex); if these are obtunded, an anaesthetist should place a cuffed orotracheal tube after inducing anaesthesia and short-acting muscle paralysis (with cricoid pressure applied). Remove any false teeth.

1 Lubricate the tube with water-soluble jelly.
2 Place a bite-block in the patient's mouth.
3 Pass the tube through the mouth and ask the patient to swallow. This is likely to induce gagging and possibly vomiting.
4 Advance the tube into stomach and confirm the position by injecting air through the tube while auscultating the stomach.
5 Place the tube below the level of the bed to siphon off the stomach contents (keep a specimen). Next, raise the tube and, using a funnel, run 100ml of lukewarm water into the stomach (Fig. 3.6). Immediately, drop the level of the funnel to siphon the contents out again (Fig. 3.7). Repeat until the returned fluid is clear.
6 Depending on the drug in question, activated charcoal in a dose of 25–100g can now be given and left in the stomach as the washout tube is removed. Activated charcoal absorbs most drugs but not inorganic salts or solvents. Repeated doses may speed elimination of the drug from the body by binding drug excreted into the gut and preventing enterohepatic recirculation.

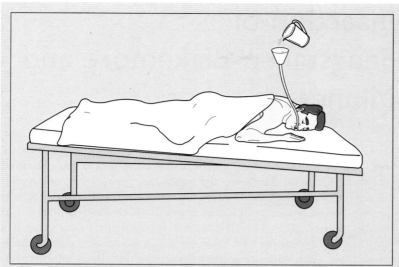

Fig. 3.6 Running lukewarm water into the stomach

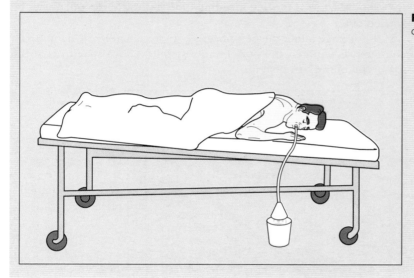

Fig. 3.7 Siphoning off the stomach contents

Complications

- Aspiration is a serious risk, particularly when the airway is compromised.
- Over-distension and perforation of the stomach can occur and the oropharynx and oesophagus can be traumatised during a difficult insertion of the tube.
- Use of cold fluids will cause a significant drop in core body temperature and large volumes of water can cause electrolyte abnormalities.

Key points

- If there is any doubt about the effectiveness of the patient's protective airway reflexes, insert a cuffed endotracheal tube before passing the stomach washout tube.

Hazards

- Aspiration of stomach contents into the lungs will result in a chemical pneumonitis with a high mortality.

177

Insertion of Sengstaken-Blakemore and Minnesota tubes

These tubes are used for tamponading bleeding oesophageal varices; both tubes have a round gastric balloon and a sausage-shaped oesophageal balloon. The Sengstaken tube has three lumina, one lumen to each balloon and a third to drain the stomach. The Minnesota tube is very similar but has a fourth lumen through which the oesophagus can also be drained (Fig. 3.8). The facility to drain the oesophagus is a significant safety feature and most clinicians would now chose a four-lumen tube. These tubes *per se* will not cure the underlying problem but they should control variceal bleeding until definitive treatment can be carried out.

In the average adult, the oesophagus is approximately 25cm long. The anastamosis between the portal and systemic venous systems is at the lower end of the oesophagus.

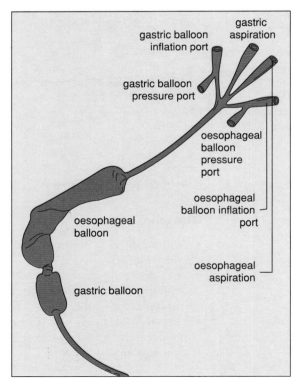

gastric balloon inflation port

gastric balloon pressure port

gastric aspiration

oesophageal balloon pressure port

oesophageal balloon inflation port

oesophageal balloon

oesophageal aspiration

gastric balloon

Fig. 3.8 A Minnesota tube

Equipment

☐ Sengstaken or Minnesota tube.
☐ 50ml syringe.
☐ 10% lignocaine spray.
☐ Water-soluble jelly.
☐ Sphygmomanometer and 3-way tap.
☐ Traction weight (300g approx.).
☐ Four heavy clamps (non-serrated).

Technique

The attempt to swallow a large tube in the presence of heavy oesophageal bleeding is likely to induce vomiting and the accompanying risk of pulmonary aspiration. If the patient is very distressed and unco-operative, do not be tempted to use sedation. If necessary, it is better to ask an anaesthetist to induce general anaesthesia and pass an endotracheal tube before attempting to insert the Sengstaken tube. However, in most cases, tube placement can be done with the patient awake. If the patient is vomiting, the lateral decubitus is the safest position to use. Make sure high flow suction equipment is immediately available.

1 Check the balloons carefully for leaks and make sure the lumina are patent. Attach the manometer to the gastric balloon pressure port and inflate the balloon, making a note of the pressure after each 50ml increment (Fig. 3.9). ► ► ►

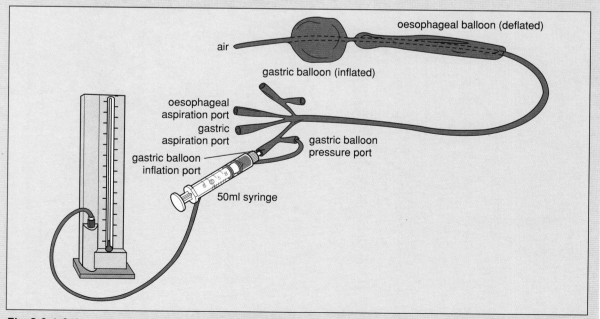

Fig. 3.9 Inflation and pressure checking of the gastric balloon

▶ ▶ ▶

The gastric balloon of the Sengstaken tube will take about 250ml, while that of the Minnesota tube will hold 400–500ml. In both cases, evacuate and clamp the balloon before insertion. Insertion is made easier if the tube is first cooled in a refrigerator.

2   Anaesthetise the oro- and nasopharynx with lignocaine spray and lubricate the tube with water-soluble jelly.

3   Find the most patent nostril and advance the tube through it. If the tube will not pass through the nose, use the mouth instead. As the tube warms up, it becomes floppy; if the tube will not pass due to floppiness, try a new, cold tube from the fridge.

4   Ask the patient to swallow and advance the tube to about 50cm. Aspirate any gastric contents through the gastric port and confirm the position by injecting air and auscultating over the stomach.

5   Connect the gastric balloon pressure port to the manometer and inflate the balloon in 50ml increments, noting the pressure after each increment. The pressures attained with the balloon *in situ* should be no more than 15mmHg greater than the pressures attained with the same volumes before insertion; higher pressures indicate that the balloon is in the oesophagus or duodenum and requires re-positioning.

6   Once the gastric balloon has been inflated fully, clamp the gastric inflation port and pull the tube back gently until it lodges at the gastro– oesophageal junction (an obvious resistance) (Fig. 3.10). Tape the tube to the nose.   ▶ ▶ ▶

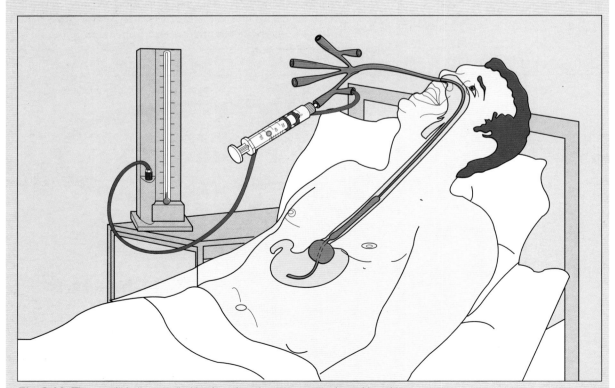

Fig. 3.10 The gastric balloon pulled back against the gastro-oesophageal junction

▶ ▶ ▶

7 Obtain an X-ray of the abdomen to confirm the position of the tube.

8 Inflate the oesophageal balloon to a pressure of 25–35mmHg, checked with the manometer attached to the oesophageal balloon pressure port. Be wary of complaints of chest pain during inflation of the oesophageal balloon. Re-check the oesophageal balloon pressure at least every three hours.

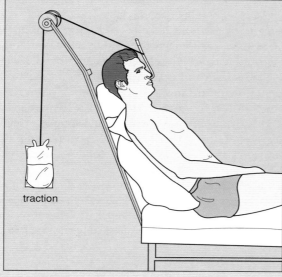

traction

Fig. 3.11 Applying traction to the tube

9 Apply traction to the tube with approximately 300g, using 300ml of saline in a fluid bag, for example (Fig. 3.11). Alternatively, apply skin traction by wrapping strong tape around the tube and sticking it to the patient's face.

10 Apply intermittent suction to the gastric lumen and continuous suction to the oesophageal lumen (Minnesota tube).

11 Oesophageal necrosis is a significant risk, therefore maintain the pressure in the oesophageal balloon at the lowest level required to stop the bleeding. Additionally, deflate the oesophageal balloon for five minutes in every six hours.

12 Resuscitate the patient with appropriate volumes of blood and fresh frozen plasma.

13 After 24 hours, deflate the oesophageal balloon and remove the traction. If this does not precipitate bleeding, leave the tube *in situ* for 24 hours before deflation of the gastric balloon and final removal. If bleeding occurs after deflating the oesophageal balloon, it can be re-inflated for 12–24 hours. Surgical intervention will be necessary after this time.

Complications

- Pulmonary aspiration is a serious risk during insertion of the tube.
- Inflation of the gastric balloon within the oesophagus may result in oesophageal rupture.
- Prolonged and/or heavy traction can cause ulceration of the nares within a few hours.
- Excessive pressure within the oesophageal balloon may cause oesophageal necrosis.

Key points

- The use of a tamponade tube for the control of bleeding oesophageal varices is only a temporising manoeuvre until definitive treatment with sclerotherapy, portasystemic shunting, or oesophageal transection can be undertaken.

Hazards

- It is dangerous to sedate a patient before inserting a Sengstaken or Minnesota tube. There is then a serious risk of pulmonary aspiration through an unprotected airway.

181

Diagnostic peritoneal lavage

Indications

Following significant blunt thoraco-abdominal trauma if:

- Abdominal examination is equivocal (findings may be obscured in the presence of rib fractures, or pelvic and lumbar spine fractures).
- Pain response is altered due to head injury, drugs (including alcohol), or paraplegia.
- Unexplained hypotension or blood loss.
- Patient cannot be easily monitored (e.g. general anaesthesia for extra-abdominal injuries or prolonged X-ray studies).

Contra-indications

Absolute
The obvious need for an immediate laparotomy.

Relative
Previous abdominal operations.
Morbid obesity.
Advanced cirrhosis.
Severe coagulopathy.
Advanced pregnancy.

Routine clinical examination of the abdomen can be extremely unreliable as a method of excluding significant intra-abdominal injury following trauma, particularly in those patients with a depressed level of consciousness who have sustained head injuries or are under the influence of drugs. Tragically, each year a number of patients die as a result of undiagnosed intra-abdominal haemorrhage.

The technique of diagnostic peritoneal lavage (DPL) involves infusion of crystalloid solution into the peritoneal cavity and examination of the returned fluid for the presence of blood. Diagnostic peritoneal lavage was described originally in 1965 and is very popular amongst trauma surgeons and emergency physicians in the United States. However, for some reason, it is not performed routinely by the majority of surgeons in the United Kingdom. Diagnostic peritoneal lavage is encouraged strongly by the Advanced Trauma Life Support (ATLS) Program and the technique described in this chapter will follow the ATLS recommendations.

The results from DPL are falsely negative in only 2% of cases. These false negatives are usually due to isolated injury of the pancreas and duodenum, which are retroperitoneal structures; or isolated injury of the small bowel, bladder or diaphragm, which tends to result in minimal haemorrhage.

Equipment

- ☐ Urinary catheter.
- ☐ Nasogastric tube.
- ☐ Antiseptic solution.
- ☐ Drapes.
- ☐ 20ml 1% lignocaine with 1:200,000 adrenaline.
- ☐ Surgical pack containing scalpel, small retractor, two artery clips and scissors.
- ☐ Peritoneal dialysis catheter.
- ☐ 1 litre warmed normal saline.
- ☐ Intravenous giving set.
- ☐ Suture for wound closure, e.g. 2/0 nylon.

Technique

Diagnostic peritoneal lavage can be performed with the patient conscious or unconscious. Place the patient in the supine position. It is essential to make sure that the stomach and bladder are decompressed with a nasogastric tube and urinary catheter, respectively, before attempting DPL. ► ► ►

▶ ▶ ▶

Diagnostic peritoneal lavage can be performed through a number of abdominal sites; the open, infra-umbilical approach is described, though a para-umbilical incision may be used. A supra-umbilical approach is used for those patients with pelvic fractures: if inserted at a lower level the peritoneal catheter may pass into a large retroperitoneal haematoma associated with the fracture.

Diagnostic peritoneal lavage is effectively a mini-laparotomy and full antiseptic precautions must be used; this includes a mask, hat and sterile gloves. Ideally, this procedure should be performed by two operators.

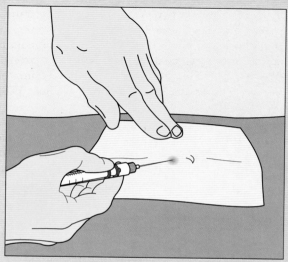

Fig. 3.12 Infiltration of DPL site with local anaesthetic

1 Clean the whole anterior aspect of the abdomen with antiseptic solution and isolate the area with drapes.
2 Inject 10ml of 1% lignocaine with 1:200,000 adrenaline in the midline, one-third the distance from the umbilicus to the symphysis pubis (Fig. 3.12). Use local anaesthetic in unconscious, head-injured patients; painful stimuli may raise intracranial pressure.
3 Make a 5cm vertical incision down to the posterior abdominal fascia, injecting additional local anaesthetic, as required (Fig. 3.13).
4 Place two clips on the fascia and get an assistant to pull up on these in order to stabilise the fascia and peritoneum.
5 Make a tiny incision through the peritoneum (Fig. 3.14).
6 Gently insert the peritoneal catheter, without the trocar, into the peritoneal cavity and guide it down into the pelvis at an angle of about 45° (Fig. 3.15).

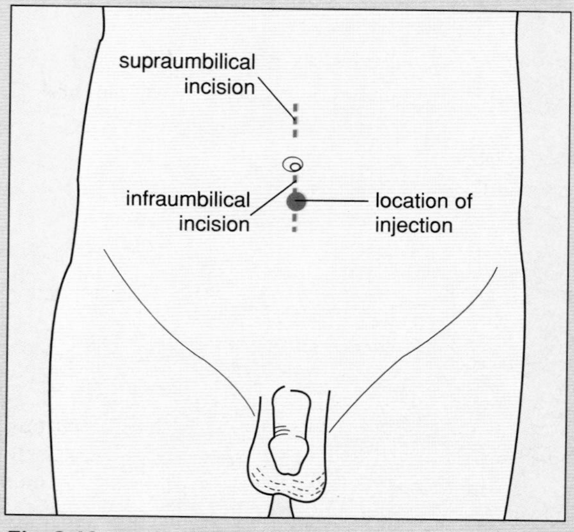

Fig. 3.13 Location of skin incision

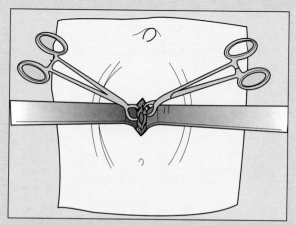

Fig. 3.14 Incision of the peritoneum

▶ ▶ ▶

7   Connect the dialysis catheter to a syringe and aspirate (Fig. 3.15). If more than 5ml of frank blood or obvious enteric contents are aspirated, the DPL is positive and the patient requires immediate laparotomy.

8   If gross blood is not obtained on aspiration, instil warmed saline (10ml/kg; up to 1litre) into the peritoneal cavity, through an intravenous giving set attached to the catheter (Fig. 3.16). Leave at least a small quantity of saline in the bag; the saline is returned later from the peritoneal cavity by a siphon effect.   ▶ ▶ ▶

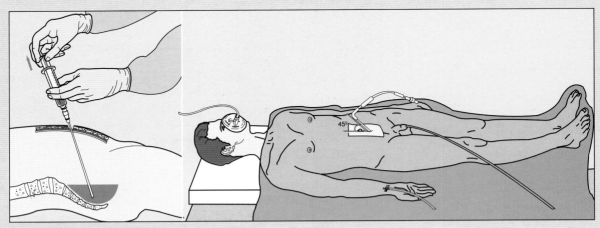

Fig. 3.15 Aspiration through the dialysis catheter

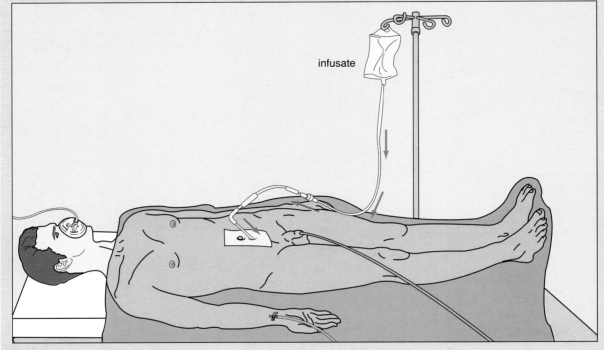

infusate

Fig. 3.16 Infusion of lavage fluid

▶ ▶ ▶

9   Distribute the fluid throughout the peritoneal cavity by agitating the abdomen gently.

10 Bring the saline bag to floor level, allowing the saline to return from the peritoneal cavity over about 15 minutes (Fig. 3.17).

11 If little or no lavage fluid returns (the average return is 650–750ml), reposition the catheter in the peritoneal cavity and place the patient slightly head up. In addition, a further 500ml of lavage fluid may be infused. If the fluid still fails to return, consider the possibility of diaphragmatic rupture.

12 Send a sample of the fluid to the haematology laboratory for measurement of red and white cell counts. A count of more than 100,000 red blood cells/mm^3 or more than 500 white blood cells/mm^3 are considered positive results and indications for laparotomy. Returned lavage fluid with a red blood cell count of 50,000–100,000 /mm^3 presents a diagnostic dilemma. If the patient is stable, leave the catheter in place and repeat the lavage after 1–2 hours. If in doubt, and the patient has other major injuries, it is probably best to perform a laparotomy, but this decision must be finally made by the surgeon responsible for the patient.

13 Remove the peritoneal dialysis catheter and suture the wound.

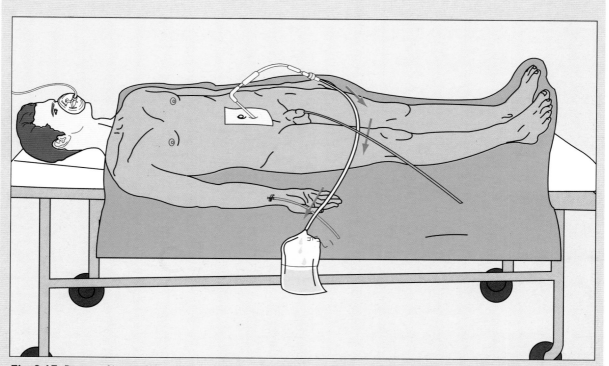

Fig. 3.17 Return of lavage fluid

Hazards

- The bladder or stomach may be perforated if a urinary catheter and nasogastric tube are not inserted before performing a DPL.

Complications

- A false positive result may occur from haemorrhage secondary to injection of local anaesthetic, or incision of the skin and subcutaneous tissues.
- The catheter may perforate the intestine, resulting in peritonitis.
- Gastric or bladder perforations are likely to occur if these organs are not decompressed adequately beforehand.
- A late complication is infection at the lavage site.

The overall complication rate for DPL is said to be approximately 1–2 per cent.

Key points

- Diagnostic peritoneal lavage is a simple procedure.
- Patient death from undiagnosed intra-abdominal haemorrhage is avoidable.
- Consider the need for a DPL in any patient who has sustained major blunt trauma.

Urethral catheterisation

Urethral catheterisation is a procedure commonly performed in the wards, operating theatre and in the critical care unit. Male catheterisation is generally undertaken by medical staff, while female catheterisation is most commonly performed by nurses. This chapter will describe insertion of a Foley catheter, the standard catheter used for continuous catheterisation. It is made of rubber, plastic, or silicone and has an inflatable balloon distally to retain the catheter in the bladder. Intermittent catheterisation, using different types of catheter, may be used for diagnostic purposes (e.g. to measure residual urine or to introduce contrast media) or for therapeutic purposes (e.g. neurogenic bladder).

Indications

In monitoring urine output:
- In critically ill patients.
- In haemodynamically unstable patients.
- During long surgical procedures.

Urinary retention secondary to:
- Spinal or epidural anaesthesia.
- Prostatic hypertrophy.
- Neurological disorders.

Incontinence, where conservative methods have failed or are inappropriate.

Contra-indications

Suspected traumatic rupture of the urethra (indicated by a high prostate, blood at the meatus or scrotal bruising).

Equipment

Urethral catheterisation pack containing:
- ☐ Drape.
- ☐ Swabs.
- ☐ Cotton wool balls.
- ☐ Forceps.
- ☐ 10ml 1% lignocaine gel.
- ☐ Dish to collect urine.
- ☐ 10ml syringe for balloon.
- ☐ Antiseptic solution.
- ☐ Appropriate size Foley catheter, e.g. 14FG for short-term drainage, 18FG silicone for long-term drainage.
- ☐ Saline for balloon inflation (if necessary).
- ☐ Sterile gloves.
- ☐ Closed system collection bag (graduated type if monitoring hourly urine output).

Technique

The patient should be supine: a male patient should have his legs slightly apart to accommodate the collection tray, a female patient should have her knees flexed and hips abducted, while keeping her heels together. Although a sterile gown is unnecessary, an aseptic technique is essential to reduce the risk of urinary tract infection.

1 Wearing sterile gloves, arrange the contents of the catheterisation pack and the Foley catheter on top of a trolley. Soak the cotton wool balls with antiseptic solution. Partially open the end of the Foley package so that the catheter can later be inserted with one hand only. Draw up 10ml of saline ready for inflation of the balloon. ► ► ►

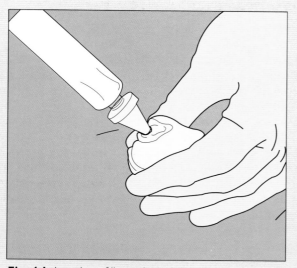

Fig. 4.1 Insertion of lignocaine gel

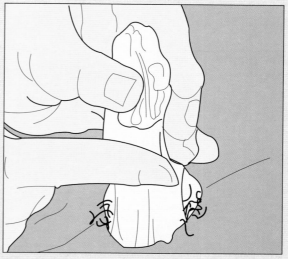

Fig. 4.2 Massage the lignocaine gel toward the perineum

► ► ►

Male

2 Place the drape around the penis (some packs have a single drape with a central hole, others have two drapes).

3 Wrap a swab around the penis and retract the foreskin, if present, with the left hand.

4 While holding the swab around the penis, clean the glans with antiseptic solution.

5 With the penis extended, gently insert the nozzle of the tube of lignocaine gel into the meatus and squeeze the contents into the urethra (Fig. 4.1). Using another swab, massage the gel down the urethra toward the perineum (Fig. 4.2). Gently squeeze the distal end of the penis for two minutes to prevent the gel pouring out and to allow time for good anaesthesia.

6 With the penis extended, insert the end of the catheter into the meatus and feed the catheter down into the urethra (Fig. 4.3). If catheter packaging is sticking to the catheter, grasp the end of the package and give it a gentle shake, while keeping a firm grip on the penis to prevent the catheter sliding back out of the urethra.

7 There is a little resistance as the catheter tip meets the external sphincter of the bladder, which is a voluntary muscle. Ask the patient to relax by inviting him to take a deep breath, and apply steady, gentle pressure. Persistent failure to pass the catheter may be due to a prominent median lobe of the prostate, bladder neck hypertrophy or creation of a false passage. If unable to pass a urethral catheter with gentle pressure, seek advice and assistance from a urologist.

► ► ►

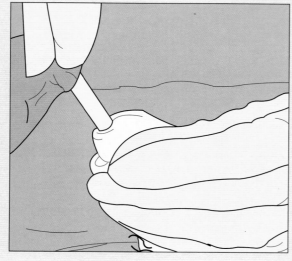

Fig. 4.3 Insertion of catheter

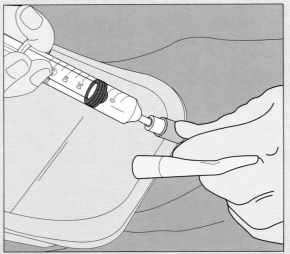

Fig. 4.4 Inflation of the balloon

▶ ▶ ▶

Do not persist if the obstruction cannot be passed. A number of catheter introducers are available, but these are best used by properly trained specialists.

8 Advance the catheter up to its hub and inflate the balloon with the appropriate volume of saline, usually 10ml (Fig. 4.4). Some catheters have their own closed system for inflation of the balloon and do not require additional saline. Pull the catheter back until the balloon stops at the bladder neck.

9 Let the proximal end of the catheter drop into the sterile collection tray and check for return of urine. If no urine is obtained at this time, it may be because the catheter is obstructed with lignocaine gel; gentle manual compression of the bladder should produce urine.

10 Connect the catheter to the urine collection bag tubing and secure the tubing to the patient's thigh with adhesive tape.

Female

2 Clean the perineum with antiseptic solution while parting the labia with the left hand.

3 Lubricate the catheter tip with lignocaine gel and insert it gently into the urethra. The female urethra is only 3–4cm long.

4 If the catheter is held up at the bladder neck, try redirecting it slightly more anteriorly.

5 Once in the bladder, inflate the balloon with saline (as above).

6 Let the proximal end of the catheter drop into the sterile collection tray and check for return of urine. If no urine is obtained at this time, it may be because the catheter is obstructed with lignocaine gel; gentle manual compression of the bladder should produce urine.

7 Connect the catheter to the urine collection bag tubing and secure the tubing to the patient's thigh with adhesive tape.

Complications

- The commonest complication is failure to pass the catheter into the bladder (a rare problem in women). This may be because of a urethral stricture, prostatic hypertrophy, or bladder neck hypertrophy. Persistent attempts to pass the catheter may traumatise the urethra with the creation of a false passage.
- A stricture may occur as a late complication.
- Haemorrhage and infection.
- Urinary tract infections are common with long-term catheterisation.

Key points

- Use plenty of lignocaine gel and allow time for it to take effect.
- During catheter insertion, use gentle pressure only.
- Do not make repeated insertion attempts; request advice from a specialist urologist.

Hazards

- Urinary catheter introducers can cause severe urethral trauma and should be used only by doctors with appropriate training.

Suprapubic catheterisation

Suprapubic catheterisation involves the passage of a catheter through the anterior abdominal wall and into the bladder. In the past, the technique was used for draining the bladder only in circumstances where urethral catheterisation was contra-indicated or not possible. However it has become more popular recently, partly because it is more comfortable for patients, particularly females requiring long-term catheterisation. Although it can be performed as an open or a closed technique, the latter is by far the commonest and is the method described here. Various types of suprapubic introducers and catheters are available, but a technique using the Lawrence introducer will be described.

Indications

Acute or chronic retention.
Ruptured urethra (e.g. in association with a fractured pelvis).
After vaginal, urethral or bladder neck surgery.
Long-term catheterisation for incontinence.

Contra-indications

Absolute

Inability to aspirate urine from proposed site of catheterisation.
Known or suspected carcinoma of the bladder.

Relative

Previous lower abdominal or pelvic surgery (abdominal contents may be tethered to the abdominal wall).
Coagulopathy.
Gross haematuria (the narrow lumen tends to block off).
Pregnancy.

Equipment

- ☐ Antiseptic solution.
- ☐ Swabs.
- ☐ Drapes.
- ☐ 20 ml 1% lignocaine with 1:200,000 adrenaline.
- ☐ 10 ml syringe and 21G needle
- ☐ A scalpel and no. 11 blade.
- ☐ Introducer with trochar (Fig. 4.5).
- ☐ Rubber catheter (e.g. 12FG) for short-term or silicone catheter for long-term.
- ☐ Collection tubing and bag.

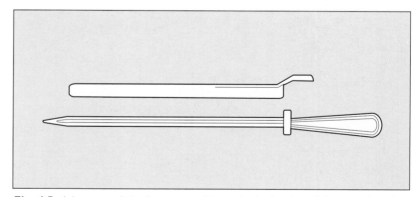

Fig. 4.5 A Lawrence introducer comprising a plastic sheath and sharpened trochar

Technique

The patient should be supine before performing suprapubic catheterisation. Ensure that the bladder is full and easily percussible above the pubis. Shave a small area of skin just above the centre of the symphysis-pubis. ▶ ▶ ▶

▶ ▶ ▶

1 Clean the lower abdomen with antiseptic solution and drape the area.

2 Determine a point 3cm above the symphysis pubis in the midline and infiltrate lignocaine into the skin and down into the bladder (Fig. 4.6a). Aspirate urine to confirm the position. If urine cannot be aspirated, aim the needle more caudad (Fig. 4.6b). If this fails, consider obtaining an ultrasound examination to confirm that the bladder is full.

3 Using the scalpel, make a 1cm vertical incision through the skin and subcutaneous tissue down to the bladder wall.

4 Push the introducer, with a twisting motion, through the incision and, aiming at about 30° from the vertical, toward the pelvis, push through the fascia and into the bladder (Fig. 4.6c). The introducer will 'give' as it enters the bladder. Use the left hand to eliminate excessive travel of the introducer.

5 Remove the trochar with the right hand, while anchoring the sheath with the left. Place a finger over the sheath to reduce the loss of urine (Fig. 4.6d). Feed the urinary catheter down through the sheath into the bladder and immediately fill the retaining balloon with saline (Fig. 4.6e) and ensure free flow of urine. Attach the collection bag tubing. ▶ ▶ ▶

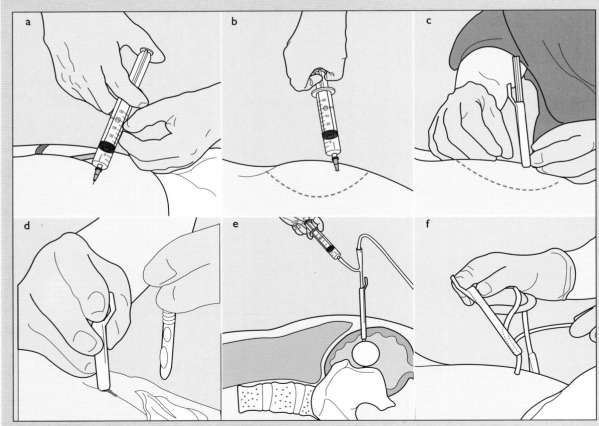

Fig. 4.6 a Infiltration of local anaesthetic **b** Aspiration of urine **c** Placement of introducer
d Stopping flow of urine from sheath **e** Retaining balloon filled with saline **f** Removal of the sheath

▶ ▶ ▶

6 Pull the sheath up out of the bladder and remove it by pulling away the tear-off strip (Fig. 4.6f).

7 Place a simple dressing on the puncture site.

Complications

- Perforation of another viscus is an obvious risk, hence the importance of ensuring aspiration of urine before undertaking this procedure.
- The catheter may be misplaced into the peritoneal cavity and this is likely to have occurred if urine fails to drain.
- Local and systemic infection are additional complications of suprapubic catheterisation.
- Bleeding is rare.

Key points

- Patients with hyper-reflexic, neuropathic bladders will usually require a general anaesthetic for suprapubic catheterisation.

Hazards

- Trauma to other intra-abdominal structures may occur if suprapubic catheterisation is attempted when the bladder is not palpable.

Peritoneal dialysis

Indications

Chronic renal failure.
Acute renal failure:
• Potassium >6.0mmol/l.
• Urea >35mmol/l.
• Creatinine >500μmol/l.
• Acidosis.
Water overload.
Drug overdose (limited benefit).
Patients requiring dialysis where
systemic anticoagulation is
contra-indicated.

Contra-indications

Intra-abdominal sepsis.
Recent abdominal surgery.
Previous extensive abdominal
surgery (adhesions).
Chronic obstructive pulmonary
disease.
Distended bowel.
Late pregnancy.

Acute renal failure is a common problem in the critical care unit and is associated with a high mortality. Conventional haemodialysis causes rapid fluid and electrolyte shifts which are poorly tolerated by critically ill patients. Peritoneal dialysis is better tolerated by these patients and can be undertaken in any hospital by intensive care doctors and nurses without specialised training in renal medicine. Until recently, peritoneal dialysis was the therapy of choice for critically ill patients in acute renal failure. However, there are now available a number of continuous renal replacement therapies (see p. 197), which are well tolerated by potentially haemodynamically unstable patients and which offer higher clearance of small molecular weight molecules. Thus, peritoneal dialysis is now less frequently used in the critical care unit, although it is still commonly used for chronic renal failure.

In the critical care unit patient with acute renal failure, the standard biochemical determinants for starting any form of renal replacement therapy are listed under 'Indications'. In the critically ill patient, other factors, such as fluid overload or pulmonary oedema, may indicate earlier renal replacement therapy.

Peritoneal dialysis uses the peritoneal membrane as the dialysing surface, supplied by a splanchnic blood flow of 1200ml/min. Water moves across this semi-permeable membrane by osmosis, while solutes move primarily by diffusion. In the hypercatabolic patient, peritoneal dialysis alone is likely to be inadequate.

Equipment

☐ Antiseptic solution.
☐ Drapes.
☐ 20ml 1% lignocaine with 1:200,000 adrenaline.
☐ Surgical pack containing scalpel, small retractor, two clips and scissors.
☐ Peritoneal dialysis catheter.
☐ Heparinised saline (500 units in 500ml).
☐ Warmed peritoneal dialysis fluid (e.g. Boots no. 61, 62 or 63).
☐ Heparin.
☐ Intravenous giving set with double spike.
☐ Suture for wound closure, e.g. 2/0 nylon.
☐ Dressing.

Technique

The patient should be supine. Ensure the bladder is empty and, if present, aspirate the nasogastric tube. The technique for inserting the dialysis catheter is similar to that described for diagnostic peritoneal lavage (p. 182). ► ► ►

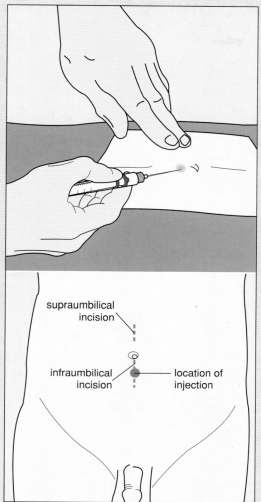

1 Clean the whole anterior aspect of the abdomen with antiseptic solution and isolate the area with drapes.

2 Infiltrate 10ml of 1% lignocaine with 1:200,000 adrenaline 5cm below the umbilicus in the midline from the skin down to the peritoneum (Fig. 4.7).

3 Make a 5cm vertical incision through the linea alba down to the posterior abdominal fascia, injecting additional local anaesthetic, as required.

4 Place two clips on the fascia and get an assistant to pull up on these in order to stabilise the fascia and peritoneum.

5 Make a tiny incision through the peritoneum (Fig. 4.8).

6 Gently insert the peritoneal catheter, without the trocar, into the peritoneal cavity and guide it down into the pelvis at an angle of about 45° (Fig. 4.9).

7 Suture the wound and secure the catheter.

8 Connect the fluid giving set to the catheter and run in 500ml of heparinised saline. Then drop the bag below the level of the patient and check for free return of fluid.

9 Select the appropriate dialysis fluid (Table 4.1) and ensure it has been warmed to body temperature. The osmolality of the three commonly available dialysis fluids is determined by the varying sodium and dextrose content; all are hyperosmolar compared with plasma. Adding 500 units heparin to each litre of dialysis fluid helps to prevent blockage of the catheter by fibrin plugs. Most patients are adequately dialysed with no. 61 fluid (Table 4.1), but 2 litre exchanges may be required initially.

10 Run in the dialysis fluid rapidly; this usually takes about 10 minutes. Leave the fluid in the peritoneal cavity for 30 minutes, then allow 20 minutes to drain. This results in hourly cycles and makes fluid balance calculations easier. The volume of returning dialysate is variable but is likely to be about 10% greater than that infused.

11 If more rapid fluid removal is required, use no. 62 fluid (Table 4.1) in place of no. 61 on every other or every third exchange. The high glucose content of no. 62 fluid may result in hyperglycaemia and the need for sliding scale intravenous insulin. ▶ ▶ ▶

supraumbilical incision

infraumbilical incision

location of injection

Fig. 4.7 Infiltration of peritoneal dialysis site with local anaesthetic

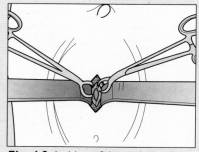

Fig. 4.8 Incision of the peritoneum

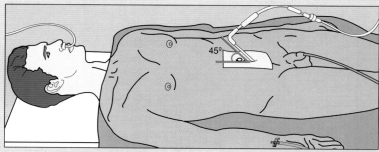

45°

Fig. 4.9 Insertion of peritoneal dialysis catheter

	No. 61	No. 62	No. 63
Na (mmol/l)	140	140	130
Cl (mmol/l)	100	100	90
Ca (mmol/l)	1.8	1.8	1.8
Mg (mmol/l)	0.75	0.75	0.75
Lactate	45	45	45
Dextrose	1.36%	6.36%	1.36%
Osmolality mosmol/l	364	643	343

Table 4.1

Contents of Boots peritoneal dialysis fluids*

* The content of dialysis fluids from other manufacturers may differ from these

▶ ▶ ▶

12 Recheck the plasma potassium frequently. Hyperkalaemia is usual in acute renal failure, consequently the dialysate fluids contain no potassium. Once the plasma potassium is in the normal range, prevent hypokalaemia by adding potassium 3–4 mmol/l to the dialysate.

Hazards

- There is a risk of perforation of the bladder if it is not emptied before inserting the peritoneal dialysis catheter.
- The volumes of fluid involved with peritoneal dialysis are large and accurate fluid balance is essential.
- The use of no. 62 fluid is likely to result in hyperglycaemia.
- The patient may become severely hypokalaemic if potassium is not added to the dialysate as soon as the potassium is in the normal range.

Complications

- At the time of catheter insertion, there is a risk of perforation of the bladder or bowel. Unrecognised placement in the bladder will be recognised by the sudden appearance of a large volume of fluid in the urinary catheter bag.
- Bleeding is common and the dialysate is often tinged red in the first 24–48 hours. Persistent or heavier bleeding indicates significant damage to a vessel and may require surgery.
- Leakage of dialysate around the catheter is a common complication. A well-placed suture may resolve the problem but failing that, the catheter should be replaced.
- The risk of catheter blockage by fibrin plugs is reduced by adding heparin to the dialysate but the tip can also become blocked by bowel or omentum, and may require re-siting.
- Peritonitis is a serious and not uncommon complication of peritoneal dialysis. Culture of dialysate should be done routinely every 1–2 days. Established infection is indicated by abdominal pain and clouding of the returning dialysate and is treated with the appropriate systemic or intraperitoneal antibiotics.
- Intraperitoneal fluid splints the diaphragm and will reduce the functional residual capacity. This may result in basal atelectasis and hypoxia.

Key points

- Most patients can be dialysed adequately with no. 61 fluid using 1 litre or 2 litre hourly exchanges.
- Use no. 62 for more rapid fluid removal and no. 63 if the patient is hypernatraemic.

Haemofiltration and haemodiafiltration

Although peritoneal dialysis is a relatively easy procedure to manage in the critical care unit, the clearances produced will be inadequate for hypercatabolic patients. Furthermore, recent abdominal surgery will contra-indicate peritoneal dialysis. Standard pumped haemodialysis induces sudden changes in intravascular volume, plasma osmolality, arterial oxygen tension and blood pressure, all of which are poorly tolerated by critically ill patients. In contrast, haemofiltration works by the principle of slow continuous ultrafiltration and avoids rapid osmotic shifts. The patient's blood passes through an extracorporeal circuit which includes a filter. An ultrafiltrate of plasma is produced by hydrostatic pressure exerted across a semipermeable membrane. Solutes, such as urea, move across the membrane by convection, the amount depending upon the size of the molecules, the membrane permeability, the hydrostatic pressure, and the ultrafiltration rate. Ultrafiltrate volumes are of the order of 10–20 litres/24 hours and the patient's circulating blood volume is maintained by intravenous replacement with a fluid that has an electrolyte composition similar to that of plasma.

Haemofiltration may be performed through a venovenous circuit which requires a pump (continuous venovenous haemofiltration, CVVH), or through an arteriovenous circuit which utilises the patient's own arterial blood pressure to drive blood through the filter (continuous arteriovenous haemofiltration, CAVH). In comparison with CAVH, CVVH results in higher flows and produces more ultrafiltrate; indeed, effective CAVH may be impossible in hypotensive patients. In addition, CVVH may be performed through a single, large-bore, double-lumen venous catheter. However, the requirement for a pump makes CVVH more complicated to set up and demands specialised training.

Solute clearance can be increased by infusing dialysis fluid through the ultrafiltrate compartment of the haemofilter in a counter-current direction to the blood flow. Solute will then move across the membrane by diffusion, as well as by convection. The relatively slow flow of dialysis fluid through the filter (15–30ml/min) allows almost complete equilibration of small molecules (e.g. urea) between plasma and dialysis fluid. This technique is known as continuous arteriovenous haemo-dialysis (CAVHD) or continuous venovenous haemodialysis (CVVHD). The advantages and disadvantages of these two circuits are as discussed above.

The indications for starting continuous renal replacement therapy (CRRT) are listed below. In critically ill patients, fluid management is made considerably easier if CRRT is started relatively early in the course of acute renal failure. In addition, there is some evidence that when used in patients with septic shock, continuous haemofiltration may remove a number of vasoactive mediators from the circulation.

Indications

Acute renal failure:
- Potassium >6.0mmol/l.
- Urea >35mmol/l.
- Creatinine >500μmol/l.
- Acidosis.

Pulmonary oedema/fluid overload.

Drug overdose (drugs with a long half-life and a small volume of distribution).

Contra-indications

Lack of trained medical and nursing staff.

Significant hypotension (mean arterial pressure <60mmHg) will necessitate the use of pumped systems.

Equipment

- ☐ Gloves and gown.
- ☐ Antiseptic solution.
- ☐ Drapes.
- ☐ 10ml 1% lignocaine with 1:200,000 adrenaline.
- ☐ Three 10ml syringes.
- ☐ 25G needle.
- ☐ Two 21G needles.
- ☐ Dialysis catheter kits: two single-lumen kits (each with: 7–8FG catheter, Seldinger wire, thin-walled needle, dilator, syringe, no. 11 scalpel blade) or one double-lumen kit.
- ☐ 10ml heparinised saline x2.
- ☐ Two clamps (for the catheters).
- ☐ Silk sutures 2/0.
- ☐ Haemofilter (flat plate or hollow fibre).
- ☐ Extracorporeal circuit tubing.
- ☐ 2 litres normal saline containing 5000 units heparin/litre (for priming).
- ☐ 3,000 units heparin for systemic anticoagulation.
- ☐ 10,000 units heparin in saline for pre-filter infusion and volumetric pump.
- ☐ Dialysis fluid no. 61 (for CAVHD) and volumetric pump(s).
- ☐ Replacement fluid and volumetric pump.
- ☐ Blood pump (for venovenous systems).

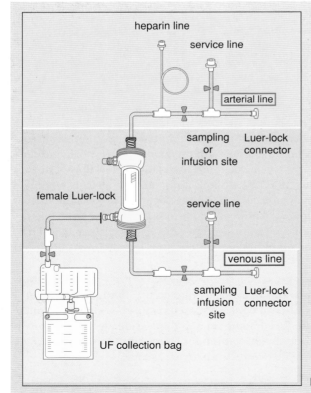

Technique

The technique for CAVH and CAVHD is described. Venovenous systems are similar but include a pump with high pressure and air alarms. For the arteriovenous systems, vascular access can be via a Scribner shunt or femoral catheters. The silastic Scribner shunt is inserted usually by a surgeon, using either the posterior tibial artery in the leg or the radial artery in the arm. This is the method of choice where long-term vascular access is required. Insertion of femoral catheters is described below. For venovenous systems, a double-lumen catheter can be inserted in a major vein (e.g. femoral, internal jugular or subclavian) using the Seldinger technique (p. 12), or single-lumen catheters can be placed in two separate veins.

The extracorporeal system and haemofilter must be assembled according to the manufacturer's instructions (Fig. 4.10) and primed with 2 litres normal saline containing 5000 units heparin/litre. Make sure all air

▶ ▶ ▶

Fig. 4.10 The assembled circuit and filter for CAVH

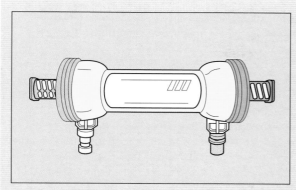

Fig. 4.11 A hollow fibre haemofilter

▶ ▶ ▶

bubbles are removed. The haemofilter has an arterial inlet port (red) and a venous outlet port (blue) at either end, and two ultrafiltrate ports on the side (Fig. 4.11). The arterial and venous sides of the circuit also are colour-coded. When using CAVH, the ultrafiltrate port toward the arterial end of the filter should remain capped off. Clamp the haemofilter to a drip stand at the patient's level. Place the filtrate collection container below the level of the haemofilter.

For arteriovenous techniques, it is best to use the femoral artery and vein on the same side, but failing that use femoral vessels on opposite sides. If neither of these options are available it is possible to use a femoral artery and a subclavian or internal jugular vein. For cannulation of femoral vessels on the right side, the patient should be supine with the right leg abducted slightly.

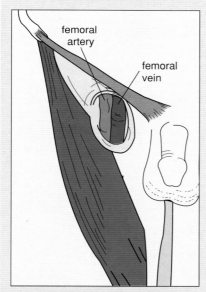

Fig. 4.12 Anatomy of the femoral artery and vein

1 Shave any hair from the right groin.
2 Clean the insertion site thoroughly with antiseptic solution and drape the area.
3 Palpate the femoral arterial pulse at the midpoint of a line drawn between the anterior superior iliac spine and the symphysis pubis. The femoral artery and vein lie in the femoral sheath, just below the inguinal ligament, with the vein medial to the femoral artery (Fig. 4.12). Infiltrate 5ml of local anaesthetic at each insertion site 3cm below the inguinal ligament, 1cm medial to and directly over the femoral pulse .
4 Insert the venous catheter first: attach a 10ml syringe to the thin-wall needle supplied in the catheter kit. Puncture the skin over the femoral vein and advance the needle at 45° and cephalad, while gently aspirating on the syringe.
5 On puncturing the femoral vein, detach the syringe taking care not to dislodge the needle. Insert approximately 10cm of the guidewire through the needle (soft end first). Remove the needle without dislodging the guidewire. If instead, the femoral artery is punctured, proceed in a similar fashion and place the arterial catheter first.
6 Using the scalpel blade, make a small incision through the skin and subcutaneous tissue adjacent to the wire. Feed the dilator and catheter over the wire and, with the right hand, push them down into the vessel, while the left hand applies gentle pressure on the overlying skin (Fig. 4.13). The latter will help to prevent the guidewire rucking up outside the vein which can be a problem when placing large-bore cannulae.
7 Remove the dilator and guidewire, leaving the catheter in the vein. Flush the catheter with 5–10ml heparinised saline and apply a clamp.
8 Repeat steps 4–7 for the femoral arterial catheter.
9 Systemically heparinise the patient with 3000 units heparin intravenously. ▶ ▶ ▶

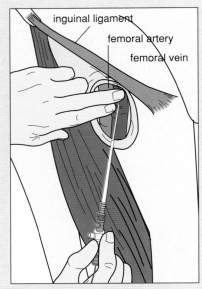

Fig. 4.13 Insertion of a femoral dilator and catheter

▶ ▶ ▶

10 Connect the heparin (10,000 units in 1litre saline) infusion line to the arterial side of the circuit. Set the volumetric pump to give 1ml/kg/h (10 units/kg/h).

11 Make sure all tubing clamps on the extracorporeal circuit are closed and that all Luer lock fittings are screwed together tightly. Connect the arterial end of the extracorporeal circuit to the femoral artery catheter and fully tighten the connector locking ring.

12 Remove the clamp on the arterial catheter and open the roller clamps on the extracorporeal circuit. Arterial blood will enter the circuit and saline prime will drain from the venous end. Reapply the arterial clamp when most of the prime has drained and then connect the venous line to the venous catheter. This reduces the volume of prime infused to the patient.

13 Remove the two catheter clamps and open the venous and arterial roller clamps. Open the side clamp on the heparin infusion line and turn on the volumetric pump to start the infusion.

14 Allow the blood to flow through the haemofilter for 3–5 minutes before opening the clamp on the ultrafiltrate tubing.

CAVH.

15 To decrease the ultrafiltration rate, raise the collection container. To increase the ultrafiltration rate lower the collection container.

16 Determine the 24 hour fluid balance required and calculate the hourly loss required, e.g. 2000ml/24h = 83ml/h. The volumetric pump for the replacement solution can be adjusted each hour to administer the appropriate volume of fluid based on the previous hour's fluid balance (taking into account all fluids, including ultrafiltrate). Urea clearance is increased if the replacement fluid is infused into the arterial side of the circuit before the filter (predilution) (Fig. 4.14); this reduces the blood viscosity and increases flow across the filter.

CAVHD

17 See Fig. 4.15. Attach a 1litre bag of dialysis fluid to a volumetric pump. Set the pump to 999ml/h. To maximise the urea clearance, use a double giving set with 2 litre of dialysis fluid running through two pumps. Attach the ultrafiltrate tubing, with the clamp closed, to the side port on the arterial end of the haemofilter. Connect the dialysing fluid administration set to the side port at the venous end of the haemofilter. Open the tubing clamp on the ultrafiltrate line and start infusing the dialysis fluid. This will be running counter to the blood flow. Connect the replacement fluid infusion into the venous side of the circuit (post-filter).

18 Adjust the heparin infusion to maintain the activated clotting time (ACT) or partial thromboplastin time (PTT) 1.5–2.0 times the baseline value.

19 A significant drop in the ultrafiltrate rate suggests that the haemofilter has clotted and both it and the circuit need replacing. Red blood cells will appear in the ultrafiltrate if there is a significant leak in the haemofilter. Again, the filter and circuit will need replacing. ▶ ▶ ▶

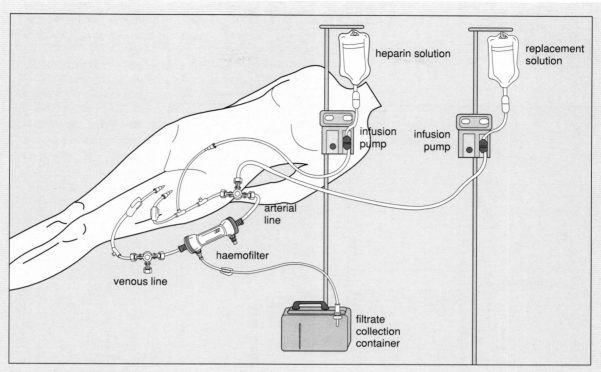

Fig. 4.14 CAVH with predilution

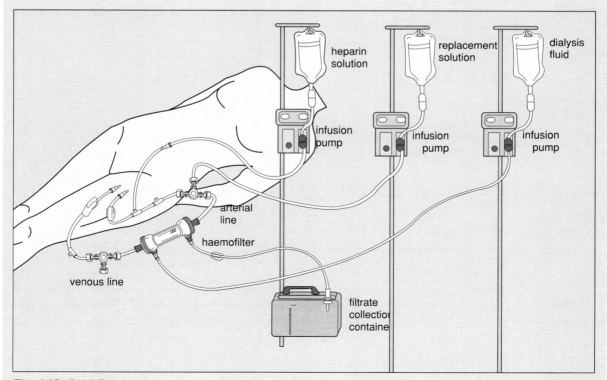

Fig. 4.15 CAVHD

▶ ▶ ▶

CVVH or CVVHD

20 Venovenous techniques require the use of a blood pump which incorporates pressure and air/foam sensors. Assemble the pump and tubing according to the manufacturers instructions. The specific details of this are outside the scope of this book but an example of a pump and circuit arrangement is shown in Fig. 4.16. When using a blood pump the replacement fluid should be infused after the filter. When the pump is started, increase the flow gradually, up to 200ml/min, to minimise the risk of hypotension.

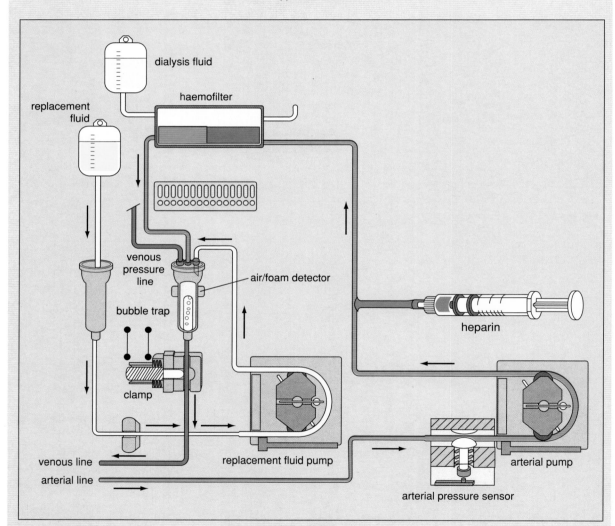

Fig. 4.16 Blood pump and circuit for CVVHD. The 'arterial' line refers to blood coming from the patient

Complications

- Filtrate output, particularly in the first hour, may be high and can result in hypotension unless adequate replacement fluids are given immediately. Fluid balance can be a significant problem and requires the constant attention of suitably trained nurses. During CAVHD, control of fluid balance can be made easier by placing a volumetric pump on the ultrafiltrate outflow tubing. This pump is set to its maximum rate (usually 999ml/h) while the pump controlling the in-flow of dialysis fluid is set at a lower rate, calculated from the required negative fluid balance. Electrolyte imbalance is an obvious potential complication and will need careful monitoring (every 4 hours in the first 24 hours). Hypophosphataemia can occur during CAVHD.
- Patients on CAVHD may become hyperglycaemic and may require an insulin infusion, particularly if the infusion rate of the dialysis fluid is 2 litre/h.
- Frequent clotting of the haemofilter can be a problem in some patients. At best, the filter has a life span of about three days, but frequently they will clot in less than 24 hours. Strict monitoring of the ACT or PTT and the addition of epoprostenol may prolong filter life.
- Rarely, the relatively large catheter in the femoral artery may cause peripheral ischaemia. Unrecognised disconnection may result in exsanguination but the use of Luer lock connections should minimise this risk.

Key points

- Urea clearance during CAVH can be improved by infusing the replacement fluid before the haemofilter.
- CAVHD will produce higher urea clearance than CAVH.
- The addition of a pump is needed for CVVH and CVVHD; both will produce higher urea clearances than their unpumped, arteriovenous counterparts. However, the use of pumped systems requires further training.
- Patients undergoing CAVHD with blood urea levels above 25mmol/l will require a dialysis infusion rate of 2 litre/h.

Hazards

- Large volumes of ultrafiltrate are produced during CAVH and meticulous fluid balance is essential.
- During the first 24 hours in particular, plasma electrolytes must be monitored closely.

Ultrasound examination of the abdomen
(Dr David Tarver MRCP, FRCR)

Ultrasound scanning (US) is a diagnostic technique using the reflection of high frequency acoustic waves from tissue interfaces to generate a sectional image of the part of the body under examination. The frequency of the energy used is above the range of human hearing and is, therefore, termed ultrasound. The generation of ultrasound waves utilises a property of some crystalline materials (e.g. lead zirconate titanate) called the piezoelectric effect. If a high electric potential difference is applied across such a crystal it will expand. Conversely, if the polarity of the potential difference is reversed, the crystal will contract. Therefore, if an alternating potential difference is applied at a frequency of 1 million cycles/second (1MHz), the crystal will expand and contract (oscillate) at a frequency of 1MHz. The oscillation generates acoustic waves with the same frequency. Any individual crystal will have an inherent resonance frequency at which oscillations are optimised, thereby generating acoustic energy in the surroundings most efficiently. A basic ultrasound probe is designed to generate ultrasound waves of one particular frequency and contains a piezoelectric crystal designed to resonate at that frequency.

When a pulse of ultrasound waves enters the body, the energy encounters many tissue interfaces, each of which will cause reflection of some of the energy and allow transmission of the remainder. The remaining energy will subsequently encounter deeper tissue interfaces at which a proportion again will be reflected. Since the velocity of acoustic waves in human tissues is constant, the time at which the energy returns to the US probe after its original transmission is a measure of the depth of the tissue interface below the probe. Returning ultrasound energy is detected by the converse property of a piezoelectric crystal, whereby if the crystal is compressed it will generate a potential difference and if the crystal is exposed to oscillating compressions, such as returning acoustic energy of its resonant frequency, an oscillating potential difference will be generated. An ultrasound probe functions by alternating short pulses of ultrasound with longer periods of 'silence' during which reflected energy is detected. The pattern of ultrasound reflections is used to generate a grey scale image of the section of the body beneath the probe.

The spatial resolution of the image is directly related to the frequency of the ultrasound energy, whereas the depth of penetration of the energy is inversely related to the frequency. Therefore, the frequency of ultrasound used for medical examination is a compromise between adequate penetration and spatial resolution. For abdominal ultrasound, a frequency of approximately 3MHz is suitable for adults and 5MHz for children.

Ultrasound probes are of the sector, linear or curvilinear variety. Sector or curvilinear probes transmit fan-shaped ultrasound beams which examine a relatively large area of the body and are therefore the most suitable type for abdominal examination.

ADVANTAGES OF ULTRASOUND

- Ultrasound provides excellent differentiation of soft tissue structures which cannot be achieved from plain X-ray examination.
- Ultrasound equipment is relatively mobile and portable units are available. This allows the scanning equipment to be moved to the patient, who may be medically unstable and connected to relatively immobile monitoring and support equipment.
- Medical US has no known adverse side effects; it is, therefore,ideal for patients who may need repeated imaging. It is safe in young or pregnant patients and in patients with an unknown history. There is no risk to other patients and staff in the critical care unit.
- Basic US equipment is relatively inexpensive.

DISADVANTAGES OF ULTRASOUND

- The technique is very operator-dependent and requires considerable expertise. In most centres in the UK, abdominal ultrasound is performed by radiologists with ultrasound training. However, non-radiological medical personnel perform US in some centres, particularly in the USA.
- Sensitivity of US for intra-abdominal pathology may be limited by:
  obesity
  intra-abdominal gas which will block transmission of ultrasound waves
  relative inaccessibility of some parts of the abdomen to scanning (e.g. hypochondrial regions)
  insensitivity of some serious pathology to US (e.g. hollow viscus perforation in the absence of free intraperitoneal fluid).
- Optimum visualisation of some regions of the abdomen (e.g. splenic region) may require turning the patient. This is not always possible with critically ill patients in critical care units
- US requires application of mild but significant pressure on the abdominal wall. This may be distressing for conscious patients with abdominal trauma or painful abdominal conditions.

It is important that the ultrasonographer is aware of his or her own limitations, and the limitations of the technique, in order to avoid being lulled into a false sense of security if the US detects no abnormality.

ULTRASOUND AND PATIENT CARE

Indications

Abdominal trauma.
Ruptured aortic aneurysm.
Renal failure.

Acute abdominal trauma

This is a common indication for abdominal ultrasound in critical care units and in some centres is performed in the resuscitation area.

The spleen is frequently injured in significant blunt abdominal trauma. The location of the spleen deep to ribs can make visualisation difficult. However, it is important to systematically examine all regions of the spleen, if possible, to avoid missing serious pathology. The sonographic findings in trauma include parenchymal cleft-like tears, capsular tears, subcapsular collections (haematoma), intraparenchymal haematoma or haemoperitoneum at perisplenic or remote abdominal locations (Figs. 4.17, 4.18). Several studies have confirmed the high sensitivity of US for detecting haemoperitoneum associated with significant splenic injury. However, the presence or absence of haemoperitoneum should be viewed with caution for the following reasons:

- US is not 100% sensitive for detecting free intraperitoneal fluid, particularly if the fluid remains in a perisplenic location.
- There may be no haemoperitoneum in the presence of significant splenic trauma if the splenic capsule remains intact.
- Even in the presence of splenic trauma, free fluid may be due to other associated injuries, such as bowel rupture or pancreatic trauma, the splenic injury being surgically insignificant.

The detection of the splenic parenchymal injury itself can be unreliable with US, due to the small size of some lesions, restricted visualisation of the splenic region and minimal difference in echogenicity between normal and traumatised parenchyma in the acute stage.

US is an acceptable modality for rapid evaluation of splenic trauma in emergency situations, but decisions between surgical and conservative management should not be based primarily on the results of US.

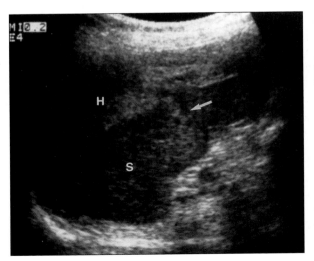

Fig. 4.17 US of traumatic splenic rupture (arrow)
S = spleen H = perisplenic haematoma

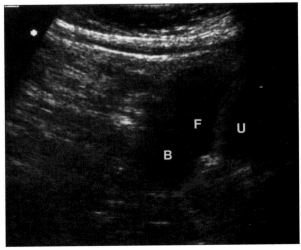

Fig. 4.18 US of free intraperitoneal fluid
F = free fluid B = bowel loops U = urinary bladder

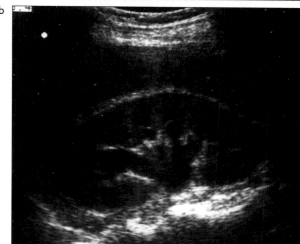

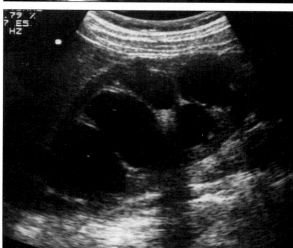

Other abdominal organs may be injured either in isolation or in addition to splenic injury. US is a useful modality for the detection of hepatic or renal rupture or haematoma. Visualisation of these organs often is more reliable and complete than the spleen. US may also detect retroperitoneal haematoma and aortic injury (see below).

Ruptured aortic aneurysm

US is a sensitive modality for assessing aneurysmal dilatation of the abdominal aorta (luminal diameter greater than 2.5cm in the upper abdomen). US may also detect aneurysmal rupture as a periaortic collection (haematoma) or free intraperitoneal fluid. However, if clinical suspicion of rupture of an aneurysm is high, particularly in a patient with a known aortic aneurysm, the patient should proceed directly to surgery. The absence of detectable haematoma or free fluid does not exclude rupture and the time required to perform a scan can delay surgical intervention sometimes with fatal consequences.

Renal failure

Acute renal failure can occur for several reasons in patients in critical care units. Renal failure is broadly divided into obstructed and non-obstructed groups with very different management implications.

Ultrasound is an excellent modality for assessing the presence or absence of obstruction. The normal renal collecting system is an elongated hyperechoic (bright) area in the centre of the kidney surrounded by the hypoechoic (dark) renal parenchyma (Fig. 4.19a). The normal calyceal spaces should be barely visible in the centre of the collecting system. The presence of a fluid-filled hypoechoic cleft in the centre of the collecting system, progressing to communicating cyst-like spaces, indicates hydronephrosis (Figs. 4.19b, 4.19c). The presence of actual renal cysts can produce a confusing and potentially misleading appearance. Also, reversible mild collecting system dilatation can be caused by a full bladder and should not be confused with obstruction. The presence of non-obstructed renal failure can be inferred from the demonstration of a normal calibre collecting system, in appropriate clinical circumstances, providing enough time has elapsed for an obstructed system to distend. In addition, the unobstructed failing kidney can be swollen or atrophic and alterations can occur in parenchymal echogenicity, producing either darker or brighter renal parenchyma than normal.

Fig. 4.19 US of renal outflow obstruction: normal kidney (**a**); moderate hydronephrosis (**b**); advanced hydronephrosis (**c**)

Equipment

☐ A mobile real-time US scanner with a 3MHz sector or curvilinear probe or a 5MHz probe for children.

☐ Aqueous US gel to prevent reflection of ultrasound from skin surface.

Technique

For abdominal scanning, no advance preparation is absolutely necessary, although a six-hour fast with clear fluids only by mouth is an advantage. For pelvic scanning, a very full bladder is required to displace gas-filled bowel and provide an acoustic 'window'. If the patient is catheterised, the catheter can be clamped to allow the bladder to fill. Alternatively, the bladder can be filled retrogradely to enable the scan to be performed more promptly.

1 Place the patient in a supine position and expose the abdomen.
2 Apply US gel copiously to the skin.
3 Examine the entire abdominal wall and flanks in longitudinal and transverse planes, applying light pressure only with the probe.
4 Pay particular attention to the solid upper abdominal organs.
5 Adjust the plane of section from the orthogonal planes for optimal visualisation of particular organs (e.g. to obtain longitudinal sections of the kidneys or common bile duct).
6 Specifically examine the pelvis (particularly the pouch of Douglas in women), the subhepatic space and the subphrenic space for free intraperitoneal fluid.
7 If the condition of the patient permits, raise the patient's left and right sides to aid scanning of the flanks. This improves visualisation of the kidneys, spleen, subphrenic spaces and superior parts of the liver. Controlled deep inspiration can also improve visualisation of these structures by flattening the diaphragm and pushing them inferiorly for improved probe access.

Key points

- The technique is mobile and readily available.
- Good differentiation of soft tissues.
- It is safe.
- The technique is very operator-dependent and requires training and experience
- There is a potentially significant false-negative rate.

Central Nervous System

Lumbar puncture

In general medical practice, lumbar puncture is used for both diagnostic and therapeutic purposes and some of these are listed below. Lumbar puncture is used in anaesthetic practice for subarachnoid block and this technique is further covered on pp. 234–239. The technique of the puncture is similar for the two types of practice, so anaesthetists may wish to read the following section, before going on to p. 234.

Successful lumbar puncture requires placement of an appropriate size needle in the lumbar subarachnoid space, below the caudal limit of the spinal cord (Fig. 5.1). This section describes puncture in two patient positions, the lateral decubitus and the sitting; lateral and midline approaches to the space are used. There are other patient positions and approaches that are equally useful in some circumstances. However, these two positions and two approaches are the most commonly used.

Indications

Diagnosis of central nervous system (CNS) disease.
Management of CNS disease including tumours of the lymphoreticular system.
Removal of cerebrospinal fluid (CSF) for intracranial pressure (ICP) control.
Measurement of intrathecal pressure.
Radio-diagnosis of CNS disease.
Subarachnoid neural block.

Contra-indications

Absolute
Known raised ICP due to lesions occupying intracranial space.
Local sepsis at site of puncture.
Unwilling patient.

Relative
Coagulation disorders.
Systemic sepsis.
Progressive neurological disease (for spinal anaesthesia).

Equipment

☐ Antiseptic solution.
☐ 1% lignocaine for skin infiltration.
☐ Appropriate skin and spinal needles plus syringes.
☐ Manometer tubing.
☐ Sterile sample collection bottles.
☐ Adhesive dressing for puncture site.

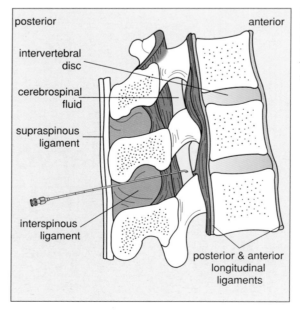

posterior   anterior

intervertebral disc

cerebrospinal fluid

supraspinous ligament

interspinous ligament

posterior & anterior longitudinal ligaments

Fig. 5.1 The lumbar spine seen in lateral section with spinal needle puncture of the subarachnoid space

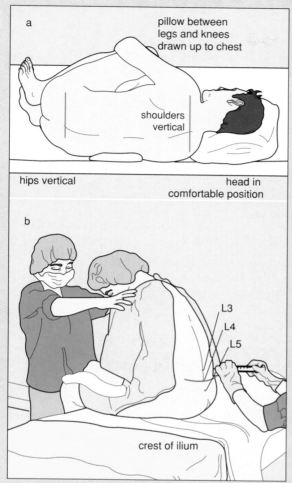

Fig. 5.2 The patient may be positioned in either (**a**) the lateral decubitus or (**b**) the sitting position

a — pillow between legs and knees drawn up to chest
shoulders vertical
hips vertical
head in comfortable position

b — L3 L4 L5
crest of ilium

Technique

The procedure should be explained to the patient, or the parent/guardian, as it may be necessary for an assistant to provide sedation or general anaesthesia in the young or the confused. A rapid and safe puncture demands a co-operative and immobile patient.

The choice of position is a matter of physician preference: in paediatric patients, for example, it may be useful to ask an assistant to hold the child in the fetal position. In adults, the puncture can be performed in the lateral decubitus position or in the sitting position (Fig. 5.2). It is important that the patient understands the position that is required, and that an immobile target is preferable to a moving one. In the sitting position, it is helpful if the patient is allowed to lean over a table, with the feet resting on a low stool. For patients in the lateral decubitus position, it is helpful to place a small towel under the lower flank if the lateral approach to the subarachnoid space is to be used as this tends to 'open up' the space.

The theca is usually punctured below the lower end of the spinal cord to avoid cord damage, thus the lumbar interspace 2/3, 3/4 or 4/5 is the usual site. A line drawn between the posterior superior iliac spines (Tuffier's line), will cross the L3/4 interspace or the 4th lumbar spine (Fig. 5.3).

The choice of spinal needle is dependent on several factors: age of patient, predicted difficulty of puncture and reason for puncture. 22G (rarely bigger) needles are useful for removal and manometry of CSF because they permit a good flow of fluid; they are also useful in patients with difficult punctures because they are more rigid than smaller gauge needles. 25G or 26G needles are appropriate for paediatric patients and for the performance of spinal anaesthesia; they have the disadvantage of being relatively flexible but are associated with a lower incidence of postspinal headaches (see 'Complications'). It is useful to insert an introducer needle before using a 25G or 26G needle as this may provide greater rigidity; some kits provide such an introducer needle, but a standard 18G 3.5cm needle is adequate.

1 Identify the intended interspace, in relation to Tuffier's line. Mark this point with a pen.
2 Don sterile gloves and a sterile gown. Clean and drape the back in an area with a 6–8cm radius around the mark.
3 Infiltrate local anaesthetic into the skin, subcutaneous tissues and the supra- and interspinous ligaments. Wait a few moments for this to take effect. ▶ ▶ ▶

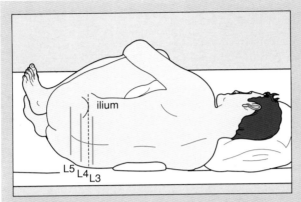

Fig. 5.3 Tuffier's line joins the posterior superior iliac spines and crosses the spine at the level of the L3/4 interspace

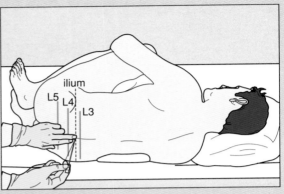

Fig. 5.4 The spinal needle should be directed 10° cephalad

▶ ▶ ▶

4 Select an appropriate needle, together with introducer if necessary. Ensure that the hub of the needle will fit the manometer tubing, if pressure manometry is to be performed.

Midline approach

5 Identify the middle of the chosen interspace in the midline, insert the spinal needle or introducer through the skin and direct it 10° cephalad (Fig. 5.4). It may be useful to advance the needle with one hand and use the other hand to restrain the needle close to the skin. The introducer needle should be inserted until ligamentous resistance is felt and the spinal needle is then inserted through it. Make sure the bevel of the spinal needle is facing laterally.

6 Continue to advance the spinal needle, until a loss of resistance is felt. This will usually indicate that the ligamentum flavum and dura have been penetrated.

7 Withdraw the stylet and wait for CSF to drip from the hub. Flow through 22G needles is brisk but a 25G or 26G needle allows only slow flow of CSF. Cerebrospinal fluid is typically 'crystal-clear' and will test positive for glucose. The presence of blood or pus may alter its colour.

8 If CSF does not appear, replace the stylet and advance the spinal needle a little further.

9 If bone is encountered, withdraw the needle and direct it slightly more cephalad.

Lateral approach

5 Confirm the midline of the chosen interspace and then identify a point 1.5cm lateral to the midline. In the lateral decubitus position, this should be the upper side (Fig. 5.5). A towel placed under the dependent flank is particularly helpful with this approach.

6 Advance the introducer or spinal needle, in a direction 10° cephalad and 20° towards the midline, until the resistance of the ligamentum flavum is felt. If bone is encountered, direct the needle slightly more cephalad, but not towards the midline (Fig. 5.6). ▶ ▶ ▶

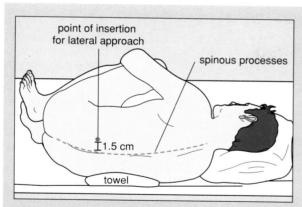

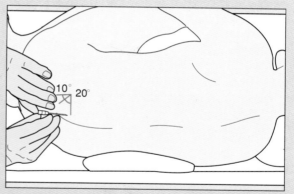

Fig. 5.5 The position for a lateral approach to the subarachnoid space: the needle should be inserted 1.5cm lateral to the midline, on the upper side

Fig. 5.6 The needle is directed 10° cephalad and 20° towards the midline

▶ ▶ ▶

7 When the resistance of the ligamentum flavum is felt, proceed as above.

This technique is useful in the obese patient and in patients with ankylosis of the spinous ligaments, as identification of these ligaments is not required.

Hazards

- Post-spinal headache.
- Local infection or haematoma formation.
- Meningitis, arachnoiditis and neuritis.
- Nerve or spinal cord damage.
- Backache and nerve root pain.

Complications

- Failed puncture is the commonest problem. This can be reduced by rechecking the patient position to ensure maximal flexion of the thoracolumbar spine. This will 'open up' the interspaces. It may be necessary, for paediatric patients, to get an experienced nurse to curl the patient up into this position. The problem of bony resistance can usually be overcome by confirming that the puncture is in the midline of the interspace and that the needle is directed cephalad. If this fails, consider the lateral approach.
- Post-spinal headache is a distressing problem that tends to affect young ambulant patients after lumbar puncture. Use of 25G or 26G pencil point needles (Whiteacre or Sprotte) and adequate hydration after the procedure reduces the incidence of post-spinal headache. Some patients who develop this problem will require an epidural blood patch; see p. 240 on epidural anaesthesia.

Key points

- Good patient position, especially lumbar flexion, is essential for successful puncture.
- Full aseptic precautions should always be observed.
- The lateral approach may be useful in the obese patient.
- An introducer needle is helpful for needles smaller than 24G.
- If bone is encountered, direct the needle in a cephalad direction.
- If cephalad direction is unhelpful, try a lateral approach, especially in patients with bony ankylosis of the spine.

Intracranial pressure monitoring
(Tom Kneuth MD)

Within the non-compliant skull, any increase in the volume of brain tissue, cerebrospinal fluid or blood is partially compensated by decrease in the other components. Intracranial pressure (ICP) remains within normal limits until a critical volume is reached, at which point any further increase in volume results in a rapid rise in ICP and a concomitant decrease in cerebral perfusion pressure (CPP). Hypoperfusion with global cerebral ischaemia and brain tissue herniation with localised ischaemic brain damage are the deleterious consequences of increased ICP and must be avoided.

When the Glasgow Coma Scale (GCS) score is above 8, changes in the neurological examination, particularly in the level of consciousness, provide an adequate indication of the ICP. Below a GCS score of 8, or in patients who are sedated and/or paralysed when clinical signs cannot be evaluated, ICP monitoring devices are needed to detect changes in ICP.

Mechanical, haemodynamic and drug therapy are used to maintain the ICP below the critical threshold of 15–20mmHg and continuous monitoring is necessary to evaluate the effects of therapy. Three basic types of monitoring devices are available, each of which has inherent risks and advantages. The intraventricular catheter (IVC) gives the most accurate and reliable measurements but imposes the greatest risk of infectious complications. The subarachnoid bolt is simple to insert and decreases the risk of complications, but readings can be unreliable and it is used less frequently. The extradural transducer is the most commonly used device today because of its ease of insertion, accurate readings and low complication rate.

Equipment

- ☐ 1% lignocaine with 1:200,000 adrenaline for local anaesthesia.
- ☐ Scalpel.
- ☐ Artery forceps.
- ☐ Drill.
- ☐ Catheter (no. 5 or no. 8 paediatric feeding tube will suffice. (Standard IVC kits are also satisfactory).
- ☐ Transducer and monitor.
- ☐ Bone wax.
- ☐ Normal saline (without preservative).
- ☐ 3/0 silk and 3/0 nylon suture.

Technique

Place the patient in the supine position and shave an area of the scalp on the right side. The area should be large enough to provide a sterile field and to allow application of an occlusive dressing at the end of the procedure. Prepare the scalp with antiseptic solution and apply the drapes.

Intraventricular cannula

1 Anaesthetise the skin and underlying subcutaneous tissues and periosteum over the coronal suture in line with the ipsilateral pupil (Fig. 5.7).

2 Make a 3cm incision, carrying it down to the periosteum. Scrape the periosteum away with the periosteal elevator (Fig. 5.8).

3 Drill a hole through to the inner table of the skull, being careful to avoid laceration of the dura. This can be prevented by setting the drill bit so that only enough to penetrate the skull protrudes.

4 Pass a small haemostat through the incision subcutaneously to a point 10–15cm laterally. Make a small stab incision over this point and pass the distal end of the catheter (feeding tube) through the stab wound and out through the original incision (Fig. 5.9).

5 Make a small cut in the side of the catheter and insert the tip of the stylet of the ventricular needle so that it can be used to guide the catheter into place (Fig. 5.10). ▶ ▶ ▶

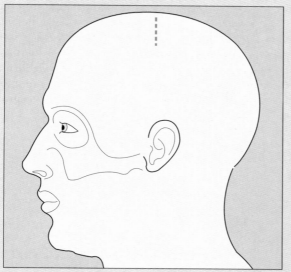

Fig. 5.7 Infiltration of the skin and subcutaneous tissues

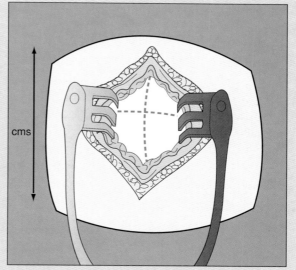

Fig. 5.8 Skin incision for placement of intraventricular cannula

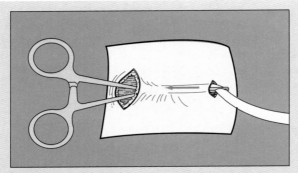

Fig. 5.9 Passage of catheter from stab wound to incision

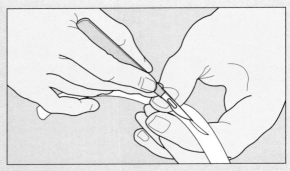

Fig. 5.10 Incision of catheter to accomodate ventricular needle

▶ ▶ ▶

6 Slowly introduce the catheter until fluid is obtained (5cm in the adult). Aim for the inner canthus of the ipsilateral eye and antero-posteriorly at a point 1cm anterior to the external auditory meatus (Fig. 5.11). Make sure that there are no kinks in the catheter.

7 Close the incision and coil the excess catheter on the scalp and secure it with suture in three places to prevent inadvertent dislodgement (Fig. 5.12). Apply an occlusive dressing and attach the catheter to the transducer.

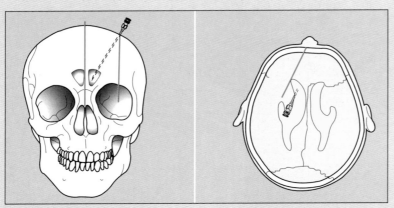

Fig. 5.11 Direction for placement of intraventricular catheter

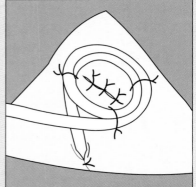

Fig. 5.12 Skin closure and fixation of catheter

Subarachnoid bolt

1 The landmarks for the insertion of the subarachnoid bolt are identical to those described for the intraventricular cannula.

2 Make a 4cm incision in line with the ipsilateral pupil and retract the skin with a mastoid retractor.

3 Remove the periosteum using a scalpel blade.

4 Make a hole using a drill that matches the size of the device being placed (0.6cm is usual). Use bone wax to stop bone bleeding.

5 Open the dura, including the arachnoid dura, using a no. 11 scalpel blade. Estimate the depth of the hole using a ventricular needle to determine how far to insert the bolt without impacting on the brain. ▶ ▶ ▶

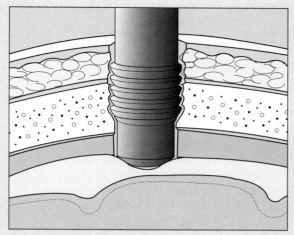

Fig. 5.13 Subarachnoid bolt in position

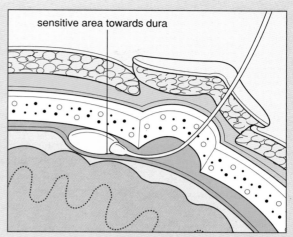

sensitive area towards dura

Fig. 5.14 Fibre-optic sensor in place

▶ ▶ ▶

6 Screw the bolt in place (Fig. 5.13).
7 Close the skin on either side of the bolt.
8 Fill the bolt with sterile saline to ensure that there is no air in the system to dampen the waveform. Attach the bolt to the transducer and ensure that all couplings are tight.
9 Apply an occlusive dressing.

Extradural transducer

1 The location, incision and burr hole for the extradural transducer are identical to those described for the subarachnoid bolt.
2 Free the dura from the table of the skull to avoid a wedge effect.
3 Insert the fibre-optic sensor so that it lies completely under the bone (Fig. 5.14).
4 Anchor it in place at the skin.
5 Close the skin and apply an occlusive dressing.

Another commonly used transducer is the Camino fibre-optic catheter. The sensor is at the tip of the catheter, which is inserted through the skull in a similar manner to the subarachnoid bolt.

Complications

• Infection.
• Intracerebral haemorrhage.

Hazards

- With the subarachnoid screw and the subdural cannula, correlation with ventricular pressures can be spurious and extraction of CSF is not possible.
- Maintenance of calibration can be problematic.
- Frequent clogging is a problem with the subarachnoid screw.

These technical problems can lead to incorrect management based on inaccurate measurements if the clinician relies solely on the ICP values. To avoid this hazard, before making major management changes, factors that can mislead ICP interpretation should be assessed and additional information should be sought including:

- Patency of the airway.
- Position of the head and neck.
- Level of the transducer.
- Transducer zero and calibration.
- Ventilator setting and respiratory pattern.
- Body temperature.
- Blood pressure.
- Arterial blood gas measurement.
- Serum electrolytes measurement.
- Computed tomography (CT) scan.

Key points

- ICP monitoring has become a routine part of the management of head-injured patients in whom clinical neurological examination cannot be relied upon as a guide for management.
- With the fibre-optic catheters, the procedure is simple and safe and the measurements are reliable. Although not a hazard of the monitoring device itself, the primary hazard of monitoring can be therapy based solely on the values obtained without an appreciation of the overall condition of the patient.
- Abnormal readings should trigger further investigation and be used only to complement clinical and diagnostic findings.
- Physicians and nurses need to understand the benefits and limitations of the systems to ensure safe and meaningful ICP monitoring.

Burr hole craniotomy
(Tom Kneuth MD)

Indications

Acute extradural and subdural haematomas in a patient with rapidly deteriorating neurologic function.

Drainage of chronic subdural haematomas.

Access for ICP monitoring.

Ventricular drainage.

Drainage of cerebral abscesses.

Cerebral biopsy and tumour diagnosis.

Contra-indications

For a non-neurosurgeon: a stable patient when neurosurgical consultation is reasonably available.

Overwhelming infection.

Coagulopathy.

Morbidity and mortality from intracranial hypertension and brain herniation due to intracranial haematomas are preventable if recognised early and treated aggressively. It is therefore incumbent upon all surgeons to be familiar with the life-saving technique of burr hole insertion and the elevation of a craniotomy flap for the emergency evacuation of subdural and extradural haematomas. This skill is especially important for surgeons working in rural or remote areas, where a neurosurgeon is not immediately available and the delay inherent in transportation to a neurosurgical facility could result in the patient's rapid demise. It should be stressed, however, that the only indication for which a non-neurosurgeon should consider this technique is when the patient is deteriorating rapidly and a neurosurgeon is not available.

A single burr hole does not provide enough exposure to make it worthwhile, even as a stopgap measure, in treating a traumatic intracranial haematoma. In this setting, burr holes are of value only as a diagnostic procedure in preparation for an immediate craniotomy. With the wide availability of CT, exploratory burr holes are rarely needed. The main indication is to provide access for ventricular drainage or ICP monitoring, but burr holes are also occasionally adequate for drainage of abscesses and chronic haematomas and for biopsy of cerebral tumours.

Equipment

- ☐ Hair shaving kit.
- ☐ Suction.
- ☐ Scalpel.
- ☐ Bulb syringe.
- ☐ Small self-retaining retractor.
- ☐ Dural hook.
- ☐ Periosteal elevator.
- ☐ Vicryl suture.
- ☐ No. 3 Penfield dural elevator.
- ☐ Skin staples.
- ☐ Gigli saw or power craniotome.
- ☐ Drill set.
- ☐ Diathermy apparatus.
- ☐ Hudson brace.
- ☐ Rane clips.
- ☐ Artery forceps.
- ☐ 4/0 suture.

Technique

Full preoperative neurological assessment is required. Hypoxaemia and hypotension must be stabilised before a meaningful examination is possible. Urgent CT scanning is imperative for accurate diagnosis. A non-contrast CT is adequate in most cases and a minimum of four axial views are usually required to demonstrate the parasagittal sulcus, the lateral ventricles, the middle fossae and the posterior fossa. In a rapidly deteriorating patient, a single axial cut at the level of the lateral ventricles will detect the majority of mass lesions requiring immediate craniotomy. Cerebral arteriography is a reasonable alternative if CT scanning is unavailable. If these diagnostic facilities are unavailable, exploratory burr holes are begun on the same side as the dilated pupil.

As well as the burr hole, the surgeon should be prepared to perform the craniotomy, which should be done only in the operating room.

When an exploratory burr hole is indicated, the patient is placed in a supine position with easy access to both sides of the head. Exploration is undertaken on the side of the dilating pupil, on the side of any unilateral fracture, or contra lateral to progressive motor weakness or posturing. When CT scanning has localised the haematoma to one side, the head is turned 45° to expose the appropriate side of the scalp. A roll is placed under the shoulder to prevent undue stress on the cervical spine.

1   Induce general anaesthesia with tracheal intubation and intermittent positive pressure ventilation.
2   Shave the hair completely; prepare the scalp with antiseptic solution and drape in a sterile fashion.
3   Plan a scalp flap that will provide generous access to the lesion. The width of the base of the flap should approximate to its length and should not be narrower than the widest point of the flap. Mark the skin with methylene blue or a similar marker using the sagittal suture, the coronal suture and the zygomatic arch as landmarks. Begin 1cm in front of the ear so that the superior temporal artery is preserved and 1cm above the zygomatic arch so that the facial nerve is not injured. Draw a question mark going above the ear up to 3cm lateral of the midline and to a point in front of the coronal suture (Fig. 5.15). ▶ ▶ ▶

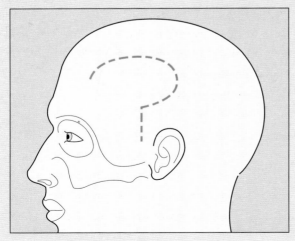

Fig. 5.15 Skin markings for scalp flap

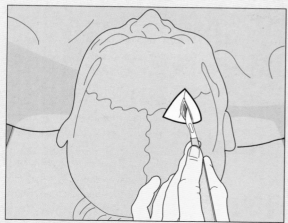

Fig. 5.16 The initial incision in a patient deteriorating rapidly

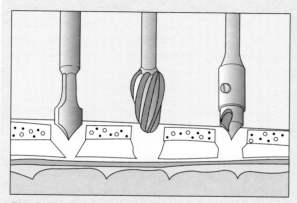

Fig. 5.17 Cutting a burr hole

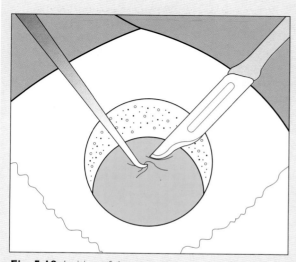

Fig. 5.18 Incision of dura mater

▶ ▶ ▶

Burr hole

4 If the patient has been deteriorating rapidly, the portion of the incision anterior to and above the ear should be opened quickly first. Make a 2cm incision down to the bone (Fig. 5.16). Use a self-retaining retractor to open the wound widely.

5 Scrape the periosteum to each side using a periosteal elevator.

6 Using a Hudson brace, cut the hole in two stages. First, drill a small hole through the inner table with a skull perforator. Use extreme caution to avoid penetration into the brain. Once the inner table is penetrated, use a conical burr or a Soutar's drill to enlarge the hole (Fig. 5.17) in the inner table. Be careful to avoid separating the dura from the bone since this may result in extradural venous bleeding.

7 Elevate the dura with a sharp hook and incise it with a small scalpel blade (Fig. 5.18). Enlarge the incision in a cruciate fashion using scissors.

8 This completes the burr hole. Multiple diagnostic burr holes might be useful only in rare situations in which no diagnostic tests are available and the patient is showing progressive deterioration without focal signs such as in a frontal or occipital haemorrhage. Similarly, contralateral burr holes after a completed craniotomy are indicated only when the surgeon strongly suspects a previously undiagnosed contralateral mass (i.e. when intraoperative swelling in a normal looking hemisphere might be due to an enlarging contralateral haemorrhage). Most often, when clinical signs suggest a unilateral mass and the first burr hole is unrevealing, the surgeon should proceed with the craniotomy rather than multiple burr holes.

Craniotomy

9 Incise the skin as marked.

10 Use special galeal clips (Rane clips) or Dandy haemostats to minimise bleeding from the subgaleal space (Fig. 5.19). ▶ ▶ ▶

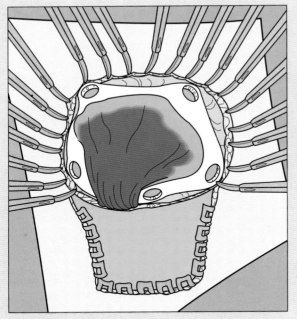

Fig. 5.19 Galeal haemostatic clips and burr hole sites

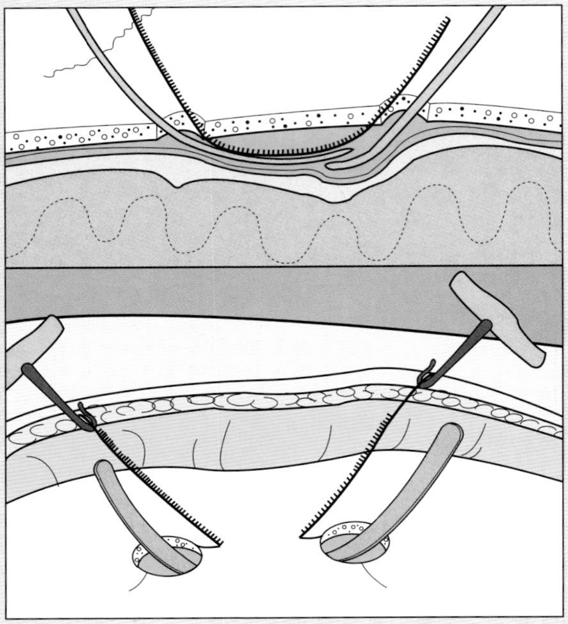

Fig. 5.20 Interconnection of burr holes using Gigli saw

▶ ▶ ▶

11 Strip the scalp flap from the underlying pericranium and temporalis fascia by gentle sharp dissection and retraction.

12 Using the diathermy coagulation point, incise the temporalis fascia and muscle in the line of the intended bone flap, except inferiorly, where a pedicle of pericranium and temporalis muscle is left uncut to retain blood supply to the bone.

13 Drill five burr holes over the frontal, parietal and temporal bones (Fig. 5.19). Placing burr holes close to each other (6–7cm) makes the craniotomy easier.

14 Using a no. 3 Penfield dissector, dissect the dura off the under surface of the skull. In case of an epidural bleed, this has already been done by the haematoma.

15 Connect the burr holes by cutting the bone between them with either a power-driven craniotome or a Gigli saw, which is passed between the holes using a malleable saw guide (Fig. 5.20).

16 Elevate the flap using a periosteal elevator and a no. 3 Penfield instrument (Fig. 5.21), using care to avoid penetrating the dura. If an epidural haematoma is present, elevation of the bone flap brings it into view.

17 At this point, obtain haemostasis. In most cases, the middle meningeal artery is the source of the bleeding and should be suture-ligated with 3/0 vicryl. Small, bleeding dural vessels should be obliterated by coagulation with a bipolar diathermy. Stop bleeding from the bone with bone wax.

18 Evacuate the haematoma by irrigation using a bulb syringe and normal saline solution with gentle suction. ▶ ▶ ▶

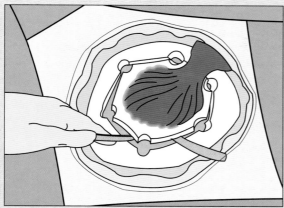

Fig. 5.21 Elevation of bone flap

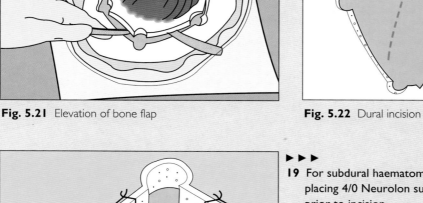

Fig. 5.22 Dural incision

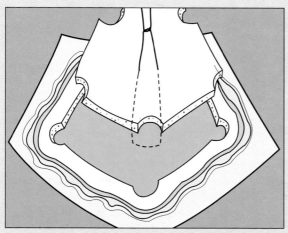

Fig. 5.23 Sutures attaching dura to pericranial tissues

Fig. 5.24 Pull through suture to attach dura to bone flap

► ► ►

19 For subdural haematomas, the procedure continues by placing 4/0 Neurolon suture in the dura to elevate it prior to incision.

20 Using a no. 15 blade make a 5–8mm incision in the dura, just enough to allow introduction of dural scissor blades. In the case of a subdural bleed, the dura will be separated from the brain by the haematoma.

21 Using the scissors, incise the dura in a H shape with the base toward the midline to avoid injury to large cortical veins, which often run from the brain onto the dura some distance from the sagittal sinus (Fig. 5.22).

22 Using warm saline irrigation under gentle pressure only, dislodge the haematoma from the brain surface. A clot that is firmly adherent to the brain surface should be left alone since dislodging it may encourage further bleeding.

23 If such bleeding is encountered, apply haemostatic foam to the surface of the brain using a cotton patch with suction applied over it. Use direct coagulation of brain vessels only as a last resort.

24 After adequate decompression, complete haemostasis and visualisation of brain pulsations, close the dura in a watertight manner using a running stitch of 4/0 Neurolon.

25 Place sutures all around the dural incision to hold the dura to the inner table of the skull to prevent a postoperative extradural haematoma. The sutures are passed through the dura right against the cut edge of the bone and tied to the adjacent pericranium or muscle (Fig. 5.23). In addition, a suture may be placed in the centre of the flap and brought up through by drilling two small holes in the bone flap. (Fig. 5.24).

► ► ►

▶ ▶ ▶

26 Replace the craniotomy flap and suture it to the adjacent bone using silk sutures passed through holes made especially for this purpose. Alternatively, the bone can be held in place using interrupted sutures through the pericranium and muscle.

27 Place a subcutaneous suction drain brought out through a separate stab incision.

28 Suture the scalp in two layers. Use 2/0 inverted Vicryl sutures for the galeal layer and staples for the skin.

Complications

- Uncontrollable bleeding.
- Infection.
- Injury to brain tissue.

Key points

- Craniotomy and burr hole evacuation of extra-dural haematomas are life-saving techniques that should be performed by a non-neurosurgeon only when the patient has signs of herniation syndrome in progress and no neurosurgeon is available. Every emergency surgeon should be prepared to perform this vital technique.
- Meticulous adherence to principles of sterility, haemostasis and critical postoperative care provide the patient with the best chance for a good recovery.

Hazards

- Inability to control bleeding from the middle meningeal artery.

Patient controlled analgesia devices

The technique of patient controlled analgesia (PCA) was first described in the 1970s. Conventional techniques of analgesia are usually based on patient request resulting in physician/nurse administration, using a variety of drugs and routes. Patient controlled analgesia developed because it was recognised that individual analgesic requirements vary widely. The technique usually involves a three-stage procedure:

- If possible, the patient is instructed in the use of PCA before operation. The patient is told that they will receive an infusion of analgesic, usually into a vein, or less often, subcutaneously. The doses delivered by this infusion will be controlled by the patient, using a demand button. This button will not deliver more than the pre-programmed amount and if the patient finds this inadequate, the pump should be reprogrammed by the nurse or anaesthetist. Patients should be advised to try to predict episodes of maximal pain, such as during physiotherapy or turning, so they can then activate the button some 10–15 minutes in advance of the pain.

- The patient's pain should be controlled by titration of intravenous opioid analgesic. This is especially important in patients with severe post-operative pain.

- The pump is set up for use (Fig. 5.25). Some clinicians prefer to use a background *intravenous* infusion of an opioid in addition to demand bolus doses. *Subcutaneous* infusions of opioids have also been used and this may be a useful alternative where intravenous cannulation is difficult, or if the patient is to receive long-term analgesic therapy. The pump is then programmed to give a bolus dose, usually 5–10% of the normal intramuscular dose. A 'lock-out' time is then programmed into the pump, which determines the minimum time between boluses. It is also possible to programme a four hour limit on the dose, with some versions of the PCA machines. The patient is instructed once more in the use of the pump.

The patient's analgesic requirement may alter over the next few hours or days and this will be reflected in the patient's button demands and pain scores. When the patient's pain decreases significantly, the PCA system can be replaced by an alternative method of analgesia.

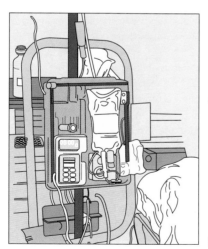

Fig. 5.25 An example of a PCA delivery system

Equipment

☐ Suitable size intravenous cannula (20–22G for adults, 22–25G for children).

☐ Container of opiod analgesic; usually a 50ml syringe of morphine in a concentration of 1mg/ml.

☐ PCA pump and patient demand button.

☐ Disposable bag and syringe for above pump.

☐ Specific opioid antagonist (optional).

☐ Y-tubing with one-way valve.

Technique

The analgesic solution should be prepared in a sterile manner, in a quantity sufficient for at least 24 hours use. Morphine and pethidine (demerol) are both popular and schemes for both agents are described.

- Morphine 50mg in 50ml of 0.9% saline; bolus dose 1mg (0.015mg/kg); lock-out five minutes, initially.
- Pethidine 1000mg in 100ml of 0.9% saline; bolus dose 10mg (or 0.15mg/kg); lock-out five minutes.

1 The syringe (or bag) containing the opioid should be labelled with the date and time of preparation.

2 Site an intravenous cannula of appropriate size, under aseptic conditions, preferably in the non-dominant arm.

3 Connect the tubing to the cannula. A one-way valve should be included in the tubing to prevent blood or other fluids backing up the intravenous line.

4 Programme the pump according to the instructions supplied. The scheme given above will be acceptable for most patients.

5 Demonstrate the action of pressing the button to the patient and ensure that a bolus dose is delivered.

6 Reset the pump recorder to zero and explain to the patient that they may now use the pump as described.

7 Secure the lock on the 'door' of the pump if it has one, to prevent tampering with the opioid infusion.

8 Write out a prescription chart for the pump and ensure that instructions for signs of opioid overdosage are included. The instructions should include a contact telephone or radiopager number, in case of problems. ▶ ▶ ▶

► ► ►

9 Visit the patient twice daily. Check the patient's pain scores, and the number of requests. Signs of inadequate analgesia include a high number of requests or high pain scores. The addition of nonsteroidal anti-inflammatory drugs (NSAIDs) will usually reduce the demand for opioids and should be prescribed concurrently unless contra-indicated.

Complications

- A common problem is blocking of the intravenous cannula, because of low flow rates. This can be prevented by the addition of a one-way valve and an additional fluid infusion through the PCA line.
- The local complications of PCA pump use are due to incorrect cannula placement and may result in infection, haematoma, extravasation and pain.
- Complications may occur because of incorrect programming of the pump resulting in an under- or overdose of analgesic. The pump itself may deliver a dose different to that programmed, although this is rare with the modern pumps. Thus, it is important to check the pump function at the beginning of the infusion. If any signs of incorrect dosage occur subsequently, the pump should be stopped and rechecked.
- Nausea is relatively common with PCA opioids and may be reduced by adding an antiemetic, e.g. droperidol 0.1 mg/ml.
- Some anaesthetists attach an ampoule of naloxone to the pump mechanism, to allow immediate treatment of opioid overdosage; 0.2–0.4mg intravenously is an appropriate prescription. It is however equally important that the responsible nurse can perform correct airway and ventilation management and support, to overcome such a problem.

Key points

- Check the intravenous site if the patient complains of inadequate analgesia.
- Add regular NSAIDs (unless contra-indicated) which can be continued once the PCA is no longer required.

Hazards

- Incorrect pump programming may cause opioid overdose.
- Do not allow another person to activate the button for the patient.

Monitoring neuromuscular blockade

After the use of neuromuscular blocking agents, it is important to confirm that adequate muscle function has returned. This may be done in several ways:

- A history of the dose, type and time of the muscle relaxant administered will indicate the likely time of return of adequate muscle power.
- Clinical signs: sustained head lift for five seconds, tongue protrusion for five seconds, sustained hand grip and normal forced vital capacity will all help to confirm adequate neuromuscular function.
- Stimulation of a peripheral motor nerve with an electrical stimulator. The contraction of the muscle group that follows may be felt, observed, or measured with an electromyograph (EMG) or a force transducer.

The clinical signs are useful in patients who are waking up, but these may not always reliably predict inadequate muscle function. More importantly, clinical signs give a poor indication of insufficient respiratory reserve. Careful measurement of forced vital capacity (FVC) may be helpful but is rarely practical in the recovering patient.

The most simple precise monitoring system is stimulation of a peripheral nerve with observation of the stimulated muscle group. Different patterns of electrical stimulation can be applied to the nerve via cutaneous electrodes. Interpretation of the observed muscle contraction helps in deciding the need for an anticholinesterase. Four patterns of stimulation are commonly used:

- Twitch–tetanus–twitch. In this method, 4 stimuli are given in 4 seconds, followed by 3 seconds of 50Hz, then another 4 stimuli in 4 seconds. This method will indicate the type of block but is poor in determining the degree of block.
- Train-of-four (TOF). Tetanic stimulation may be painful and may also alter the subsequent function of the stimulated nerve. Repeated train-of-four indicates the degree of block, by visual or electrical count of the number of twitches and the ratio of the fourth twitch strength to the first (T4:T1 ratio).
- Post-tetanic count. In the case of a very intense block, it may be necessary to apply 5 seconds of a 50Hz tetanic stimulus and then a repeated train-of-four. The count of visible twitches after this prolonged tetanic stimulus, the post-tetanic count, gives a good indication of the reversibility of the block.
- Double burst stimulation (DBS). This is a new technique designed to assess the degree of residual neuromuscular blockade. Two short bursts of 50Hz tetanus separated by 750ms are given and the response of the muscle group is observed. If there is no fade in the muscle contraction during the tetanic stimuli, then there is only a small

Indications

Assessment of neuromuscular blockade especially following:
- Prolonged anaesthesia.
- Renal/hepatic dysfunction.
- Muscle relaxant infusion.
- Novel/research neuromuscular blockers.
- Muscle or neuromuscular junction disease.

Exclusion of neuromuscular block before testing for brain stem death.

Contra-indications

Use of tetanic stimulus in awake patients.
Incorrect function of nerve stimulator.

chance of considerable residual paralysis. This method is more sensitive than the train-of-four (TOF) which may not detect residual paralysis in a substantial proportion of cases.

Equipment

☐ Peripheral nerve stimulator to deliver both 1Hz and 50Hz, at up to 50mA current: this requires a voltage of 50–300V. DBS is an optional feature that may confer more accuracy on neuromuscular block assessment.
☐ Skin electrodes with conducting jelly.
☐ Force transducer (optional).
☐ Electromyography (optional).

Technique

The battery function in the nerve stimulator should be tested either on a volunteer, or a patient who has not received muscle relaxants. However, the tetanic stimulus should never be used on a conscious patient. It is necessary to decide on the following for each patient:
• The nerve and muscle group to be stimulated (Fig. 5.26):
    ulnar nerve at the wrist and adductor pollicis
    ulnar nerve at the elbow and adductor pollicis
    facial nerve over the stylomastoid foramen and the facial muscles
    lateral popliteal nerve at the apex of the fibula and the peroneal muscles.
• The method of measuring the contraction produced:
EMG and force transduction will require calibration in the awake patient and may be subject to electrical interference in the operating theatre. Simple observations and palpation of the force of contraction is adequate for most clinical situations.

1 If a force transducer or EMG is to be used, it should be applied and calibrated before general anaesthesia and paralysis is induced.
2 Identify the surface markings of the nerve to be stimulated and clean the skin with a mild abrasive, such as fine sandpaper. Attach the electrodes to the skin, about 2–3cm apart and ensure that they are firmly applied.
3 Confirm that the nerve stimulator functions correctly and connect it to the electrodes.
4 Turn on the nerve stimulator and select a current of about 10–15mA. Apply a 2 second, 2Hz stimulus and look for contraction in the corresponding muscle group . If none is present, increase the current to the maximum, about 50mA, and after 1 minute, reapply a similar train-of-four. If no contraction is seen, go straight to (5); if contraction is seen, perform a post-tetanic count as at (6). ► ► ►

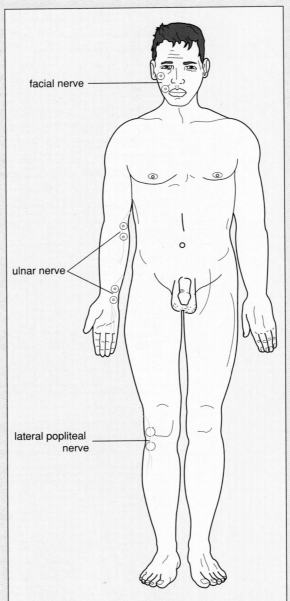

Fig. 5.26 Four possible sites for peripheral nerve stimulators: the ulnar nerve at the wrist; the ulnar nerve at the elbow; the facial nerve over the parotid gland; the lateral popliteal nerve over the head of the fibula

facial nerve

ulnar nerve

lateral popliteal nerve

▶ ▶ ▶

5 If there is no response to the above stimulus, consider the following:
  • The electrodes may not have made good contact with the skin. Resite new electrodes and repeat the above sequence.
  • The patient may have such a dense block that no response to train-of-four will occur. In this situation, perform a twitch-tetanus-twitch: give 4 stimuli at 1 Hz, then 3 seconds of tetanus, then 4 stimuli at 1 Hz.

 ▶ ▶ ▶

▶ ▶ ▶

6 Apply a 5 second stimulus at 50Hz and then immediately perform repeated train-of-four stimuli and count the number of visible muscle twitches that are seen. This number is the post-tetanic count.

7 Interpret the results in the following way:
   • Train-of-four, see Fig. 5.27.
   • Twitch-tetanus-twitch, see Fig. 5.28.
   • Post-tetanic count:
       <8, block is at this time irreversible
       8–12, block may be reversible within 10 minutes for medium duration muscle relaxants, e.g. vecuronium and atracurium.
       >12, block easily reversible.
   • DBS, absence of fade makes it very likely that the block can be safely antagonised.

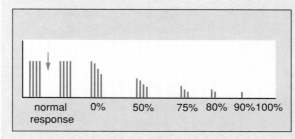

Fig. 5.27 The effect of increasing the neuromuscular junction block from 0–100% on the train-of-four twitch height

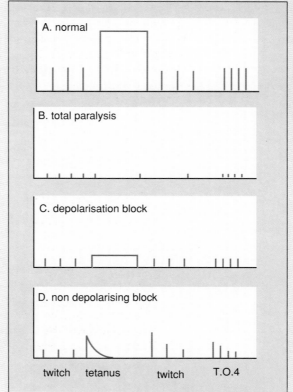

Fig. 5.28 The effect of twitch-tetanus-twitch according to the type and degree of muscular relaxation, measured by force transducer of the adductor pollicis muscle

231

Complications

- Technical problems are the commonest cause of poor results: inadequate electrode contact and low battery power are the most frequently cited. Occasionally, there will be such a dense block, that the above tests will not demonstrate any twitch, although this is unlikely. In this situation, recheck according to the above plan 20 minutes later.
- The type of muscle relaxant used will also help to determine the period of likely recovery. A faster recovery will occur following the use of the short- and medium-duration muscle relaxants such as suxamethonium, atracurium, vecuronium and ocuronium.
- Doubts have been raised concerning the correlation between the twitch pattern produced by the stimulation of a peripheral nerve and the power of the respiratory muscles. However, if clinical signs are combined with normal results for the adductor pollicis muscle, it is likely that adequate respiratory muscle power will be present.
- The current from peripheral nerve stimulators is insufficient to produce interference with cardiac pacemakers.

Hazards

- Pain from application of tetanic stimulus in an awake patient.
- False negative results .

Key points

- Check the battery, wires and electrodes before clinical use.
- Apply the electrodes according to the surface markings of a motor nerve.
- Do not apply repeated tetanic or twitch-tetanus-twitch stimuli to one single nerve.
- If twitch is absent, change sites and then use a twitch-tetanus-twitch pattern.
- Always correlate the pattern obtained with the timing and type of muscle relaxant used.

Spinal anaesthesia

Spinal anaesthesia, first described in 1898 by August Bier, is achieved by the injection of local anaesthetic into the subarachnoid space. The blockade of anterior and posterior nerve roots results in a temporary loss of motor power and sensation over a number of dermatomes.

Spinal injection of local anaesthetics, opioid analgesics or a combination of both may be used to provide analgesia for acute or chronic pain. However, this section will confine itself to the use of local anaesthetics for surgery.

The patient should be prepared in the same way as for any other regional or general anaesthetic. The patient should understand the risks and effects and should give consent for the procedure. An intravenous infusion is started and the procedure should be performed under sterile conditions.

EXTENT OF THE BLOCK

The height of the block is influenced by :
- Baricity, type and dose of local anaesthetic solution.
- Speed of injection.
- Site of injection.
- Use of barbotage.
- Moving the patient before local anaesthetic has 'fixed'.
- Use of vasoconstrictors in the local anaesthetic.

The height of the block may be increased by using hyperbaric local anaesthetic solutions prepared with dextrose solution ('heavy' solutions). A higher dose, or more rapid injection of local anaesthetic will also increase the height of the block. Gravity is an important factor; a slight head down posture, particularly when combined with a hyperbaric local anaesthetic solution, will result in a high block. Pregnancy, increasing age, short stature and kyphosis also all increase the height of the block. It is possible to produce a block that is appropriate for any surgery below the T5 level. A motor block above this level will be associated with marked hypotension and some degree of respiratory difficulty. There is great inter-patient variation to spinal blockade and even operator experience cannot always accurately predict the height of a block.

Generally, longer-acting blocks may be produced by the use of a larger (mg) dose of one of the long duration local anaesthetics. The addition of adrenaline (epinephrine) to the spinal block solutions is not widely favoured now, because of the risk of spinal cord ischaemia.

CHOICE OF ANAESTHETIC AGENT

The choice of agent will be influenced by the duration and height of the block required, and whether or not a unilateral block is required.

Duration

- Rapid onset, short duration blocks: 2% lignocaine or 5% lignocaine in 8% dextrose.
- Long duration blocks: 0.5% plain bupivacaine or 0.5% bupivacaine in 8% dextrose; 0.5% amethocaine in N/2 saline or 8% dextrose.

Height

The cutaneous dermatomes are shown in Fig. 6.1.

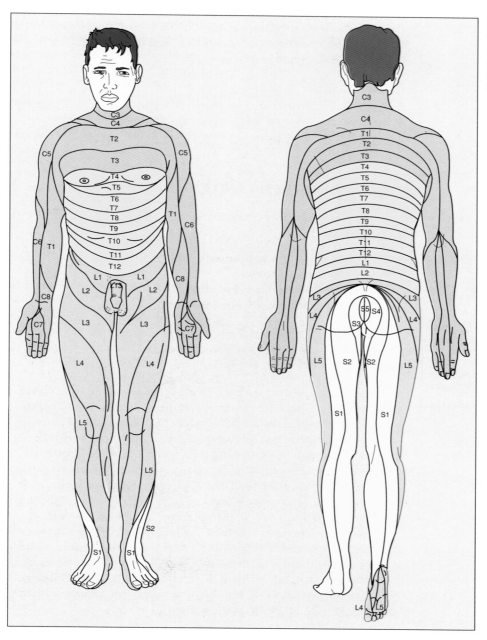

Fig. 6.1 The cutaneous dermatomes: low, medium and high blocks correspond to sacral, lumbar and mid-thoracic blocks, respectively

Saddle (sacral) block

Hyperbaric bupivacaine 1–1.5ml is given at the L4/5 interspace with the patient in the sitting position. Keep the patient in the sitting position for 10 minutes.

High lumbar blocks

A hyperbaric or isobaric solution is injected at the L2/3 interspace in the lateral position with the table slightly head up. The patient is then returned to the supine position quickly. For a block of longer duration, increase the dose of isobaric solution.

Mid-thoracic block

Inject a hyperbaric solution, e.g. 3.5–4ml 0.5% heavy bupivacaine at the L2/3 interspace with the patient in the lateral position. Quickly return the patient to the supine position.

Unilateral blocks

Inject 2–3ml of hyperbaric solutions with the patient in the lateral position on the affected side ('affected side down') and leave for 15 minutes. Return the patient to the supine position, just prior to surgery.

SPINAL ANAESTHESIA AND PATIENT CARE

Indications

Patient unwilling to have a general anaesthetic.

Anaesthesia for surgery lasting less than 2–4 hours below the costal margin, particularly when a bloodless field is important.

Post-operative pain relief (especially using spinal opioids).

Pharmacological sympathectomy for patients with poor perfusion of lower limbs.

Equipment

☐ Equipment as for lumbar puncture (see p. 210).
☐ Filtered drawing-up needle.
☐ Local anaesthetic of chosen baricity and type.
☐ Spinal needle of appropriate type and size.

Technique

The patient should be prepared in the same way as for any surgical procedure: adequate resuscitation facilities and qualified assistance are essential before the block is started. An intravenous infusion of 1000–2000ml of crystalloid or colloid solution via a wide-bore intravenous cannula is given and full monitoring of blood pressure, pulse and SpO_2 is instituted. It may be necessary at this point to sedate the patient, after a full explanation has been provided.

There are many types and sizes of spinal needles (Fig. 6.2): the smaller needles will not allow rapid flow of CSF on entering the subarachnoid space and may be difficult to site in patients with bony ankylosis. However, smaller needles are associated with a lower incidence of postspinal headache (see below) and this is an important factor in choosing a needle. Sprotte and Whiteacre needles are associated with a lower incidence of headache than Quincke needles of similar size. ► ► ►

Contra-indications

Absolute

Unwilling patient.

Local sepsis.

Hypovolaemia.

Raised ICP due to space
  occupying lesions.

Patient with a fixed cardiac output,
  e.g. severe aortic stenosis.

Relative

Systemic sepsis.

Coagulation disorders.

Chronic backache.

Stable neurological disease.

Agitated patients.

Procedure expected to last more
  than two hours.

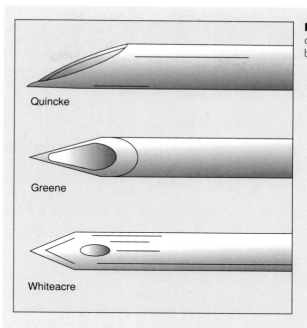

Fig. 6.2 Types of spinal needle bevel

Quincke

Greene

Whiteacre

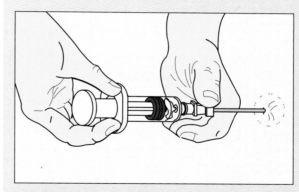

Fig. 6.3 The left hand restrains the spinal needle while the syringe containing local anaesthetic is attached

▶ ▶ ▶

1 The patient should be placed on a trolley which can be easily tilted into the head-down position. The patient is put into the chosen position for lumbar puncture, which will be determined by the intended spread of block. The lumbar puncture is then performed in the same way as for a diagnostic puncture, see p. 210.

2 When the subarachnoid space has been punctured, replace the central guide in the hub of the spinal needle, to temporarily occlude the flow of CSF. Then, remove it and attach the syringe containing the local anaesthetic.

3 Hold the spinal needle with one hand (Fig. 6.3) to steady it. With the other hand, gently draw back on the plunger of the syringe, to confirm free flow of CSF. Aspiration of CSF causes swirling patterns as it mixes with the local anaesthetic. If this does not occur, rotate the spinal needle 90° and repeat the process. If this fails, withdraw and re-insert the spinal needle. ▶ ▶ ▶

▶ ▶ ▶

4   Do not draw back more than 0.1–0.2ml of CSF, unless barbotage is to be used. Barbotage is the practice of producing a higher block by mixing CSF with the local anaesthetic solution.

5   Ask the patient to remain very still and then inject the local anaesthetic over 20 seconds. If there is resistance to injection, stop immediately and re-aspirate CSF into the syringe. If it is impossible to aspirate CSF, remove the syringe and rotate the spinal needle 90°. If this fails, re-insert the needle and inject the *remainder* of the local anaesthetic.

6   At the end of the injection, remove the syringe and needle together and put an adhesive dressing over the puncture site.

7   The patient should be placed in a position appropriate for the type of block (see above). The desired block will normally be achieved within 10 minutes.

Complications

Hypotension is a common problem with spinal anaesthesia. It is a result of sympathetic blockade, causing vasodilatation. The higher the block the greater the degree and duration of hypotension. Blocks above T5 may also cause bradycardia secondary to cardiac sympathetic inhibition. Short stature, pregnancy and increasing age also make high blocks more likely.

Hypotension may be attenuated by pre-loading with 1–2 litre of crystalloid solution intravenously. Measurement of systemic blood pressure using an automated non-invasive blood pressure device should be performed every 2–3 minutes initially. The development of hypotension requires a rapid infusion of 500ml of fluid and the use of a vasoconstrictor. Appropriate drugs include ephedrine 5mg, methoxamine 2mg, or phenylephrine 20mcg, administered as boluses as required. Treat any bradycardia with atropine 0.3–1.0mg. The patient's posture should not be changed, although *all pregnant patients should either be in the left lateral tilt or full lateral position*, to prevent the syndrome of supine hypotension, due to inferior vena cava compression. The patient may develop nausea (with or without vomiting) just prior to the development of hypotension.

Blocks above T10 cause a progressive loss of intercostal muscle power, although this is unlikely to be a problem in healthy patients, where intercostal function is not important at rest. There is also a slight increase in physiological deadspace. Sensory blocks of the thoracic segments may cause a feeling of dyspnoea, but the patient can be reassured if they are asked to take a large breath. Anaesthesia that extends into the cervical region will cause progressive phrenic nerve block. This will cause a decreased tidal volume and may result in respiratory failure in patients with limited reserve. Such high spinal blocks, associated with loss of motor power in the hands (C7, T1) will be characterised by marked hypotension, a soft voice and progressive dyspnoea. The patient should be pre-oxygenated and given a small dose of an induction agent, followed by a muscle relaxant. The trachea should be intubated and mechanical ventilation commenced. Then, the hypotension should be aggressively treated as above. The high block will decrease after 1–2 hours depending on the dose and type of local anaesthetic used.

Post-spinal headache is one of the most distressing complications of dural puncture. The headache is typically occipital and usually develops within 24 hours of dural puncture. It is more common in young patients and is more likely to develop after puncture with a large-gauge, cutting needle. The sitting position typically makes the headache worse, but keeping the patients supine after dural puncture does not reduce the incidence of post-spinal headache.

The treatment depends on the duration and severity:

- Mild headaches may be managed with increased fluid intake and simple analgesics such as dihydrocodeine and paracetamol.
- An epidural blood patch is indicated for those patients with severe headaches, especially if associated with photophobia and malaise. This procedure involves two physicians, one of whom punctures the epidural space while the other takes 10–20ml of sterile blood for epidural injection. A blood patch will cure over 90% of such headaches.

Other complications include: backache, urinary retention, local infection and haematoma. Cranial nerve palsies, arachnoiditis and meningitis are rare.

Key points

- Ensure adequate assistance and correct equipment before starting.
- Have a fast running intravenous infusion in place before starting.
- Position the patient appropriately for the type of block required.
- Use a small pencil point needle to reduce post-dural puncture headache.
- Use accompanying sedation/general anaesthesia where appropriate.

Epidural anaesthesia and analgesia

Many types of drugs have useful activity when introduced into the epidural space:

- Local anaesthetics will produce sensory, motor, and sympathetic neuronal blockade.
- Narcotic analgesics produce spinal analgesia, as well as respiratory depression and sedation.
- Alpha 2 adrenoceptor agonists cause hypotension (or abolition of the pressor response), sedation and analgesia.
- Ketamine produces sedation and analgesia.
- Glucocorticoids such as methylprednisolone or triamcinolone, in a preservative-free form, may be used for their anti-inflammatory properties.

Operative and post-operative analgesia may be provided by a mixture of a local anaesthetic and an opioid analgesic, or local anaesthetic alone. The agents may be given by injection through the epidural needle, or more often by infusion via a catheter placed in the epidural space.

RELEVANT ANATOMY

The epidural space is formed by the two reflections of the dura. It extends from the foramen magnum cranially to the sacral hiatus caudally, where it is covered by the sacrococcygeal ligament. The space is covered in its posterior part by the ligamentum flavum, which is itself separated from overlying skin by various ligaments. The anterior border of the epidural space is the posterior longitudinal ligament, which covers the posterior aspect of the vertebral bodies (Fig. 6.4). The distance from the ligamentum flavum to the dura varies from 3mm in the cervical region to 6mm in the lumbar region; the distance from the skin to the epidural space is about 3.5–5.5cm in the lumbar region and 2.0–3.5cm in the cervical region. A given volume of local anaesthetic will spread over more dermatomes in the cervical region than in the lumbar region.

The contents of the space are:

- Fat.
- Blood vessels.
- Nerve roots from the spinal cord that acquire a covering of dura as they emerge from the space.

Local anaesthetic delivered into the space will block the emerging nerves at the site of injection and, as the volume is increased, will extend further through the space in both caudad and cephalad directions.

The space has a negative pressure within it, which varies according to site: it is most negative in the cervical and thoracic regions and may even be slightly positive in the lumbar region, especially during pregnancy and in the sitting position. Identification of the epidural space during

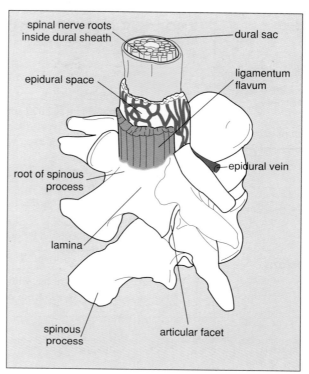

Fig. 6.4

Horizontal section of a typical lumbar epidural space and relations

Labels in figure:
- spinal nerve roots inside dural sheath
- dural sac
- epidural space
- ligamentum flavum
- epidural vein
- root of spinous process
- lamina
- spinous process
- articular facet

puncture makes use of this negative pressure: loss-of-resistance techniques or negative pressure techniques may be used. Loss-of-resistance techniques depend on the movement of air or saline from a syringe into the space, as the epidural needle tip enters the space. The use of saline has the advantage of a slightly lower incidence of accidental dural puncture, but carries the problem of being confused with CSF. The use of an air-filled syringe does not cause such confusion, but may be associated with more difficult catheter insertion. Both techniques are described and the reader should decide on their own preference. Negative pressure techniques, such as the hanging drop and Odom's indicator, are used very infrequently.

The epidural space can be cannulated at any point from the lower cervical vertebrae to the caudal (sacral) hiatus. However, the levels most often chosen are:

- Thoracic level for analgesia of structures innervated by the thoracic dermatomes.
- Lumbar level for lumbar and lower thoracic dermatomal block.
- Caudal level for sacral, lumbar and low thoracic dermatomal block.

Epidural cannulation at the thoracic and lumbar levels may be performed using either a lateral (paramedian) or midline approach and both of these approaches are described. The caudal approach to the space is a separate technique and will also be described.

THORACIC AND LUMBAR EPIDURAL PUNCTURE

Indications

Operative anaesthesia and peri-operative analgesia using local anaesthetics and/or opioid analgesics.

Injection or infusion of drugs such as steroids or alpha 2 agonists with activity in the epidural space.

Epidural blood patch.

Radiological investigation of the epidural space.

Contra-indications

Absolute

Unwilling patient.

Local sepsis.

Hypovolaemia.

Raised ICP due to space-occupying lesions.

Left-to-right cardiac shunt (air-filled syringe only).

Relative

Systemic sepsis.

Coagulation disorders.

Neurological disease.

Agitated patients.

Equipment

☐ Antiseptic solution.

☐ 2% lignocaine with 1:200,000 adrenaline.

☐ 23G needle with 2ml syringe for skin infiltration.

☐ Range of drawing-up needles.

☐ No. 11 scalpel blade.

☐ 10ml syringe, either plastic or glass.

☐ 20ml of sterile 0.9% saline.

☐ Preservative-free 1.5% lignocaine with 1:200,000 adrenaline or 0.5% bupivacaine.

☐ Suitable size Tuohy epidural needle, usually 16G or 17G for adults and large children (Fig. 6.5).

☐ Epidural catheter.

☐ Bacterial filter for catheter, with Luer lock hub.

☐ Adhesive dressing to run from puncture site over shoulder.

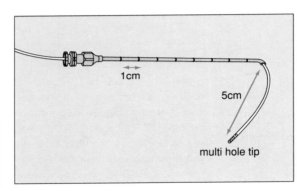

Fig. 6.5 A typical epidural catheter shown protruding from the end of a Tuohy needle

Technique

The patient should be prepared in the same way as for any surgical procedure: adequate resuscitation facilities and qualified assistance are essential before the block is started. In adults, an intravenous infusion of one litre of crystalloid or colloid solution is given via a wide-bore intravenous cannula and monitoring of blood pressure (BP), pulse and arterial oxygen saturation is instituted. A vaso-constrictor such as ephedrine 3mg/ml or methoxamine 2mg/ml should be drawn up. It may be necessary at this point to sedate the patient, after a full explanation has been given.

The patient should be placed on a flat trolley, which can be easily tilted into the head-down position. The patient is then positioned according to the type, approach and technique to be used:

- Caudal epidural is performed either in the lateral Sims (Fig. 6.6a) or semi-jack-knife prone position (Fig. 6.6b). ▶ ▶ ▶

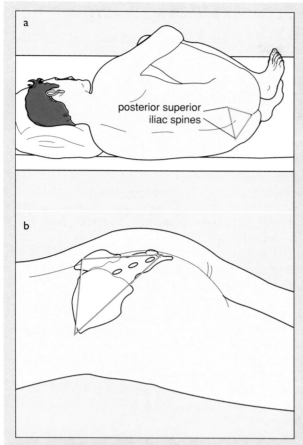

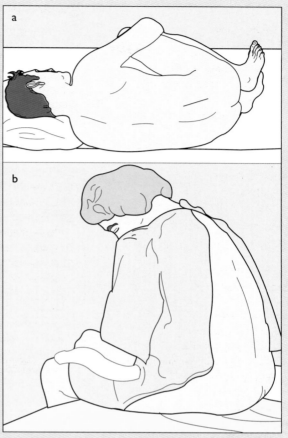

Fig. 6.6 Patient in lateral Sims position, the prone jack-knife position for caudal injection

Fig. 6.7 Patient positions for lumbar epidural

▶ ▶ ▶

- Lumbar epidural is performed either in the lateral position (Fig. 6.7a) or the sitting position. When using the latter, it is useful if the patient rests his or her feet on a stool, with the head, neck and thorax flexed (Fig. 6.7b).

- Thoracic epidural is usually performed in the lateral position. A small towel or pillow should be placed under the thorax at the chosen level, if the paramedian approach is being used, to 'open up' the intervertebral space to allow easier puncture from above (Fig. 6.8). ▶ ▶ ▶

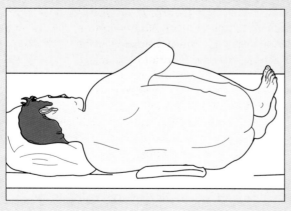

Fig. 6.8 Patient in lateral position for thoracic epidural puncture (note the small towel under the lower thorax, to open up the intervertebral space)

► ► ►

The choice of technique will determine the contents on the sterile trolley. Practitioners using the loss-of-resistance-to-saline technique will need a conventional 10ml syringe and some sterile preservative-free normal saline. Those using air will need either a glass syringe, or one of the disposable plastic syringes (loss-of-resistance devices) which are included in many commercially prepared packs.

It is then necessary to identify the intervertebral space to be punctured: the seventh cervical vertebra (vertebra prominens) is the first spinous process that is clearly palpable below the back of the cranium. The chosen thoracic vertebra may be found by counting down the spinous processes from this point. As a further reference, the lower margins of the scapulae usually lie opposite T6. The lumbar vertebra may be identified as for lumbar puncture: the line that connects the posterior superior iliac spines, Tuffier's line, indicates the L3/4 interspace or the 4th lumbar spinous process. The identification of the sacral hiatus is described in the appropriate section below.

1 Make a small pen mark over the area of the intended puncture, based on the above landmarks. Don sterile gloves and gown and prepare the area around the mark with aseptic cleaning solution.
2 Open the sterile dressing or epidural pack and check the contents. Ensure that the epidural catheter is patent, has the appropriate markings and will pass through the epidural needle.
3 Infiltrate the skin, subcutaneous tissues and interspinous and supraspinous ligaments over the chosen interspace with local anaesthetic, using first a 23G and then a 21G needle.
4 Draw up 10ml of either air or sterile saline into the appropriate syringe.

Lateral (paramedian) approach
5 Make a 0.5cm incision in the skin over the chosen interspace, at a point 2cm above the midline (Fig. 6.9). Insert the epidural needle with the bevel at 90° to the long axis of the spine and advance the epidural needle towards the space, parallel and lateral to the spinous process. When the needle contacts the vertebral lamina, direct the needle tip cephalad and medially, at an angle of about 15° to the sagittal plane and walk the needle off the lamina and into the ligamentum flavum (Fig. 6.10).
6 Remove the needle stylet and attach the syringe containing air or saline to the hub of the epidural needle. With the left hand restrain the needle by holding the wings and with the right hand put gentle pressure on the plunger of the syringe (Fig.6.11).
7 Advance the needle by gentle pressure with the left hand. The right hand should maintain pressure on the plunger, but should not be used to push the needle forwards.

Midline approach
5 Identify the interspace chosen and make a 0.5cm incision with a scalpel blade, in the space between two spinous processes. Insert the epidural needle in the midline, with the bevel facing 90° to the long axis of the spine. The needle should be directed 10–20° cephalad (Fig. 6.12). ► ► ►

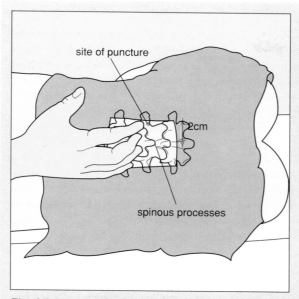

Fig. 6.9 Lateral (paramedian) approach to the epidural space; the needle is inserted 2cm lateral to the midline

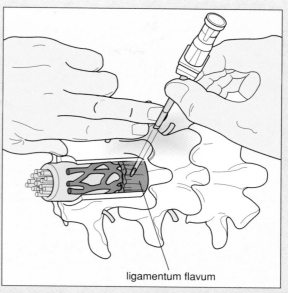

Fig. 6.10 The epidural needle has contacted the lamina, and is now directed in a medial and caudal direction

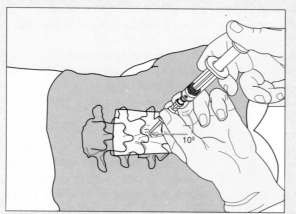

Fig. 6.11 The left hand restrains the advance of the needle, while the right hand maintains gentle pressure on the syringe plunger to identify the loss of resistance when the epidural space is reached

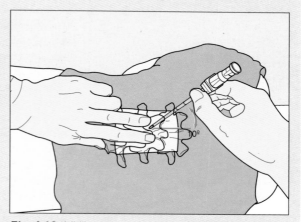

Fig. 6.12 Midline approach to the epidural space. The needle is directed 10–20° cephalad

► ► ►

6 Advance the epidural needle until it is firmly held in the interspinous ligament in the midline. This can be confirmed by the tendency of the needle to remain rigid when in the ligament; needles sited outside the ligament tend to flop easily.

7 Remove the stylet from the needle and attach the syringe containing air or saline to the hub of the needle. Restrain the needle with the left hand and put gentle pressure on the plunger with the right hand. The left hand should then advance the needle, while the right hand maintains pressure on the syringe plunger.   ► ► ►

► ► ►
Both approaches

8 As the needle reaches the ligamentum flavum, there will be an increase in resistance to the air or fluid flow from the syringe. The epidural space is directly beneath the ligamentum flavum, and it will require little advance with the needle to reach the space. Continue to advance the epidural needle using firm pressure with the right hand on the syringe hub. Entry of the needle tip into the epidural space is indicated by a sudden 'give' in resistance to the plunger and several ml of fluid or air may enter the space.

9 Stop advancing the needle and rotate it so that the bevel faces cephalad. Confirm that air/fluid still leaves the syringe freely: if it does not, withdraw the needle slightly and re-advance it in the same way as described for the loss-of-resistance technique.

10 Remove the syringe and check that fluid or blood does not come back into the hub: if it does, proceed as below (specific problems).

11 Hold the needle firmly with the right hand and insert the distal end of the epidural catheter into the needle. Advance the catheter gently until the 20cm mark is level with the hub. The 20cm mark is usually indicated by four close hatched circles on the catheter. The catheter should enter freely and excessive force should not be applied (Fig. 6.13). If the catheter will not thread beyond the first long mark (indicating that the catheter has not passed beyond the needle tip) the needle should be re-inserted after removing the needle and catheter as one. *Do not remove the catheter through the needle, as the needle point may shear off a portion of catheter.*

12 Note the point on the epidural needle where it penetrates the skin: the Tuohy needle will have centimetre markings along its length. Hold the catheter with the left hand and withdraw the needle over the catheter, making sure to push on the catheter as the needle is removed. When the needle has come out, withdraw the catheter until 4cm remains inside the space, i.e. the needle depth at insertion plus 4cm.

13 Connect the proximal end of the catheter to the locking system and the bacterial filter. Attach a sterile transparent dressing over the catheter entry site (Fig. 6.14) and run adhesive tape over this dressing up the patient's back and over the shoulder. ► ► ►

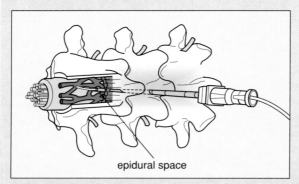

Fig. 6.13 The epidural catheter is advanced up the needle, which is firmly held in place

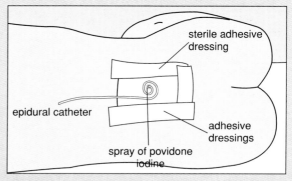

Fig. 6.14 The epidural puncture site is covered with a sterile transparent dressing

▶ ▶ ▶

14 Allow the patient to turn supine and then measure the blood pressure.

15 Attach a 2ml syringe to the filter and aspirate gently to see if fluid or blood appears in the catheter:

• If clear fluid is aspirated freely, test it for glucose by putting a small drop onto a blood sugar testing stick. A positive result indicates CSF and the catheter should be removed.

• If blood is aspirated, inject 10ml of saline through the catheter: wait 10 minutes and then repeat the aspiration. If blood recurs, remove the catheter.

• If no fluid flows, inject a test dose. The test dose must be able to detect either intravascular cannulation or intrathecal placement. An appropriate dose for a lumbar epidural is 3ml 0.5% bupivacaine with 1:200,000 adrenaline:

a rise in heart rate on the ECG of more than 20/min, within 90 seconds, indicates intravascular cannulation

inability to flex the hips after 10 minutes indicates an intrathecal puncture

a negative test does not exclude incorrect placement, but makes it very unlikely.

Level of catheterisation

• Lumbar catheters can be inserted with either a lateral or midline approach, in the lateral or sitting position.

• Thoracic catheters are best inserted in the lateral position using a lateral approach: the angle of the spinous processes is very steep in the thoracic region and midline puncture is difficult (Fig. 6.15).

• Cervical epidural cannulation is best performed in the sitting position using a midline approach.

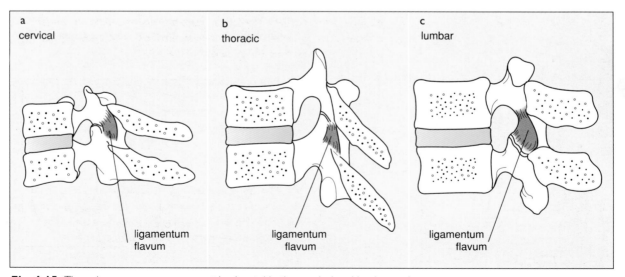

a cervical

b thoracic

c lumbar

ligamentum flavum

ligamentum flavum

ligamentum flavum

Fig. 6.15 The spinous processes are most horizontal in the cervical and lumbar regions

247

CAUDAL EPIDURAL INJECTION

Caudal injections deliver local anaesthetic into the epidural space through the sacrococcygeal membrane, at the lowermost level of the epidural space. The dura normally ends at the second sacral segment, but may extend as low as the fourth sacral segment in adults; the mean distance from hiatus to dura is 4–5cm but the range is wide in adults. In children the distance from the hiatus to the dura is much more constant and caudal techniques are particularly effective in this age group. Injection is usually by a single bolus from a needle, although it is possible to insert a catheter in the same way as for the levels described above.

Indications

To provide analgesia and anaesthesia covering the sacral and lumbar dermatomes.

Contra-indications

As for epidural puncture.

Equipment

- ☐ Antiseptic solution.
- ☐ 2% lignocaine with 1:200,000 adrenaline.
- ☐ 25G needle with 2ml syringe for skin infiltration.
- ☐ 0.25% bupivacaine.
- ☐ 21G needle (for adults).
- ☐ 23G needle (for children).
- ☐ 10ml or 20ml syringe.

Technique

Position the patient in the lateral Sims position or a semi-jack-knife prone position (Fig. 6.6). Don sterile gloves and gown, and clean and drape the skin over the upper part of the buttocks.

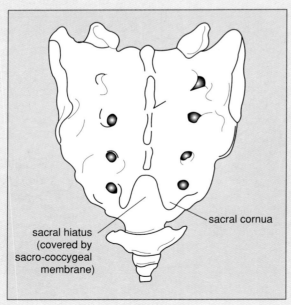

sacral cornua

sacral hiatus (covered by sacro-coccygeal membrane)

Fig. 6.16 The anatomy of the sacral canal

1 With the tip of the right index finger pointing caudad, palpate the coccyx. The sacral cornua will lie over the proximal phalanx of the operator's finger, 3–5cm from the tip of the coccyx (Fig. 6.16). The hiatus lies between the two cornua.

2 Infiltrate the skin and subcutaneous tissues over the hiatus with local anaesthetic.

3 Attach a 21G needle (adults) or 23G needle (children) to a 2ml syringe and insert the needle at an angle of about 80° to the long axis of the back, through the hiatus in a cephalad direction. 'Give' is felt as the needle enters the hiatus.

4 Immediately depress the syringe and needle, so that they lie parallel to the sacral canal, with the needle tip pointing cephalad (Fig. 6.17). Advance the needle about 1cm and then aspirate gently on the 2ml syringe: ► ► ►

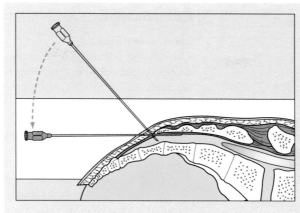

Fig. 6.17 The needle is directed more horizontally as the sacral canal is entered (note the proximity of the dura to the sacral hiatus)

▶ ▶ ▶

    • If blood or fluid appears, then remove the needle and syringe and re-insert as above.

    • If no fluid appears, attach a syringe containing local anaesthetic (see below) and inject a small volume of local anaesthetic while palpating over the sacrum. There should be little resistance to flow and no subcutaneous swelling. If this occurs, stop the injection and re-insert the needle. Appropriate total doses are shown below.

5 Remove the needle and apply a sterile adhesive dressing to the puncture site. Return the patient to the supine position and observe the pulse and the BP for the next 20 minutes.

CHOICE OF AGENT AND DOSE FOR EPIDURAL INJECTIONS

Caudal route

In adults, 20–30ml of 0.25% bupivacaine is usually sufficient.
In children the volume depends on the extent of block required:

- Sacral segments: 0.5ml/kg 0.25% bupivacaine plain.
- Lumbar segments: 0.75ml/kg 0.25% bupivacaine plain.
- Low thoracic segments: 1ml/kg 0.25% bupivacaine plain, to a maximum of 20ml.

Lumbar and thoracic route

- Bolus dose: 1.0–1.5ml 0.25–0.5% bupivacaine per dermatome to be blocked. In adults, preservative-free diamorphine 2mg or fentanyl 50–75mcg (in 10ml of saline) may be given as a single bolus in addition to the local anaesthetic.
- Infusion: 0.125–0.167% bupivacaine plain 2–10ml/h in adults according to height of block (diamorphine 0.1–0.2mg/ml or fentanyl 2–5mcg/ml may be added).

Complications

Local anaesthetics

The most important side effect of epidural anaesthesia with local anaesthetics is the production of a high block with associated hypotension and bradycardia.

This can be attenuated by i.v. infusion of 1–2 litres of crystalloid or colloid fluid before instituting the block and cautious injection of local anaesthetic.

Treatment consists of the administration of oxygen via a non-rebreathing mask, return to a supine position (left lateral tilt in parturients) and a rapid infusion of a bolus of colloid or crystalloid (dose 10ml/kg). Ephedrine in 6mg boluses may be necessary. Methoxamine 2mg is a useful alternative but is not recommended in the parturient because of its effect on the placental circulation. (Elevating the legs is useful, but it should not delay any of the other measures listed.)

High spinal block may occur after overdosage via the epidural space, or injection after accidental unrecognised dural cannulation. The priorities for treatment are:

- Ventilation with a face mask with 100% oxygen.
- Orotracheal intubation and ventilation should be rapidly instituted if the block extends as far as the level of C3. This should be facilitated by the cautious use of an intravenous induction agent and suxamethonium.
- Aggressive management of hypotension, which will include the use of infusions of fluid, inotropes and vasoconstrictors.

High blood levels of local anaesthetic arise from accidental intravenous injection or inappropriately high doses. Such levels produce generalised CNS excitation, followed by depression, which usually respond to discontinuation of the injection, high inspired oxygen concentration and benzodiazepines intravenously.

Common but less serious side effects include urinary retention and missed segments.

Opioid analgesics

Epidural opioids have a number of side effects of which the most dangerous is respiratory depression. This should be managed by ventilation by self-inflating bag valve mask device, or automatic resuscitator, followed by reversal with boluses of intravenous naloxone 0.04mg. This is a rare but dangerous side effect and is often preceded by the development of drowsiness and nausea.

Other side effects include urinary retention, pruritis and nausea and vomiting. Many of these side effects can be managed by the cautious use of naloxone intravenously, using a dose that is small enough to not reverse the analgesia.

The development of an epidural haematoma or abscess is an exceedingly rare but serious complication.

Failure to thread catheter

If the catheter will not pass beyond the tip of the Tuohy needle, try reinsertion of the needle and catheter followed by injection of 10ml of normal saline to attempt to 'open up' the epidural space. If the catheter does not even pass beyond the tip of the needle, it should be gently withdrawn and the hub of the needle rotated slightly and catheterisation re-attempted after injection of 10ml of saline.

Fluid from the Tuohy needle

Clear fluid emerging from the needle after loss of resistance to air indicates dural puncture. Fluid from the needle following a *saline* injection is more vexing: if the fluid flow continues, is warm or tests positive for glucose, then a dural tap has occurred. The procedure for dural tap (see below) should then be followed.

If the fluid flow stops, then attach a 2ml syringe to the hub of the needle and aspirate gently: if fluid flows freely, a dural tap has occurred. If fluid does not flow, then insert a catheter and continue as at step 15, p. 247.

Accidental dural puncture

Leave the needle in place and re-insert the hub. Insert another epidural needle in an adjacent interspace. After threading the catheter into the epidural space through the second needle, remove the first needle and then perform a test dose as above. Observe the height of block following this test dose carefully, as an unexpectedly high block may occur. It may be necessary to reduce the size of subsequent top-up doses.

Difficulty injecting into catheter

Check that the connecting mechanism joining the catheter to the filter is not too tight and attempt to repeat the injection. If this does not work, withdraw the catheter 2cm and attempt an injection of 10ml of saline. If this fails, it is necessary to remove the catheter and re-insert it at a different interspace.

Key points

- Establish a reliable intravenous fluid infusion before epidural puncture.
- Ensure that vasoconstrictors, ventilation and intubation equipment are immediately available.
- Have an assistant who is competent in resuscitation.
- Thoracic epidural puncture is best performed via a paramedian approach.
- If a test dose is used, ensure that the results are fully observed and understood.

Hazards

- Dural puncture.
- Epidural haematoma.
- Epidural abscess.

Brachial plexus block

The brachial plexus is derived from the anterior primary rami of C5–T1. These five roots form three trunks which split into anterior and posterior divisions, which in turn unite to form three cords. These cords form the main nerve supply of the arm as the ulnar, radial, median and musculocutaneous nerves (Fig. 6.18). Additionally, the shoulder joint receives a direct supply from the circumflex humeral nerve arising from the posterior division before it continues as the radial nerve, the skin over the shoulder derives its sensation from the supraclavicular branches of the cervical plexus and the skin of the axilla and inner aspect of the upper arm is supplied from the intercostobrachial nerve (T2 and T3).

The roots of the brachial plexus lie between the scalene muscles in the neck in close relationship to the vertebral artery and stellate ganglion. As the plexus descends it comes into apposition with the subclavian artery and vein and the dome of the pleura in the supraclavicular region (Fig. 6.19). In the axilla components of the plexus surround the subclavian artery and vein.

The plexus and major vessels (Fig. 6.20) lies within a sheath of fibrous tissue which is derived from the prevertebral fascia. Local anaesthetic injected within this sheath should spread to affect all elements of the plexus at that level.

The brachial plexus is approached at one of three levels during its course. Each route has particular advantages and disadvantages.
The commonest approaches are:
- The interscalene approach.
- The supraclavicular approach.
- The axillary approach.

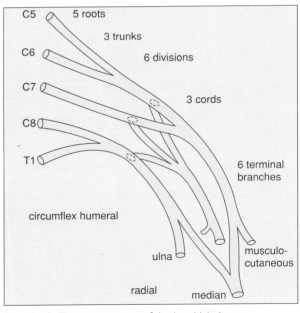

Fig. 6.18 The components of the brachial plexus

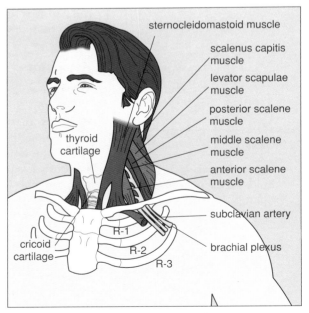

Fig. 6.19 The anatomy of the brachial plexus

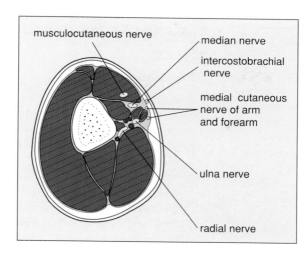

musculocutaneous nerve

median nerve

intercostobrachial nerve

medial cutaneous nerve of arm and forearm

ulna nerve

radial nerve

Fig. 6.20 The axillary brachial plexus in cross section

The interscalene block offers reliable analgesia for the structures supplied by the nerves derived from C5–C7 spinal roots including the deep tissue of the shoulder and radial aspect of the forearm. It is, however, less reliable in providing analgesia for the lower roots of the plexus which include some areas supplied by the ulnar nerve along the medial aspect of the forearm and hand. There is little danger of penetrating the pleural dome and creating a pneumothorax with the interscalene approach.

The supraclavicular block should cover all roots of the plexus and offers the best chance of a complete block. However, it carries with it a danger of penetration of the dome of the pleura and creation of a pneumothorax which can have serious consequences, particularly in patients receiving intermittent positive pressure ventilation or those with a reduced respiratory reserve.

The axillary block is the simplest and safest technique and is probably most suitable for the occasional user. There is little chance of pleural penetration. However, the approach is unreliable for producing analgesia of the shoulder joint and upper arm as the circumflex humeral and musculocutaneous nerves often escape from the effect of the local anaesthetic solution. Injury to the upper arm may make it difficult to position the patient correctly for the block to be performed.

The onset of analgesia may be slow with all approaches (20–30 minutes). Motor block usually occurs before sensory block. Lignocaine with a vasoconstrictor may produce reliable analgesia for about 45 minutes, and bupivacaine for 3 hours or more. The duration of action can be increased by inserting a cannula or catheter and administering the local anaesthetic solution by continuous infusion. However, great care must be taken not to exceed the safe dose for the patient calculated on a weight basis. Similar doses are required whichever approach is used although lower doses may suffice in the supraclavicular approach.

Short bevel needles should be used as penetration of the fascial sheath is more perceptible and damage to the nerve is less likely. The patient should be warned of paraesthesia occurring as the needle approaches the nerve. Some operators chose to use a peripheral nerve stimulator to aid with identification of the correct needle placement, but many patients find this distressing and uncomfortable.

Indications

Analgesia for surgical procedures below the elbow, particularly in patients who may be at risk from gastric regurgitation or from general anaesthesia or who require early ambulation.

Temporary benefit from sympathetic disorders such as limb causalgia or Raynaud's phenomena.

As a diagnostic aid to determine if the patient's pain is central or peripheral, and to ascertain potential movement of wrist and finger joints limited by pain alone.

Contra-indications

Local sepsis at the injection site.
Known bleeding diasthesis.
Injury to the shoulder or upper arm precluding satisfactory positioning.
Operations contemplated on the upper arm or requiring a tourniquet applied to the upper arm for a prolonged period of time.
Unco-operative patients.

THE AXILLARY BRACHIAL PLEXUS BLOCK

Equipment

☐ Antiseptic solution.
☐ Short bevel 22G needles or 22G cannula.
☐ 2ml, 5ml and 20ml syringes.
☐ 1.5% lignocaine with 1:200,000 adrenaline or 0.25–0.5% bupivacaine with 1:200,000 adrenaline.
☐ 30cm lightweight intravenous extension tubing with Luer lock connections.
☐ Brachial plexus catheter (optional).
☐ Peripheral nerve stimulator (optional).
☐ Syringe pump (optimal).
☐ Resuscitation equipment.

Technique

1　Place the patient in the supine or recumbent position with the upper arm abducted and externally rotated and the forearm flexed to 90° at the elbow (Fig. 6.21).
2　Identify and mark the axillary artery as high up in the axilla as possible.
3　Clean and drape the axilla and surrounding area.
4　Don gloves and gown.　►►►

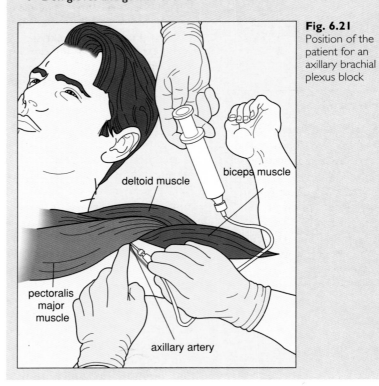

Fig. 6.21
Position of the patient for an axillary brachial plexus block

deltoid muscle

biceps muscle

pectoralis major muscle

axillary artery

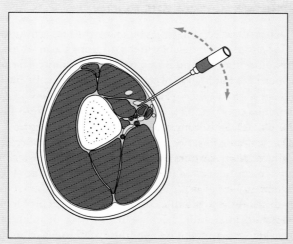

Fig. 6.22 The needle 'swings' with the arterial pulse

▶ ▶ ▶

5 Infiltrate the skin and subcutaneous tissues with a tiny (0.5ml) amount of 1% lignocaine.

6 With a finger on the axillary artery insert the needle attached to the length of intravenous extension tubing at angle of 30° to the skin parallel to the artery and just above it pointing towards the back of the humeral head (Fig. 6.21). A 'pop' or 'give' may be felt as the needle penetrates the neural sheath and the patient may complain of paraesthesia. The needle should oscillate with the arterial pulse (Fig. 6.22).

7 Leaving the needle *in situ*, an aspiration test is performed with a syringe attached to the distal end of the extension tubing.

8 If aspiration is negative, 30–40ml of the chosen local anaesthetic solution is injected. (Note: maximum dose of bupivacaine is 2mg/kg and of lignocaine with adrenaline is 7mg/kg.)

9 Severe pain on injection may indicate intraneural injection. Relocate the needle immediately.

10 Some clinicians prefer to move the needle during the procedure to deposit the local anaesthesia above, below and in front of the artery.

11 If the artery is punctured the needle should be withdrawn or advanced until aspiration is negative, before the local anaesthetic solution is injected.

12 If a cannula or brachial plexus catheter is used it may be advanced once the indwelling needle has penetrated the sheath, and a continuous infusion of 5–6ml/h of the local anaesthetic solution may be used for more prolonged procedures after the initial bolus dose.

13 Wait for up to 30 minutes for signs that the block has worked.

Hazards

- Arterial or venous puncture with intravascular injection of the local anaesthetic solution.
- Systemic toxicity due to overdose of local anaesthetic.
- Intraneural injection.
- Ineffective or incomplete block.

Key points

- Calculate the safe total dose of local anaesthetic based on the patient's weight (see step 8 above).
- An assistant competent in resuscitation should monitor the patient's vital signs throughout the procedure.

INTERSCALENE BLOCK

The interscalene block is relatively reliable at blocking the cervical roots, and so is favoured for surgery on the shoulder and upper arm. It also carries little risk of pneumothorax, and is said to be technically easier in the obese patient, where the landmarks of the other routes may be hard to confirm.

The technique depends on the injection of local anaesthetic into the roots of the brachial plexus, as they emerge in the interscalene groove: this is formed by the scalenus anterior and scalenus medius muscles. These two muscles have their origins on the anterior and posterior tubercles of the transverse processes of the lower cervical vertebrae (Fig. 6.23). The block needle must be directed into the groove, or onto the transverse process, to produce a reliable, successful block. The block should not be performed bilaterally, because of the risk of bilateral phrenic nerve palsy, which can precipitate respiratory failure in patients with limited respiratory reserve.

Indications

As for axillary block: the interscalene approach is favoured where block of the cervical roots is important

Contra-indications

As for axillary block

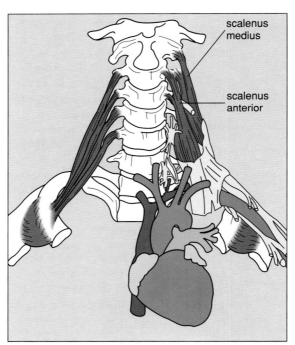

scalenus medius

scalenus anterior

Fig. 6.23 The roots of the brachial plexus emerge in the interscalene groove, between the scalenus anterior and medius muscles

Equipment

☐ The equipment list is as for the axillary route
☐ 20–40ml of local anaesthetic is required for an adult patient: the higher dose is required in patients who need an extensive or long duration block

Technique

1 Lie the patient supine on the bed, with the head turned slightly away from the side to be blocked. The arm on the chosen side should lie at the side, and the shoulder should be depressed slightly.

2 Identify the cricoid cartilage, which is level with the C6 vertebra, and then draw a line around to the posterior border of the sternocleidomastoid, on the chosen side.

3 Ask the patient to sniff: this will identify the interscalene groove, which is seen as an indentation just behind the posterior border of sternocleidomastoid: the intersection of the groove and a line drawn from the cricoid, is over the site of the transverse process of C6. Indeed, in thin or anaesthetized patients, the bony transverse process can be felt subcutaneously (Fig. 6.24). Mark this point.

4 Don sterile gloves, and clean and prepare the area identified above.

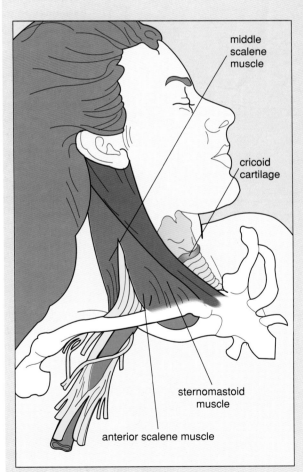

Fig. 6.24 An imaginary line is drawn from the cricoid cartilage, to intersect the surface marking of the interscalene groove: this represents the site of insertion of the needle for interscalene brachial plexus block

middle scalene muscle

cricoid cartilage

sternomastoid muscle

anterior scalene muscle

257

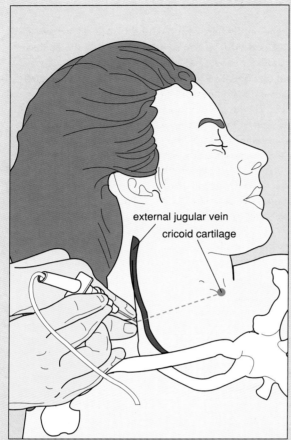

external jugular vein

cricoid cartilage

Fig. 6.25 The block needle is directed into the interscalene groove in a backwards, inwards and slightly caudal direction: this direction favours contact with the transverse process of C6

▶ ▶ ▶

5   Infiltrate 2–4ml of 1% lignocaine with adrenaline into the subcutaneous tissues over the mark: aspirate frequently, as the external jugular vein lies near to this point

6   Select a 32mm 23G block needle, and attach extension tubing to the needle. A peripheral nerve stimulator may be used, if so desired. A syringe containing local anaesthetic is then connected to the proximal end of the extension piece.

7   Insert the needle perpendicular to the skin. Direct it medially, backwards, and slightly caudally, to meet the 'transverse' process (Fig. 6.25).

8   If paraesthesia occurs, particularly in the arm or shoulder, then the plexus has been reached. If paraesthesia does not occur, but the bone of the transverse process of C6 is reached, the needle should be withdrawn slightly. If the needle is inserted more than 3cm, it is either too posterior or anterior, and should be withdrawn and re-inserted. The transverse process is very superficial even in obese patients.

9   Steady the needle with the left hand, and aspirate gently with the right hand on the syringe plunger: if any fluid, either blood or clear CSF returns, withdraw and re-insert the needle. If the aspiration is negative, inject local anaesthetic gently. After completing the injection, massage the site to promote distal spread along the plexus. The volume of local anaesthetic depends on the block required. If it is necessary to block the lower trunks of the brachial plexus, 40ml of 0.375% bupivacaine or 1% lignocaine 1:200,000 adrenaline should be used in an adult patient, while 20ml is appropriate for less extensive blocks in the adult.

Complications

The complications of the interscalene route relate to the close proximity of the intervertebral foramina, and the dura.

- Accidental epidural and spinal anaesthesia have been reported, and should be immediately treated as for high spinal block (see the first part of this section).
- Accidental injection into the vertebral artery will be followed by unconsciousness and convulsions, and should be treated symptomatically.
- Block of the phrenic, recurrent laryngeal, or cervical sympathetic nerves may occur; they will not cause particular problems in healthy patients, but the patient should be warned of the associated symptoms.
- Chronic toxicity from absorption of local anaesthetic is not a problem usually, as the block does not require high volumes of local anaesthetic.

SUPRACLAVICULAR BLOCK

The supraclavicular approach is the most technically difficult of the approaches to the brachial plexus, because of the relations to a hidden structure, the first rib. The technique has the advantage that the trunks of the plexus are closely arranged at this point, and so a low volume of local anaesthetic will therefore produce a rapid onset of block. It is uncommon to miss segments, if the block is correctly performed. The main disadvantage of the block is the risk of pneumothorax, because of the close relation of the pleura to the site of injection: this is perhaps the only reason why the route is not the approach of choice to the plexus in all cases.

This approach to the plexus is contra-indicated in patients with severe respiratory disease, in whom a pneumothorax would be a considerable problem. It is also more difficult in the obese individual, and those with poor anatomical landmarks: the other two approaches are more prudent in these patients. The block should never be performed bilaterally, as the hazards associated with bilateral phrenic nerve palsy or pneumothoraces are too great.

Indications

As for interscalene block. This block is favoured for patients where it is important to block all the segments

Contra-indications

As for interscalene block. The block should not be performed bilaterally, or in patients with severe respiratory disease

Equipment

☐ The same equipment is used as for all other types of brachial plexus block: a lower volume of local anaesthetic (20ml) is usually adequate

Technique

The trunks of the plexus are blocked at the point that they cross the first rib: the trunks run over the lateral margin of the rib, and this point is marked on the skin by the midpoint of the clavicle. Further, the subclavian artery, which can be felt behind the midpoint of the clavicle, has the brachial plexus as a posterior and lateral relation (Fig. 6.26). Therefore, the approach is to identify the subclavian artery at the midpoint of the clavicle, and then direct the block needle down behind the artery, in a slightly medial direction: backwards, inwards and downwards. If paraesthesia occurs, then the plexus has been reached. More often however, the first rib is reached, and the needle is then 'walked' in an antero-posterior direction along the rib to elicit paraesthesia: medial direction risks pleural puncture. The success of the technique is dependent on either finding the first rib or the subclavian artery or both, as these are the most valuable landmarks for this block.

1 Position the patient supine, without a pillow. Allow the ipsilateral arm to fall to the side, and get the patient to take a deep breath in against a closed glottis: this will indicate the supra-clavicular fossa (Fig. 6.27).

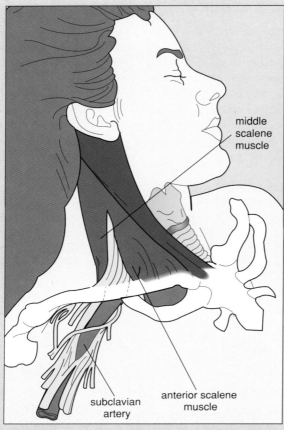

Fig. 6.26 The relation of the first rib to the subclavian artery and the brachial plexus trunks

middle
scalene
muscle

subclavian
artery

anterior scalene
muscle

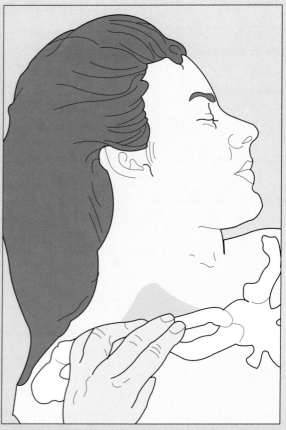

Fig. 6.27 The patient is asked to take a deep breath, to demonstrate the supra-clavicular fossa

▶ ▶ ▶

2 Palpate the clavicle, and identify the midpoint: this usually lies about 2cm lateral to the clavicular head of sternocleidomastoid. Attempt to identify the pulsation of the subclavian artery in the supraclavicular fossa, posterior to the midpoint of the clavicle: if this cannot be felt, then direct a line 2cm backwards from the midpoint of the clavicle, as this is where the artery should be palpable (Fig. 6.28).

3 Don sterile gloves, and clean and prepare the area over the supraclavicular fossa. Take a 32mm 23G block needle, which may be attached to a nerve stimulator if desired. Attach an extension tubing to the hub, and fix a 20ml syringe primed with local anaesthetic to the other end.

4 If the artery is palpable, place the tip of the index finger of the left hand onto the artery. Infiltrate the skin with local anaesthetic just posterior to the artery. Advance the block needle just posterior to the finger tip: if the artery is not located, then the needle should be inserted at the point identified earlier, 2cm posterior to the midpoint of the clavicle. Direct the needle backwards, inwards, and downwards: the inward direction is very slight (Fig. 6.29). ▶ ▶ ▶

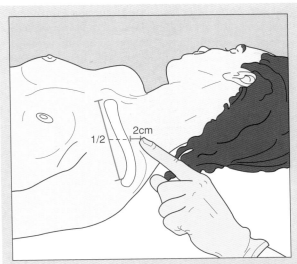

Fig. 6.28 In patients in whom the subclavian artery is impalpable, a point 2cm posterior to the midpoint of the clavicle is identified for puncture

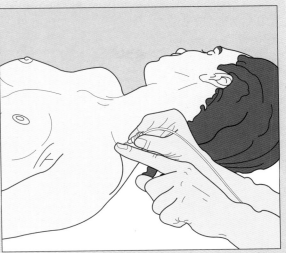

Fig. 6.29 The block needle is directed just posterior to the subclavian pulsation, in a backwards, inwards and downwards direction

▶ ▶ ▶

5 If paraesthesia is elicited, then steady the needle with the left hand, and aspirate the syringe with the right hand. After negative aspiration, inject 20ml of local anaesthetic.

6 If the rib is contacted, then direct the needle both anteriorly and posteriorly along the rib, to search for paraesthesia: do not direct the needle more medially. If this fails, then try a more posterior entry to the skin. If the artery is hit, then simply withdraw the needle, and direct the needle more posteriorly: accidental arterial puncture has actually identified one of the landmarks, and it is a useful guide to the position of the plexus. If the needle does not elicit any of the above results, then try a more posterior approach: if this fails, it is appropriate to use a different approach to the brachial plexus.

Complications

- The most important complication of this technique is accidental pneumothorax. This may be heralded by coughing during needle insertion, and the needle should be immediately withdrawn and inserted more laterally: in this situation, or if the patient has symptoms of a pneumothorax, a chest X-ray should be performed immediately after the block, unless immediate needle decompression is required.

- In all other cases, the X-ray should not be performed until 2–4 hours after the block, as the pneumothorax may take some time to develop. Indeed, in some patients, it may not be detectable radiologically until 12–24 hours after the block. The treatment is dependent upon the size of the air pocket: generally, patients with respiratory disease, or any sign of dyspnoea or hypoxia must have an underwater seal chest drain inserted immediately. There is little place for conservative management of anything but the smallest pneumothorax.

- Phrenic nerve palsy is common (60–80%) but rarely causes problems, except in patients with respiratory disease. Treatment is symptomatic, and usually consists of supplemental oxygen alone. Horner's syndrome and neuritis require nothing more than expectant treatment.
- Systemic toxicity is rare with this approach, and is usually due to accidental vascular injection: this should be managed symptomatically. Oxygen and anti-convulsants are the first line of treatment.

Key points

- Select the best block for the patient, and the surgical procedure.
- Remember the anatomical landmarks, and if the block proves difficult, re-insert the needle, and follow the guidelines.
- Use a correctly insulated nerve stimulator needle where possible.
- Wait at least 30 minutes before confirming that a block has failed: if paraesthesia has been obtained, successful block is very likely.

Hazards

- Pneumothorax has serious sequalae in patients with respiratory disease.

Intercostal nerve block

Indications

To provide initial and short term analgesia for patients with fractured ribs and chest trauma.

To provide analgesia for patients with fractured ribs and chest trauma requiring chest physiotherapy and breathing exercises in the early stages after injury.

To provide analgesia for cleaning and suturing of chest wall injuries.

To provide postoperative analgesia for patients with thoracotomy or subcostal surgical incisions.

Contra-indications

Local sepsis or severe oedema at proposed injection site.
Known bleeding diathesis.
Unco-operative patient.

The intercostal nerves are derived from the thoracic anterior primary rami and classically run laterally beneath the lower border of each rib accompanying the intercostal vascular bundle. The nerve lies deep to the external and internal intercostal muscles and superficial to the subcostal muscle posteriorly and the intercostalis intimus anteriorly (Fig. 6.30).

Each nerve gives off two branches: a lateral cutaneous branch in the mid axillary line and an anterior cutaneous branch at the lateral border of the sternum. The lateral branch has anterior and posterior branches and the anterior branch has medial and lateral branches. Together they supply the skin over the particular thoracic segment. If all components of the nerve are to be blocked, then the injection site must be posterior to the origin of the lateral cutaneous branch.

Anatomical studies have shown that in some cases the main nerve breaks up into three or four bundles. This may give rise to a number of instances of incomplete block when a single injection of local anaesthetic is given. Additionally, in some patients the intercostalis intimus consists only of separate fasciculi which allows local anaesthetic to permeate via the subpleural space to adjacent segments and produce a more extensive block than planned.

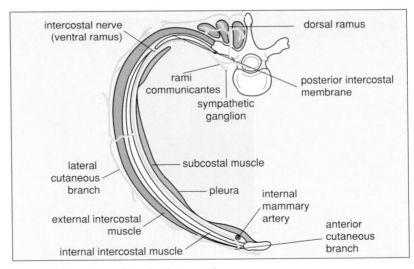

Fig. 6.30 Anatomy of a typical intercostal nerve

Equipment

☐ Antiseptic solution.
☐ 2ml and 5ml syringes.
☐ 23G needles.
☐ 1% lignocaine with 1:200,000 adrenaline or 0.25% bupivacaine with 1:200,000 adrenaline.
☐ Resuscitation equipment.

Technique

1 Ideally the patient should be placed sitting over the edge of the bed with arms folded across each other, and resting on a table just above hip height to abduct the scapulae (Fig. 6.31).

2 However, the block may also be performed with the patient in the prone or lateral position.

3 Identify and mark the posterior angle of the appropriate ribs which lie 2–5 cm behind the mid axillary line.

4 Don sterile gloves and gown.

5 Clean and drape the skin around the appropriate area.

6 Using a 23G needle infiltrate the skin and subcutaneous tissues over the lower border of the rib near its posterior angle with the chosen local anaesthetic solution.

7 Advance the needle vertically until it impinges onto the bony surface of the rib. Note the depth at which bone is encountered. Inject 0.5ml of local anaesthetic to render the periosteum insensitive.

8 Withdraw the needle 1–2mm and advance it again to 'walk down' the rib surface until the intercostal space is encountered at the lower border of the rib.

9 Advance the needle to lie just below the rib about 3mm deeper than the point of contact with bone so that it lies beneath the external and internal intercostal muscles but does not penetrate the pleura (Fig. 6.32).

10 After negative aspiration inject 3–5ml of the chosen local anaesthetic solution.

11 Repeat the procedure at other desired levels.

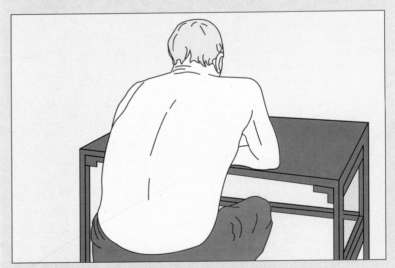

Fig. 6.31 The ideal position for a patient having an intercostal block

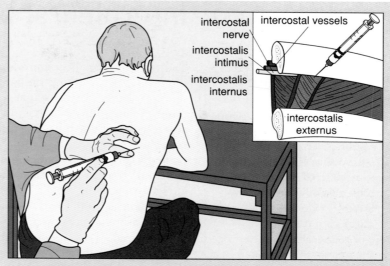

Fig. 6.32 The needle position for an intercostal block

Complications

- Accidental creation of a pneumothorax due to lung puncture. The patient should breathe shallowly during insertion of the needle and if possible hold his breath during the injection.
- Local bleeding due to penetration of the intercostal vascular bundle (usually easily controlled by direct pressure).
- Systemic toxicity due to overdose of local anaesthetic or adrenaline solution. This can easily occur if several intercostal nerves are to be blocked for multiple bilateral rib fractures. Bupivacaine provides the most satisfactory long-acting block but prilocaine is safer for poor risk patients and those in whom multiple bilateral blocks are needed.

Key points

- Ensure that the patient is correctly positioned.
- Carefully check the total dose of the local anaesthetic to be given to ensure that it is within the recommended safe range for a patient of that weight.
- An assistant competent in resuscitation should monitor the patient's vital signs throughout the procedure and afterwards for one hour if multiple blocks have been used.
- A chest X-ray should be taken after the procedure to check for the presence of a pneumothorax.

Hazards

- There is extensive absorption of anaesthetic from the intercostal site; calculate the maximum permitted dose carefully.

Interpleural block

This technique has been introduced relatively recently and operates on the principle of bathing the intercostal nerves with local anaesthetic solution as they exit the spinal column and lie exposed in front of the posterior intercostal membrane (Fig. 6.33). The method has some advantages over the thoracic epidural block in that hypotension does not occur as the sympathetic chain is relatively unaffected. However, it is of limited use in bilateral chest injuries because of the high doses of local anaesthetic agent required, and it appears to diminish in effectiveness after 12–36 hours.

An epidural catheter is introduced via a Tuohy needle into the interpleural space and after an initial bolus dose of local anaesthetic is administered, a continuous infusion can be established to maintain analgesia. The catheter can be introduced through any intercostal space but generally the fifth to eighth space is selected. A space distant from a penetrating injury or chest drain should be used.

Indications

To provide initial and short term analgesia for patients with fractured ribs and chest trauma.

To provide analgesia for patients with fractured ribs requiring chest physiotherapy and breathing exercises in the early stages after injury.

To provide analgesia for cleaning and suturing of chest wall injuries.

To provide post operative analgesia for patients with thoracotomy or subcostal surgical incisions.

Contra-indications

Major haemothorax.
Pyothorax.
Open pneumothorax.
Pleural adhesions.
Known bleeding diathesis.
Unco-operative patient.

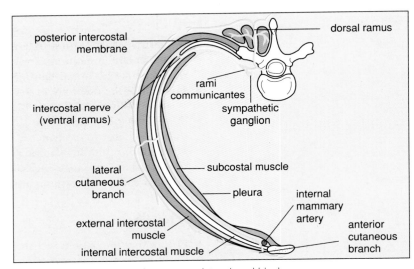

Fig. 6.33 The anatomy relevant to an interpleural block

Equipment

☐ Antiseptic solution.
☐ 2ml, 5ml, 10ml and 20ml syringes.
☐ 23G needles.
☐ Scalpel blade.
☐ Tuohy needle.
☐ Epidural catheter and bacterial filter.
☐ 5ml 1% lignocaine.
☐ 20ml 0.5% bupivacaine or 50ml 0.125% bupivacaine for infusion.
☐ Adhesive tape.
☐ Continuous infusion syringe pump.
☐ Resuscitation equipment.

Technique

1 Place the patient in the lateral position with the upper arm elevated and rotated across the chest (Fig. 6.34).

2 Identify and mark a suitable intercostal space (usually between the fifth and eighth).

3 Don sterile gloves and gown.

4 Clean and drape the area.

5 Using a 23G needle infiltrate the skin and subcutaneous tissues over the upper border of the selected rib using 1% lignocaine.

6 Make a tiny incision (2mm) in the skin with the point of a scalpel blade.

7 Advance the Tuohy needle through the incision into the subcutaneous tissues (Fig. 6.35).

8 Attach a 10ml syringe with a freely moving plunger containing 5ml of air to the hub of the Tuohy needle.

9 Using the loss-of-resistance method advance the tip of Tuohy needle until it enters the interpleural space. Frequently a 'pop' is also felt as the needle penetrates the parietal pleura.

10 In the spontaneously breathing patient, the negative pressure generated in the interpleural space during inspiration may draw the syringe plunger in spontaneously as the needle penetrates the parietal pleura.

11 In the patient receiving intermittent positive pressure ventilation, the loss of resistance should be identified by gentle pressure with the palm of the hand on the syringe plunger as the needle enters the interpleural space. ► ► ►

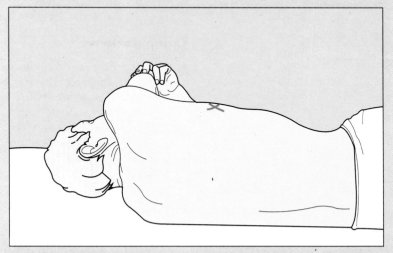

Fig. 6.34 The position of the patient for an interpleural block

▶ ▶ ▶

12 Advance an epidural catheter through the Tuohy needle, 5–10cm into the interpleural space.

13 Withdraw the Tuohy needle over the catheter and tape the catheter securely in position.

14 After negative aspiration, inject 15–20ml 0.5% bupivacaine or other chosen local anaesthetic into the catheter.

15 Connect the catheter to a syringe pump via a bacterial filter.

16 5–10ml/h 0.125% bupivacaine is given by continuous infusion to maintain analgesia.

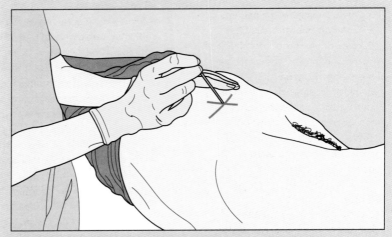

Fig. 6.35 The position of the Tuohy needle for an interpleural block

Complications

- A pneumothorax may occur if the Tuohy needle or catheter penetrates the lung. This risk is obviously higher in patients receiving intermittent positive pressure ventilation with high mean intrathoracic pressures.
- High bolus doses or very fast infusion rates may result in systemic toxicity due to overdose of the local anaesthetic agent.
- Haemorrhage may occur if the intercostal vascular bundle is penetrated with the Tuohy needle.

Key points

- Carefully check the total dose of the local anaesthetic to be given to ensure that it is within the recommended safe range for a patient of that weight.
- An assistant competent in resuscitation should monitor the patient's vital signs throughout the procedures, and afterwards during the infusion.
- A chest radiograph should be taken after the procedure to exclude the presence of a pneumothorax.

Hazards

- There is a high risk of pneumothorax with positive pressure ventilation especially if PEEP is used.

Block of the femoral nerve and the lateral cutaneous nerve of the thigh

Indications

To provide analgesia for patients with fractures of the middle third of the femur (femoral nerve only).

To provide analgesia for superficial wound debridement and suturing of the medial aspect of the thigh (femoral nerve) or the lateral aspect of the thigh (lateral cutaneous nerve of the thigh) or the anterior aspect of the thigh (both).

To provide analgesia for the harvesting of small areas of skin for grafting from the thigh.

Contra-indications

Infection adjacent to the proposed injection site.

Known bleeding.

Severe oedema in the region of the proposed injection site.

Unco-operative patient.

The femoral nerve is formed from branches derived from L2–L4 nerve roots. It supplies the musculature of the anterior compartment of the thigh and the skin over the anterior medical aspect of the leg from a point 6–8 cm below the inguinal ligament to the medial malleolus at the ankle (Fig. 6.36). It also conducts sensation from the periosteum of the middle third of the femur and the adjacent deep structures.

The femoral nerve emerges from the lateral border of the psoas muscle in the iliac fossa and appears in the thigh beneath the inguinal ligament just lateral to the femoral artery. The femoral artery and vein are enclosed in a fascial sheath. The femoral nerve lies lateral and slightly behind this sheath. At this point it is readily accessible for injection of local anaesthetic (Fig. 6.37).

The lateral cutaneous nerve of the thigh is formed from branches of L2 and L3 and supplies sensation to the antero lateral aspect of the thigh (Fig. 6.36). The nerve emerges from the psoas muscle and enters the thigh from the iliac fossa through the inguinal ligament, 2cm medial to the anterior superior iliac spine. It divides into anterior and posterior branches 2–4cm below the inguinal ligament. It is thus accessible for injection of local anaesthetic at a point 2cm medial to and 2cm below the anterior superior iliac spine (Fig. 6.37).

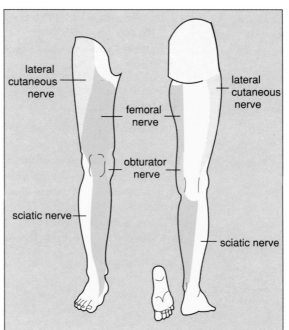

Fig. 6.36 The sensory nerve supply of the leg

lateral cutaneous nerve

femoral nerve

obturator nerve

sciatic nerve

lateral cutaneous nerve

sciatic nerve

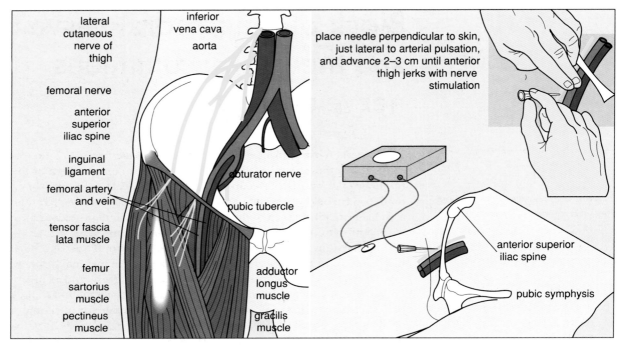

Fig. 6.37 The relevant landmarks for blocks of the femoral and lateral cutaneous nerve of the thighs

Equipment

☐ Antiseptic solution.
☐ 2ml, 5ml and 20ml syringes.
☐ 23G and 21G needles.
☐ 1% lignocaine with 1:200,000 adrenaline; 0.25% or 0.5% bupivacaine with 1:200,000 adrenaline.
☐ Peripheral nerve stimulator generating 0.2mA of electrical current.

Technique

1 Place the patient supine with the thigh slightly abducted and externally rotated.
2 Identify and mark the position of maximum pulsation of the femoral artery (femoral nerve) and a point 2cm medial and below the anterior superior iliac spine (lateral cutaneous nerve of the thigh) with a waterproof marker.
3 Don sterile gloves and gown.
4 Clean and drape the skin around the area of the groin. ▶ ▶ ▶

▶ ▶ ▶

To block the femoral nerve

5   Palpate the femoral artery and maintain the finger in position.

6   Insert a 5cm 23G needle vertically through the skin 1.5–2.0cm lateral to the finger palpating the artery, infiltrating the skin and superficial tissues with 1–2ml of anaesthetic solution.

7   Advance the needle 1.5–3.0cm and feel the 'pop' as it pierces the fascia lata.

8   Continue advancing for a further 0.5–1.0cm feeling for penetration of the iliac fascia.

9   If a peripheral nerve stimulator is to be used, attach one lead to a short bevel needle placed near the nerves and the other to an ECG electrode attached to the thigh. Observe twitching of the quadriceps muscle in response to a current of 0.2mA. The patient may also report paraesthesia felt on the anteromedial aspect of the thigh. Adjust the position of the needle until the signs are elicited.

10 When the needle is in a satisfactory position aspirate to ensure that it is not within a blood vessel and then inject 10–15ml of the preferred anaesthetic solution.

11 It may be necessary to inject an additional 5ml in a fan distribution to cover branches of the femoral nerve which have emerged just above the injection site.

To block the lateral cutaneous nerve

5   Identify a point 2cm medial and 2cm below the anterior superior iliac spine.

6   Insert a 5cm 21G needle at this point, infiltrating the skin and subcutaneous tissues with 1–2ml of anaesthetic solution.

7   Advance the needle vertically for 2–3 cm until a 'pop' is felt as the fascia lata is pierced.

8   After negative aspiration, inject 5–10ml of the anaesthetic solution in a fan distribution vertical to the inguinal ligament.

9   Check for successful block after five minutes.

Hazards

- Accidental injection into an artery or vein.
- Intraneural injection (heralded by severe pain on injection).
- Overdose of local anaesthetic solution.

Key points

- Accurate identification of the landmarks is essential. A peripheral nerve stimulator may be helpful in identifying the femoral nerve.
- Both nerves may branch above the point of needle insertion and further proximal or lateral infiltration may be required.
- The lower and upper thirds of the femur are not covered by the femoral nerve and so analgesia will not be provided for fractures at these sites.

Intravenous regional anaesthesia (Bier's block)

Indications

Single limb injury requiring surgical manipulation or intervention.

Carpal tunnel or Dupytren's contracture surgery.

Adjunct to injection of guanethidine for chronic pain control.

Contra-indications

Absolute

Unwilling or uncooperative patient.

Unreliable tourniquet.

Known allergy to local anaesthetics.

Absence of resuscitative skills or equipment.

Relative

Infections in the affected limb.

Sickle cell disease/trait.

Procedures lasting more than one hour.

Injuries above the knee or elbow.

Intravenous regional anaesthesia (IVRA) is a useful anaesthetic technique, for procedures on the upper or, less frequently, the lower limb. It provides analgesia for procedures lasting up to an hour; the tight tourniquet is increasingly painful after this time. As with all types of regional and general anaesthetic, there is a need to ensure that the patient is adequately fasted before the block is performed; suitable resuscitation equipment should be kept available during the entire procedure.

Equipment

☐ Resuscitation equipment and tilting trolley.
☐ Antiseptic solution.
☐ 40–50ml of 0.5% prilocaine or 0.5% lignocaine.
☐ Two small intravenous cannulae (e.g. 20G or 22G Venflon).
☐ Esmarch bandage.
☐ Pneumatic tourniquet of adequate size for affected limb.

Technique

The procedure should be explained to the patient and full consent obtained. The patient should be on a tilting trolley, in a supine position for lower limb blocks, or sitting for upper limb blocks. The operator should measure the patient's blood pressure and then attach suitable monitoring, avoiding the application of leads or probes to the affected limb.

An i.v. cannula is then secured in the non-affected hand and flushed with heparinised saline. A second cannula is then placed in the affected limb: this should be as small as possible and should be sited as far distally on the limb as is possible. This is also flushed with heparinised saline.

1 Select an appropriate tourniquet for the chosen limb. Confirm that the tourniquet functions correctly: automatic versions should maintain a constant selected pressure and manual devices should not demonstrate any leak following inflation.

2 Wrap one turn of a soft dressing around the circumference of the limb. Apply the tourniquet to the upper part of the limb, over this dressing, but do not inflate the tourniquet (Fig. 6.38). ▶ ▶ ▶

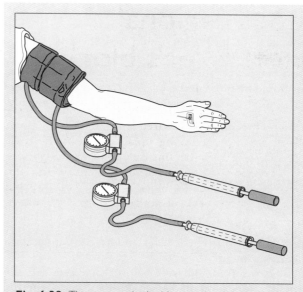

Fig. 6.38 The pneumatic double tourniquet is applied high up on the affected arm or leg

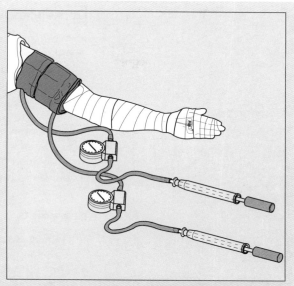

Fig. 6.39 The limb is exsanguinated by application of an Esmarch-type bandage and then the upper pneumatic tourniquet is inflated while the bandage remains in place

▶ ▶ ▶

3 Elevate the arm or leg, for 2–3 minutes. It is useful to apply an Esmarch-type bandage, in non-painful conditions, to exsanguinate the limb. In other situations, apply pressure over the brachial artery, while the arm is elevated: this will assist in exsanguination.

4 With the limb elevated, inflate the upper cuff on the pneumatic tourniquet, to 100mmHg above the patient's systolic blood pressure (Fig. 6.39).

5 Remove the bandage and allow the limb to return to a comfortable position.

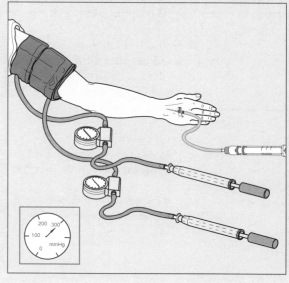

6 Check that the distal pulse in the limb has disappeared. If it has not, then deflate the cuff and recheck the equipment and start again at step 1.

7 Inject local anaesthetic into the limb and note the time. 35–45ml of local anaesthetic is adequate for an upper limb, while 50ml should be used for the lower limb (Fig. 6.40).

8 The tourniquet should remain inflated for at least 20 minutes after the time of injection. It may be wise to perform several cycles of deflation/inflation at the end, to allow for a slow systemic release of local anaesthetic.

9 Cuff pain may become a problem after 20–30 minutes. It may be alleviated by inflating the lower cuff of a double cuff (if used) *before* deflating the upper cuff.

Fig. 6.40 Local anaesthetic is slowly injected into the cannula, after tourniquet inflation

Complications

- Acute or chronic leak of local anaesthetic past the cuff may be followed by signs of systemic toxicity: drowsiness, convulsions, twitching, and cardiac depression. The injection should be stopped and the patient should be given 100% oxygen via a tight fitting face mask. Drugs to treat CNS excitation may be necessary, including anti-convulsants.
- Local sepsis may make the block ineffective and an alternative method of anaesthesia should be sought.
- Inadequate block is usually due to inadequate limb exsanguination and is rarely improved by a second dose of local anaesthetic.

Key points

- IVRA is a useful, safe, local anaesthetic block and has wide application in the emergency department.
- The cuff should be carefully checked before each use and the anaesthetist should understand the mechanism of action of the particular pneumatic cuff.
- Place the cannula as far distally as possible in the limb; avoid the antecubital fossa or veins above the knee.
- An inadequate block may occur if the limb is not completely exsanguinated; it is important to correctly apply the technique of limb elevation as described above.
- Check the cuff pressure repeatedly during injection and stop the injection if the patient becomes drowsy or confused.

Hazards

- Premature deflation of the tourniquet may result in serious local anaesthetic toxicity.

Guidelines for adult cardiopulmonary resuscitation

Over the past 25 years guidelines have been set for cardiopulmonary resuscitation by authoritative bodies such as the American Heart Association, the Heart and Stroke Foundation of Canada, the Australian Resuscitation Council, the Resuscitation Council (UK), the Scandinavian Resuscitation Council, the South African Resuscitation Council and, most recently, the European Resuscitation Council.

International consensus for both basic and advanced life support has been reached in broad principle although each continent has minor variations related to ethnic principles, resource availability, differences in local practice and legal constraints. It is likely that worldwide agreement will be achieved in the near future.

Guidelines are based on scientific evaluation of research and practice and are updated every five years or earlier to take account of new developments and audit of performance and outcome.

The examples given below of guidelines for basic and advanced life support reflect the most recent recommendations of the European Resuscitation Council which have been adopted by the European Nations, China and many other countries. They are reproduced by kind permission of the European Resuscitation Council.

BASIC LIFE SUPPORT

The guidelines for basic life support (Fig. 7.1) reflect the need for a rapid overall assessment of airway, ventilation and pulse prior to starting cardiopulmonary resuscitation (CPR).

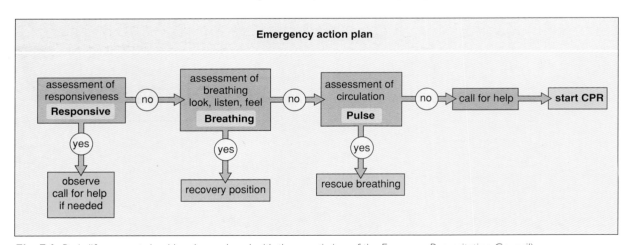

Fig. 7.1 Basic life support algorithm (reproduced with the permission of the European Resuscitation Council)

If a pulse is present but the patient is not breathing, then artificial ventilation should be started immediately in an attempt to reoxygenate the patient prior to calling for help as soon as possible.

In the event of there being no pulse, help should be called for immediately because, without the early assistance of an advanced life support team, particularly with a defibrillator, there is little chance of a favourable outcome. The precordial thump is recommended in the pulseless patient particularly if the event is witnessed. It is not recommended for application by lay citizens.

ADVANCED LIFE SUPPORT

The guidelines for advanced life support (Fig. 7.2) place special emphasis on the need for early defibrillation in patients with ventricular fibrillation for it is this group which will produce the majority of survivors. The guidelines are geared to the use of an automated external defibrillator (AED). CPR cannot be performed during ECG analysis by this device and so the three shocks indicated should follow in rapid sequence without CPR until defibrillation is successful. If a manual defibrillator is being used, CPR may be applied during the charging period.

The guidelines advocate a 'loop' sequence consisting of an intervention such as intravenous cannulation or airway control with a tracheal tube, after the three initial shocks followed by adrenaline 1mg, 10 sequences of CPR and three further defibrillatory shocks. At least three 'loops' should be followed before abandoning resuscitation. Resuscitation should not be abandoned if ventricular fibrillation still persists after three 'loops'. At this stage anti-arrhythmic drugs such as lignocaine, bretylium or amiodarone may be considered. Alkalising agents such as sodium bicarbonate are generally not considered until 20 minutes after the arrest and then are best administered in a measured dose calculated in response to arterial blood gas analysis. Intravenous calcium is reserved for patients with hypocalcaemia or hyperkalaemia.

In apparent asystole, emphasis is placed on the need to distinguish this rhythm from very fine ventricular fibrillation and if there is any doubt, defibrillation should be attempted. Adrenaline is the recommended drug and reoxygenation is of paramount importance. Cardiac pacing should be considered if there is any evidence of spontaneous electrical activity.

In electromechanical dissociation (also known as pulseless electrical activity), there is a need to consider a potentially remedial cause such as tension pneumothorax or cardiac tamponade. Otherwise adrenaline is the mainstay of treatment.

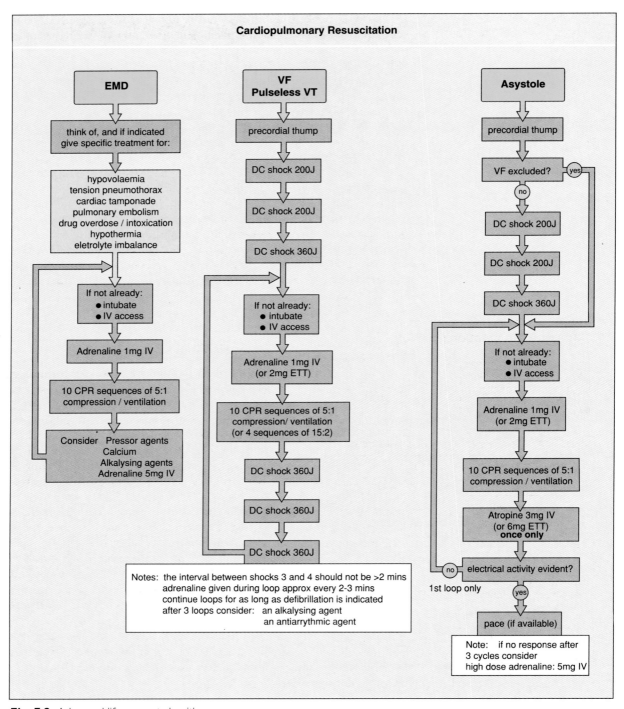

Fig. 7.2 Advanced life support algorithm
(reproduced with the permission of the European Resuscitation Council)

Guidelines for paediatric cardiopulmonary resuscitation

In 1994, the European Resuscitation Council followed up their publication of the 1992 guidelines for adult cardiopulmonary resuscitation by producing guidelines for paediatric resuscitation.

Cardiac arrest in neonates, infants and children is nearly always secondary to asphyxia and is rarely primarily cardiac in origin. The priorities in the guidelines for paediatric resuscitation, therefore, centre around airway management and re-oxygenation rather than defibrillation as in adults. Ventricular fibrillation is rare in children; asystole is more common but this rhythm may carry a better prognosis than in adults.

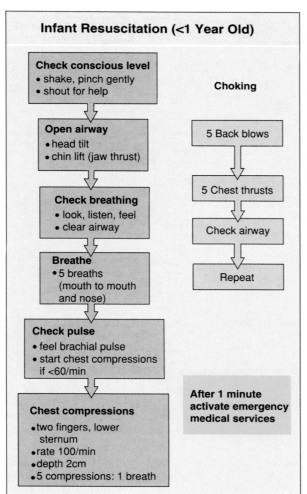

Fig. 7.3 Basic life support for infants

BASIC PAEDIATRIC LIFE SUPPORT

Slightly different guidelines are produced for infants under one year old (Fig. 7.3) and for children over one year. (Fig. 7.4).

For infants, the brachial pulse is considered the best one to palpate and it is recommended to start chest compressions if the pulse rate is below 60/min. Chest compressions in an infant are performed by two fingers placed over the lower sternum. A compression depth of 2cm and a rate of 100/min is recommended.

In children over one year, the carotid pulse is recommended for palpation and chest compressions are started only if the pulse is absent. Compression is performed using the heel of the hand. A compression depth of 3cm and a rate of 100/min is recommended.

The guidelines for both neonatal and child basic life support also incorporate an algorithm for the management of choking. (Figs. 7.3, 7.4). Back blows and chest thrusts are recommended for all ages. Abdominal thrusts are recommended in children over one year old only if back blows and chest thrusts are not successful.

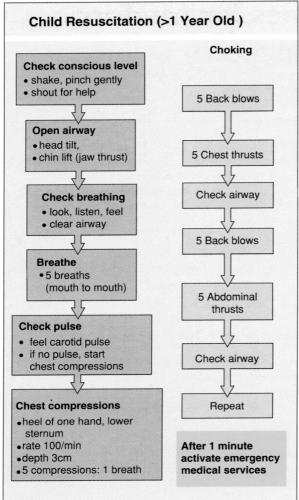

Fig. 7.4 Basic life support for children

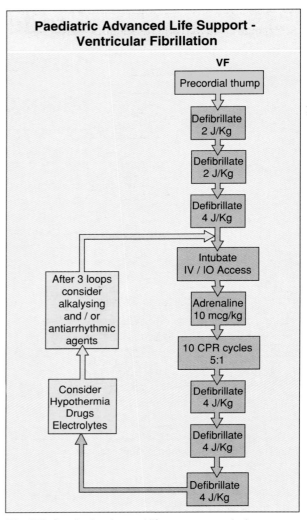

Fig. 7.5 Paediatric advanced life support: ventricular fibrillation

ADVANCED PAEDIATRIC LIFE SUPPORT

The guidelines for management of ventricular fibrillation (VF), asystole and electromechanical dissociation (EMD), also known as pulseless electrical activity (PEA) are shown in Figs. 7.5–7.7. In neonates and small children, intravenous access may be particularly difficult and intraosseous access is a useful alternative (see p. 20). Drugs are rapidly effective given via this route although the intravenous route is preferred, if possible.

If VF is present (which is rare), a precordial thump, by health care professionals only, is recommended prior to early defibrillation using two initial shocks at 2J/kg before moving to 4J/kg for further shocks. As with adults a 'loop' pattern is advocated with a short period (60 seconds) allowed for intervention, such as intubation, intravenous or intraosseous access, followed by 10mcg/kg adrenaline, 10 cycles of CPR and a series

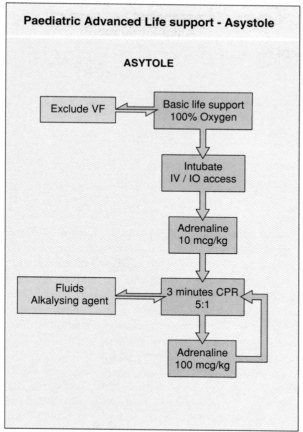

Fig. 7.6 Paediatric advanced life support: asystole

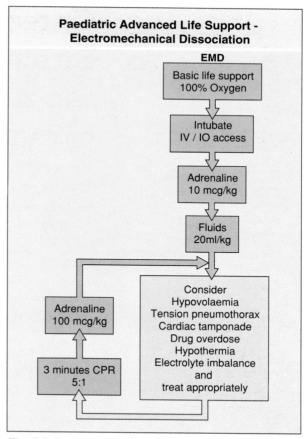

Fig. 7.7 Paediatric advanced life support: electromechanical dissociation

of three further shocks. (Fig. 7.5). Only after three loops should anti-arrhythmic or alkalising agents be considered. In infants and children, ventricular fibrillation may be precipitated by hypothermia, drug overdose or electrolyte imbalance.

In asystole, emphasis is placed on rapid re-oxygenation, intubation and then intravenous or intraosseous access to enable adrenaline to be given in an initial dose of 10mcg/kg. If this is ineffective after a further three minutes of CPR a high dose of adrenaline (100mcg/kg) is given and a 'loop' pattern followed with further CPR and adrenaline (Fig. 7.6).

The management of EMD follows similar principles to that for asystole (Fig. 7.7). The mainstays of treatment are re-oxygenation, adrenaline and CPR. In some cases EMD may be precipitated by a rapidly remediable cause such as tension pneumothorax or cardiac tamponade.

Drug overdose and hypothermia are relatively common in children and may confer a degree of cerebral protection and resuscitation should be continued for up to two hours in such cases.

Criteria for diagnosis and certification of brain death and authority for removal of cadaveric organs

Patients with severe and irrecoverable brain damage who are apnoeic and dependent on artificial ventilation in a critical care unit may be declared dead and treatment withdrawn.

Clearly it is vital that the diagnosis of brain death is confidently and accurately made before the irreversible step of withdrawing life support. For this reason, a code of practice has been established in the UK and many other countries, which sets down criteria and tests which must be fulfilled before the diagnosis can be confirmed. The examination of the patient and the specific tests must be undertaken by two separate senior doctors. One of the doctors must be the consultant in charge of the patient or the consultant in charge of the intensive care unit. The second, may be one of the above or a deputy who must be another consultant or senior registrar, or equivalent, who has been involved with the patient's management and who has been medically registered for more than five years and who has had previous training and experience with the procedures involved. Neither doctor should be a member of the transplant team. The examination and tests should be repeated on two separate occasions at an interval which should reassure all concerned.

CRITERIA

The following examination criteria should be fulfilled:
- There should be an identifiable underlying cause of brain damage, e.g. head injury or spontaneous subarachnoid or intracerebral haemorrhage.
- The patient should be in profound coma with:
  both pupils fixed and unreactive to light
  no cranial nerve motor responses
  no eye movement with a cold caloric test
  no spontaneous respiratory movements after disconnection from the ventilator for 10 minutes (with intratracheal oxygen insufflation).
- It should be confirmed that apnoea is not due to:
  cerebral depressant drugs
  neuromuscular blocking agents
  hypothermia
  metabolic or endocrine disturbances.

Only if all criteria are met should the patient be declared dead and the ventilator disconnected.

CERTIFICATION OF BRAIN DEATH

I. CRITERIA FOR DIAGNOSING BRAIN DEATH

Nature of brain damage

		Dr. A		Dr. B	
PLEASE CONFIRM WITH A SIGNATURE THAT APNOEIC COMA IS **NOT** DUE TO:	Date				
	Time				
1. Depressant drugs Name of drug ...... Dosage ...... Time given					
2. Neuromuscular blocking drugs (relaxants) Name of drug ...... Dosage ...... Time given ...... State whether peripheral nerve stimulator used					
3. Hypothermia Record temperature in degrees centigrade					
4. Metabolic or endocrine disturbances					
PLEASE CONFIRM WITH A SIGNATURE THE FOLLOWING					
1. Pupils both fixed and unreactive to light					
2. No eye movements with cold caloric test					
3. No cranial nerve motor responses					
4. No respiratory movements on disconnection from ventilator for 10 mins. with intratracheal O_2					

COMMENTS: (e.g. Biochemistry values, EEG report, Angiography report, etc.)

II. CONFIRMATION OF BRAIN DEATH

DIAGNOSIS OF DEATH

Date and Time Diagnosis is made ......

Name of Doctors: (BLOCK LETTERS) A. ...... B. ......

Signature and status of Doctors Making Diagnosis:

A. ...... Status. ......

B. ...... Status. ......

Fig. 7.8 An example form for certification of brain death

REMOVAL OF ORGANS FOR TRANSPLANTATION

Has the Form "CRITERIA FOR DIAGNOSING BRAIN DEATH" been completed YES/NO

Now complete Section I or II as indicated.

I **To be completed if the patient had requested Removal of Organs after Death.**

a. How was the request made?
Donor Card ......
Other (Specify) ......

b. Which, if any, organs were specified? ......

c. Views of relatives, if known (state relationship) ......

(Provided this is not a Coroner's Case and no objection has been raised, authorisation may now be given)

II **To be completed if there is no evidence that the patient had requested Removal of Organs after Death.**

a. Name and status of person(s) making enquiries ......

b. Name and relationship of person(s) approached ......

c. Date, time and nature of approach (personal/phone) ......

d. Views of those approached (specify any organs to which objections are raised) ......

If such reasonable enquiry as may be practical was made but views could not be obtained, state reason: ......

(Provided this is not a Coroner's Case, authorisation may now be given if there is no reason to believe that there is a relevant objection.)

N.B. Where the patient has requested removal of **ONE ORGAN** and additional or alternative organs are required, SECTIONS I AND II SHOULD **BOTH** BE COMPLETED.

III CORONER'S CASE

In all cases which come into this category, no organs may be removed without the coroners specific consent.

Name and Status of person approaching Coroner. ......

Organs specified for removal ......

Date and Time consent given ......

If consent withheld, state reasons ......

IV AUTHORISATION FOR REMOVAL OF ORGANS

If organs are to be removed, the relevant sections above must be completed prior to authorisation being requested.

Date and time authorisation given ......

How given (telephone, orally, etc.) ......

Name of designated person. ...... (Sector Administrator or Deputy)

Signature of person to whom Authorisation communicated ......

Fig. 7.9 An example form for authorisation of removal of organs for transplantation

AUTHORISATION OF REMOVAL OF ORGANS FOR TRANSPLANTATION

Organs may be removed for transplantation from patients certified brain dead provided certain additional criteria are met.

Two situations can be envisaged:

- The patient had previously requested removal of organs after death by completing a donor card or other method.
- There is no evidence that the patient had requested removal of organs after death.

In the first situation, the patient may have specified permission to remove one (e.g. kidneys) or more organs. If the case is being investigated by the Coroner, then permission should be sought before any further steps are taken. The views of the relatives should be sought and their consent agreed. If no relatives are available, then consent may be given by the Hospital Authority. If consent is received from the Coroner (if involved) and from the relatives, then authorisation may now be given and arrangements for the organ harvest may proceed.

In the second situation, if the patient is known to have expressed wishes not to have organs removed, those wishes should be respected. Where there is no evidence either way and the case is being investigated by the Coroner, then permission should be sought before any further steps are taken. The views and consent of the relatives should also be sought. If no relatives are available, then consent may be given by the Hospital Authority.

In either case, the relatives must be treated with the utmost sensitivity in a time of great distress. The approach should be made initially by the c onsultant in charge of the patient in the critical care unit and, once agreement in principle is reached, a member of the transplant team may provide further detailed information. No attempt should be made to coerce relatives into giving consent against their wishes. On the other hand, some time may be needed for them to assimilate the tragic situation and arrive at a decision which they will be content with in the future.

Examples of suitable forms for the certification of brain death and authorisation of removal of cadaveric organs for transplantation are given in Figs. 7.8, 7.9.

Advanced prehospital care 'working out of a box'

From time to time anaesthetists, accident and emergency physicians, critical care specialists, surgeons, family doctors and others may be required to provide advanced prehospital care in the field outside their normal working environment. Examples include medical services at sporting events such as motor racing, power boat racing, rugby and soccer matches and equestrian competitions; attendance to complement the paramedic ambulance services at multi-casualty incidents; cases of entrapment; escort services for national interhospital transfer of the seriously ill, by road and air; international patient repatriation by air; or management of casualties at an advanced clearing station in times of conflict.

In such cases, the doctor is expected to provide advanced life support 'out of a box' within an ambulance or at a relatively primitive medical centre or tented casualty clearing station.

The aim should be to confine procedures to those which are essential for simple life-saving resuscitation and to evacuate the patient(s) as quickly as possible to a suitable hospital which is capable of providing definitive care. It is essential to make sure that the patient is as stable as possible before transport and that adequate portable and effective monitoring equipment is available to complement continuous clinical assessment during the trip. It is not good practice to embark on an advanced procedure for an emergency occurring during transport.

This chapter outlines the procedures which may be required in advanced prehospital care and the equipment which is needed at each stage: immediate management of the patient on site, management within the ambulance and/or the local community medical centre or casualty clearing station, and monitoring devices to be used during transport.

PROCEDURES USED DURING ADVANCED PREHOSPITAL CARE

Respiratory care

- Basic airway control including oro- and naso-pharyngeal airway insertion.
- Laryngeal mask insertion.
- Tracheal intubation.
- Cricothyroidotomy.
- Basic ventilation techniques.
- Ventilation with an automatic resuscitator or transport ventilator.
- Transtracheal jet ventilation.
- Needle thoracostomy.
- Chest drain insertion.

Cardiovascular care

- Peripheral intravenous cannulation.
- Central cannulation of the internal or external jugular vein.
- Surgical cut-down venous cannulation.
- Intraosseous cannulation.
- Pericardiocentesis.
- External chest compressions.
- Defibrillation.
- Pneumatic anti-shock garment application.

Miscellaneous procedures if a prolonged period of transport is anticipated

- Gastric intubation.
- Urethral catheterisation.
- Intercostal nerve block.
- Femoral nerve block.

Equipment

Clothing

It is essential to be properly clothed for the job. Clearly this will depend on climatic conditions and the anticipated working environment. The list may include:

- ☐ Fire resistant boiler suit with knee pads and identity badge.
- ☐ Thermal underwear, socks and gloves.
- ☐ Chrome leather gloves.
- ☐ Waterproof acid-resistant boots.
- ☐ Waterproof coat and trousers (high visibility) with identity badge.
- ☐ Helmet with headlight with rechargeable battery.
- ☐ Splash resistant goggles.
- ☐ Heat packs.

Medical equipment

Equipment for advanced prehospital care should be divided into:

- ☐ Medical snatch bags.
- ☐ Equipment carried on ambulance or aircraft.
- ☐ Equipment available at medical centre or casualty clearing station.

Medical snatch bags

It is tempting to try to carry too much equipment in a medical snatch bag. This bag plus its contents should be light, compact, waterproof and, as far as possible, shock proof. All that is required in the first few minutes of any trauma emergency is control of the obstructed airway, the facility to provide artificial ventilation, and the means to arrest haemorrhage from a peripheral site and establish an intravenous access to begin transfusion.

► ► ►

► ► ►

When dealing with cardiac emergencies, a portable defibrillator and adrenaline in a preloaded syringe should be included. The following are suggested contents for a medical snatch bag:

- ☐ Oropharyngeal airways; sizes 1, 2 and 3.
- ☐ Nasopharyngeal airways; sizes 4.0mm and 6.00mm.
- ☐ Laryngeal masks; sizes 2 and 4.
- ☐ Portable hand-powered suction unit.
- ☐ Equipment for tracheal intubation:
  laryngoscope
  tracheal tubes size 4.0, 5.0 and 8.0mm
  10ml syringe
  artery clip
  lubricating gel sachet
  length of bandage to secure tube
  gum elastic bougie.
- ☐ Self-inflating bag/valve/mask.
- ☐ Compression shell dressings x3.
- ☐ Intravenous giving set.
- ☐ Intravenous cannulae sizes 14G, 16G and 20G x2.
- ☐ 10ml syringe.
- ☐ Plain blood sample tube for cross match.
- ☐ Haemaccel or Gelofusine 500ml or Hartmann's solution 1000ml.
- ☐ Swabs.
- ☐ Roll of adhesive tape.
- ☐ Neck collars; regular, tall and short.

Ambulance equipment

The ambulance should contain a more extensive array of equipment. In addition to duplicating the contents of medical snatch bags, it should also carry:

- ☐ Oxygen and equipment for its administration.
- ☐ An automatic resuscitator.
- ☐ Needles to perform needle thoracostomy.
- ☐ Further cannulae suitable for internal or external jugular vein cannulation.
- ☐ 3-way taps for insertion in the intravenous line.
- ☐ Intraosseous cannulae.
- ☐ Defibrillator/ECG.
- ☐ Cardiac resuscitation drugs in preloaded syringes.
- ☐ Pneumatic anti-shock garment.
- ☐ Pulse oximeter.
- ☐ Non-invasive blood pressure monitor.
- ☐ Entonox.
- ☐ Nalbuphine or chosen opiate analgesic.
- ☐ Diazemuls or midazolam.
- ☐ Syringes and needles.
- ☐ Salbutamol.
- ☐ Glucagon.
- ☐ Glyceryl trinitrate spray.

► ► ►

▶ ▶ ▶

☐ Limb splints.
☐ Back boards or KED or RED cervico-lumbar immobilisation splints.
☐ Badges and dressings.

Medical centre or casualty clearing station

At sporting and crowd events the ambulance rescue vehicle will normally visit the medical centre so that more detailed assessment of the patient and further stabilisation can be carried out prior to transport to definitive care.

In addition to duplication of the equipment carried in the medial snatch bag and on the ambulance, the medical centre should also hold equipment for cricothyroidotomy, transtracheal jet ventilation, chest drain insertion, surgical cut-down venous cannulation, pericardio-centesis, gastric intubation and urethral catheterisation.

On rare occasions when a prolonged transfer time to definitive care is anticipated, it may be considered prudent to include equipment for intercostal or femoral nerve block.

The equipment required for these procedures is detailed in the relevant chapters of this book.

In multi-casualty incidents, re-supply is essential and boxes containing the above equipment should be stockpiled for the event and brought to the casualty clearing station as required.

Repatriation by air

Repatriation by air is often a prolonged process and the space allocated is confined. All likely procedures necessary should be performed prior to departure. Splints must be secured and the patient should be in a stable condition.

All equipment should be carefully checked prior to departure. Electrical equipment should be powered by rechargeable batteries. The aircraft's intrinsic electrical supply generally cannot be used.

Equipment for repatriation

☐ Oxygen; calculated on the anticipated flow rate per hour and doubled to allow for unscheduled delays and unexpected increased requirements.
☐ Suction; hand or battery powered.
☐ Portable ventilator with nebuliser; oxygen powered with facility to entrain air.
☐ Intubation equipment.
☐ Intravenous giving sets, cannulae and fluids.
☐ Syringe pumps powered by rechargeable batteries.
☐ Pulse oximetry.
☐ ECG monitor.
☐ Non-invasive blood pressure monitor.
☐ Invasive blood pressure monitor.   ▶ ▶ ▶

► ► ►

- ☐ Portable defibrillator.
- ☐ Supplies of the patient's current medication.
- ☐ Sedatives, e.g. diazemuls, midazolam or temezepam.
- ☐ Analgesics, e.g. nalbuphine (morphine may present legal difficulties) and less potent oral preparations.
- ☐ Anti-emetics e.g. prochlorperazine or metoclopramide.
- ☐ Salbutamol.
- ☐ Glyceryl trinitrate spray.
- ☐ Nursing equipment such as vacuum mattress, sheets, blankets, pillows, bedpan, bottle, urinary catheter, vomit bowl, dressings, swabs, bandages and tape.
- ☐ Food and drink for patient and attendants.

Clearly the selection of equipment will depend on the patient's condition, current therapy and anticipated transit time.

Who should be taught what

Figs. 7.10–7.13 set out guidelines as to who should be taught the various practical procedures described in this book. Clearly the situation will vary with locality, with national traditions of training and practice and, most of all, with staffing levels of specialists in different hospitals.

Within some specialties there will also be variations. For example, only certain surgeons will need to be able to place an intra-aortic balloon pump, Sengstaken tube or create an arteriovenous fistulae. Certain anaesthetists not specifically involved in critical care may not be required to place tunnelled central venous lines or apply brain death criteria. Family practitioners involved in immediate care will require at least the life-support skills of a paramedic. However, those confining their practice to surgery or office work are less likely to need the skills of tracheal intubation, for instance.

Skill / group	Ambulance technician	Paramedic	Student nurse	RGN/RN	Ward sister / Head nurse	Senior nurse critical care unit	Medical student	Houseman / Intern	Family doctor	Dentist	Military doctor	Physician	Surgeon	Anaesthetist	Radiologist	Critical care specialist	Accident and emergency Physician
Peripheral IV	X	✓	✓	✓	✓	✓	✓	✓	✓	✓	✓	✓	✓	✓	✓	✓	✓
Central IV	X	X	X	X	X	X	X	X	X	X	✓	✓	?	✓	✓	✓	✓
Tunnelled IV	X	X	X	X	X	X	X	X	X	X	X	✓	✓	✓	X	✓	X
Cut down IV	X	X	X	X	X	X	X	X	X*	X	✓	✓	✓	✓	✓	✓	✓
Intraosseous cannulation	X	?	X	X	X	X	X	X	X	X	✓	✓	✓	✓	X	✓	✓
Pulmonary artery catheter	X	X	X	X	X	X	X	X	X	X	X	✓	X	✓	✓	✓	?
Arterial cannula	X	X	X	X	X	✓	✓	✓	X	X	✓	✓	?	✓	✓	✓	✓
Pericardiocentesis	X	X	X	X	X	X	X	X	X	X	✓	✓	✓	✓	✓	✓	✓
External chest compressions	✓	✓	✓	✓	✓	✓	✓	✓	✓	✓	✓	✓	✓	✓	✓	✓	✓
Internal cardiac massage	X	X	X	X	X	X	X	X	X	X	✓	✓	✓	✓	X	✓	✓
Defibrillation	✓	✓	✓	✓	✓	✓	✓	✓	✓	✓	✓	✓	✓	✓	✓	✓	✓
12 Lead ECG	X	X	X	X	✓	✓	✓	✓	✓	X	✓	✓	?	✓	?	✓	✓
Cardiac pacing	X	X	X	X	X	X	X	X	X	X	X	✓	?	✓	✓	✓	✓
Intra aortic balloon pump	X	X	X	X	X	X	X	X	X	X	X	?	✓	?	?	?	X
Pulse oximetry	✓	✓	✓	✓	✓	✓	✓	✓	✓	✓	✓	✓	✓	✓	✓	✓	✓
Pneumatic anti-shock garments	?	?	X	X	X	?	X	X	X	X	?	X	✓	✓	X	✓	✓

Figs 7.10

Accident and emergency physicians may be supported to a greater or lesser extent by surgeons, anaesthetists and radiologists in a trauma team, and by cardiologists and anaesthetists in an emergency cardiac care team. Their breadth of skills will, therefore, vary accordingly.

The ward sister or charge nurse (or head nurse) and the senior nurse in a critical care unit (intensive care unit or coronary care unit, accident and emergency department or operating department) does not necessarily need to have the technical skills involved in the procedure but requires a detailed knowledge of the equipment required and its function, and should be familiar with the techniques for monitoring of the patient afterwards.

Skill / group	Ambulance technician	Paramedic	Student nurse	RGN/RN	Ward sister / Head nurse	Senior nurse critical care unit	Medical student	Houseman / Intern	Family doctor	Dentist	Military doctor	Physician	Surgeon	Anaesthetist	Radiologist	Critical care specialist	Accident and emergency Physician
Basic airway control	✓	✓	✓	✓	✓	✓	✓	✓	✓	✓	✓	✓	✓	✓	✓	✓	✓
Simple airways	✓	✓	✓	✓	✓	✓	✓	✓	✓	✓	✓	✓	✓	✓	✓	✓	✓
Laryngeal mask	✓	✓	X	✓	✓	✓	✓	✓	✓	✓	✓	✓	✓	✓	✓	✓	✓
PTLA	X	?	X	X	X	X	X	X	X	X	X	X	X	✓	X	✓	✓
Combitube	X	X	X	X	X	X	X	X	X	X	X	X	X	✓	X	✓	✓
Tracheal intubation	X	✓	X	X	X	✓	X	X	X	?	✓	X	X	✓	X	✓	✓
Fibreoptic intubation	X	X	X	X	X	X	X	X	X	X	X	X	X	✓	X	✓	?
Double lumen intubation	X	X	X	X	X	X	X	X	X	X	X	X	X	✓	X	✓	X
Retrograde intubation	X	X	X	X	X	X	X	X	X	X	X	X	X	✓	X	✓	X
Cricothyrotomy	X	X	X	X	X	X	X	X	X	X	X	X	✓	✓	X	✓	✓
Percutaneous dilatational Tracheostomy	X	X	X	X	X	X	X	X	X	X	?	X	✓	?	X	✓	?
Tracheostomy	X	X	X	X	X	X	X	X	X	X	?	X	✓	X	X	?	X
Basic ventilation	✓	✓	✓	✓	✓	✓	✓	✓	✓	✓	✓	✓	✓	✓	✓	✓	✓
Automatic resuscitators	✓	✓	X	X	X	✓	X	X	X	X	✓	✓	✓	✓	X	✓	✓
Complex ventilators	X	X	X	X	X	X	X	X	X	X	X	X	X	✓	X	✓	X
Transtracheal jet ventilator	X	?	X	X	X	X	X	X	X	X	✓	X	✓	✓	X	✓	✓
Needle thoracostomy	X	✓	X	X	X	?	X	✓	✓	X	✓	✓	✓	✓	✓	✓	✓
Chest drain	X	X	X	X	X	X	X	X	X	X	✓	✓	✓	✓	✓	✓	✓
Bronchoscopy	X	X	X	X	X	X	X	X	X	X	?	✓	✓	✓	X	✓	?
Bronchial lavage	X	X	X	X	X	X	X	X	X	X	X	?	X	?	X	✓	X
Nebuliser use	✓	✓	X	X	✓	✓	✓	✓	✓	X	✓	✓	X	✓	X	✓	✓

Fig.7.11

Skill / group	Ambulance technician	Paramedic	Student nurse	RGN/RN	Ward sister / Head nurse unit	Senior nurse critical care	Medical student	Houseman / Intern	Family doctor	Dentist	Military doctor	Physician	Surgeon	Anaesthetist	Radiologist	Critical care specialist	Accident and emergency Physician
Lumbar puncture	X	X	X	X	X	X	✓	✓	X	X	✓	✓	✓	✓	✓	✓	✓
Intracranial pressure and CFAM	X	X	X	X	X	X	X	X	X	X	X	?	✓	?	X	✓	X
Burr holes	X	X	X	X	X	X	X	X	X	X	✓	X	✓	X	X	X	X
Patient controlled analgesia	X	X	X	X	✓	✓	X	X	X	X	✓	✓	✓	✓	X	✓	X
Monitor neuromuscular block	X	X	X	X	X	✓	X	X	X	X	X	X	X	✓	X	✓	X
Spinal blockade	X	X	X	X	X	X	X	X	X	X	X	X	X	✓	X	✓	X
Epidural blockade	X	X	X	X	X	X	X	X	X	X	X	X	X	✓	X	✓	X
Brachial plexus block	X	X	X	X	X	X	X	X	X	X	✓	X	✓	X	✓	✓	✓
Intercostal block	X	X	X	X	X	X	X	X	X	X	✓	X	✓	X	✓	✓	X
Intrapleural block	X	X	X	X	X	X	X	X	X	X	✓	X	✓	X	✓	✓	X
Femoral block	X	X	X	X	X	X	X	X	X	X	✓	X	✓	X	✓	X	✓
IVRA	X	X	X	X	X	X	X	X	X	X	✓	X	?	X	✓	X	✓

Fig.7.12

Skill / group	Ambulance technician	Paramedic	Student nurse	RGN/RN	Ward sister / Head nurse unit	Senior nurse critical care	Medical student	Houseman / Intern	Family doctor	Dentist	Military doctor	Physician	Surgeon	Anaesthetist	Radiologist	Critical care specialist	Accident and emergency Physician
Gastric tube	X	?	✓	✓	✓	✓	✓	✓	✓	X	✓	✓	✓	✓	✓	✓	✓
Gastric lavage	X	X	X	X	X	X	X	X	X	X	✓	✓	✓	✓	✓	X	✓
Sengstaken tube	X	X	X	X	X	X	X	X	X	X	X	✓	✓	X	X	✓	X
Diagnostic peritoneal lavage	X	X	X	X	X	X	X	X	X	X	✓	X	✓	✓	X	✓	✓
Arteriovenous shunt fistula	X	X	X	X	X	X	X	X	X	X	X	X	✓	X	X	✓	X
Urethral catheter	X	X	✓	✓	✓	✓	✓	✓	✓	X	✓	✓	✓	✓	✓	✓	✓
Suprapubic catheter	X	X	X	X	X	X	X	X	X	X	✓	X	✓	✓	?	✓	?
Haemofiltration	X	X	X	X	X	X	X	X	X	X	✓	✓	✓	X	X	✓	X
Peritoneal dialysis	X	X	X	X	X	X	X	X	X	X	X	✓	✓	✓	X	✓	X
Abdominal ultrasound	X	X	X	X	X	X	X	X	X	X	X	X	?	X	✓	?	?
Brain stem death criteria	X	X	X	X	X	X	X	X	X	X	✓	✓	✓	✓	X	✓	?

Fig.7.13

Further reading

1. American Heart Association. American Heart Association 1992 National Conference Standards and Guidelines for Cardiopulmonary Resuscitation (CPR) and Emergency Cardiac Care (ECC). *JAMA* 1992; **268**: 2171–2307.

2. American Society of Anesthesiologists Task Force on Management of the Difficult Airway. *Anesthesiology* 1993; **78**: 597–602.

3. American Society of Anesthesiologists Task Force on Pulmonary Artery Catheterization. Practice guidelines for pulmonary artery catheterization. *Anesthesiology* 1993; **78**: 380–394.

4. Australian Resuscitation Council. *Policy Statements of the Australian Resuscitation Council.* Sydney: Australian Resuscitation Council.

5. Baskett PJF. Difficult and impossible intubation. In Fisher M McD ed., *The Anaesthetic Crisis.* Bailliere's Clinical Anaesthesiology 1993; **7**: 261–280.

6. Baskett PJF, ed. *Resuscitation Handbook*, 2nd edition. London, Wolfe, 1993.

7. Bennett D, Boldt J, Brochard L, *et al.* European Society of Intensive Care Medicine Expert Panel. The use of the pulmonary artery catheter. *Intensive Care Med* 1991; **17**: I–VIII.

8. Benumof JL, ed. *Clinical Procedures in Anesthesia and Intensive Care.* Philadelphia: JB Lippincott, 1992.

9. Brain AIJ. The laryngeal mask – a new concept in airway management. *Br J Anaesth* 1983; **55**: 801–805.

10. Brain AIJ. The laryngeal mask airway – a possible new solution to airway problems in the emergency situation. *Arch Emerg Med* 1984; **1**: 229–232.

11. Bromage PR, ed. *Epidural Analgesia.* Philadelphia: WB Saunders, 1978.

12. Broviac JW, Cole JJ, Scribner BH. A silicome rubber atrial catheter for prolonged parenteral alimentation. *Surg Gynaecol Obstet* 1973; **136**: 602.

13. Calder I, Oudman AJ, Jackowski A, Crockard HA. The Brain laryngeal mask airway – an alternative to emergency tracheal intubation. *Anaesthesia* 1990; **45**: 137–139.

14. Ciaglia P, Graniero KD. Percutaneous dilatational tracheostomy. Results and long-term follow-up. *Chest* 1992; **101**: 464–467.

15. Committee on Trauma of the American College of Surgeons. *Advanced Trauma Life Support Instructor Manual.* Chicago: American College of Surgeons, 1993.

16. European Resuscitation Council. Guidelines for Basic and Advanced Life Support (1992). *Resuscitation* 1992; **24**: 103–123.

17. European Resuscitation Council. Guidelines for Paediatric Life Support. *Br Med J* 1994; **308**: 1349–1355.

18. Evans TR, ed. *ABC of Resuscitation*, 3rd edition. London: British Medical Journal. 1994, in press.

19. Fiser DH. Intraosseous infusion. *N Eng J Med* 1990; **322**: 1579–1581.

20. Frass M, Rodder S, Ilias W, Leithner C, Lackner F. Esophageal tracheal combitube, endotracheal airway and mask: comparison of ventilatory pressure curves. *J Trauma* 1989; **29**: 1476–1479.

21. Griffiths DM, Ilsley AH, Runciman WB. Pulse meters and pulse oximeters. *Anaesth Intens Care* 1988; **16**: 49–53.

22. Henderson JJ, Nimmo WS, eds. *Practical Regional Anaesthesia*. Oxford, Blackwell, 1983.

23. Kaye WE, Dubin HG. Vascular cannulation. In Civetta JM, Taylor RW, Kirby RR, eds, *Critical Care*. Philadelphia: JB Lippincott, 1988.

24. Lichtenstein D, Axler O. Intensive use of general ultrasound in the intensive care unit. *Intensive Care Med* 1993; **19**: 353–355.

25. Mermel LA, Maki DG. Infectious complications of Swan–Ganz pulmonary artery catheters. Pathogenesis, epidemiology, prevention and management. *Am J Respir Crit Care Med* 1994; **149**: 1020–1036.

26. Resuscitation Council UK. *Advanced Life Support Manual 1993*. London: Resuscitation Council UK, 1993.

27. Rippe JM, Irwin RS, Alpert JS, Fink MP, eds. *Intensive Care Medicine* 2nd edition. Boston: Little, Brown and Company, 1991.

28. Seldinger SI. Catheter replacement of needle in percutaneous arteriography: A new technique. *Acta Radiol* 1953; **39**: 368–376.

29. Skinner D, Driscoll P, Earlam R, eds *The ABC of Major Trauma*, 2nd edition. London: British Medical Journal, 1994, in press.

30. Stradling P, ed. *Diagnostic Bronchoscopy*, 4th edition. London: Churchill Livingstone, 1981.

31. Sutton R, Citron P, Perrins J. Physiological cardiac pacing. *Pace* 1980; **3**: 201–219.

32. The use of the laryngeal mask by nurses during cardiopulmonary resuscitation – results of a multicentre trial. *Anaesthesia* 1994; **49**: 3–7.

33. Ward CS, ed. *Anaesthetic Equipment*, 3rd edition. London: Baillière Tindall, 1992.

34. Wildsmith JAW, Armitage EN, eds. *Principles and Practice of Regional Anaesthesia*, 2nd edition. London, Churchill Livingstone, 1993.

35. Winnie AP, Rammamurthy S, Durrani Z. The inguinal perivascular technique of lumbar plexus anaesthesia, the three-in-one block. *Anesth Analg* 1973; **52**: 989–996.

Index